MW00463428

Rudy's
Ruminations On
Rheumatology

uide for The Practitioner, The Patient and The Student - Updated Version

Rudy R Greene MD

Dedicated to my friend and colleague, Larry Levin.

Thanks to my wife Leanne, Curt Anderson, Peng Fan, Frank Quismorio and Bob Shour for their kind contributions and encouragement.

Rheumatology is an ever-changing field. The publisher and author of Rudy's Ruminations on Rheumatology have made every effort to provide information that is accurate and complete as of the date of publication. However, in view of the rapid changes occurring in medical science, as well as the possibility of human error, this site may contain technical inaccuracies, typographical or other errors. Readers are advised to check with their Rheumatologist about the product information currently provided by the manufacturer of each drug to be administered to verify the recommended dose, the method and duration of administration, and contraindications. It is the responsibility of the treating physician who relies on experience and knowledge about the patient to determine dosages and the best treatment for the patient. The information contained herein is provided "as is" and without warranty of any kind. The contributors to this site, including CreateSpace, disclaim responsibility for any errors or omissions or for results obtained from the use of information contained herein.

ISBN: 0692205802
ISBN 13: 9780692205808

Library of Congress Control Number: 2014907707
Rudy Greene, Ashland, OR

Table of Contents

You are about to enter the world of rheumatology. I hope to share with you the joy of rheumatology and give you an idea of what it's all about. This book is not a textbook—it is my take on each of the more common and sometimes uncommon diseases in this fascinating and challenging but rewarding specialty. I have been practicing and teaching my craft for close to thirty years and have picked up a few insights along the way. Like many specialties in medicine, rheumatology is shrouded in mystery to the public, patients, and even most doctors. In fact, I find that many doctors will consider a rheumatology disease when nothing else fits. It's one of the factors that attracted me to this specialty—I like mysteries and intellectual challenges. Office staff members are often baffled by the diseases and medications associated with rheumatology, and this book was inspired by a group of lectures I gave to my staff to familiarize them with some of the terms, diseases, medications, and challenges they would encounter daily. Occasionally patients and new acquaintances would ask me to explain rheumatology to them, and I found it helpful but inadequate to summarize some basic concepts in simple terms. Manuals and textbooks were either tedious or too sophisticated for their consumption. As I have aged as a rheumatologist, I have found it easier and more necessary to explain each disease and medication to patients in terms they can understand despite the fact that our knowledge of each disease process has become more sophisticated and complex. I hope this book will not only be educational but entertaining and kindle interest in what I think is an important and little known or understood specialty in medicine. It is not only about concepts but people. My patients are some of the nicest, more interesting, and even bravest people you'll meet. They have become like family since I see them on a regular basis. Some of them light up my day with their successes, loves, and personalities. That's not to say that I don't see my share of angry, depressed, and even psychotic people, but they are a small minority and add spice to my day if I don't let them get to me.

Before I start I want to dispel some of the misconceptions about rheumatology. It is not just about "rheumatism" or arthritis. Most rheumatology patients' immune systems have a defect, usually linked to specific genes, causing them to overproduce certain factors in the blood that cause inflammatory cells or antibodies to attack any part of the body, including all organs, skin, blood cells, and most famously joints. Most of these diseases are systemic, so patients feel sick. The kind of arthritis these patients develop is inflammatory, which leads me to two of the biggest misconceptions. Not all arthritis is the same. Most of us as we age will develop osteoarthritis, or degenerative arthritis. It is localized and not systemic and often comes from wear and tear or trauma. The majority of our patients have inflammatory arthritis, which can have many causes. Not all arthritis is the same, nor is there one treatment that fits all. Any drug that is advertised as a panacea for arthritis is snake oil. Finally the average age of onset of many of our diseases is between twenty and forty, and they may occur in children and infants, so rheumatology is not a geriatric specialty. Although we do treat osteoarthritis, or the arthritis of older people, the majority of these patients are treated by their primary care providers or orthopedics. Years ago my day was spent 75 percent in the office and 25 percent in the hospital setting. More recently with the advent of hospitalists, the ratio is more like 99 percent and 1 percent I go to the hospital about two to three times a year. It also reflects the kind of patient I am seeing. I see far fewer of the extremely ill intensive care unit patients than I used to. The hospitalists are just one factor. I believe I am seeing patients at an earlier stage and can intercede before they deteriorate to the ICU level. The primary care docs are better informed. Also, rheumatologists have better tools to treat early disease and have more knowledge. I am better at putting out little fires rather than big ones. There is also some sense that some of the diseases may be changing—they are less severe. Finally, I practice in a small rural area without a big medical center, so the more severe cases may gravitate to big cities.

In any case, let's step into a day in my life in the office.

Introduction

The Man with
the Crooked Fingers

John, a squarely built man with a mane of gray hair and a boyish smile, is one of my favorite patients, but inevitably every visit ends with some friendly jousting about his medications. He is one of my many medication nihilists. He is a talented writer and a political activist, who always has a smile and some interesting words of wisdom for me. He has had rheumatoid arthritis (RA) for twenty years, and now at age sixty-five, he is finally accepting treatment and is more mobile and active than he has been in years. He has very little inflammation in his joints, but his hands are deformed and ravaged by years of unchecked inflammation and erosion of cartilage and bone. His mother is ninety-one and has similar hands and a similar attitude. He is much better but far from perfect. He still has some swollen joints, and his measures of inflammation are moderately elevated despite maximal doses of methotrexate (the most common drug in RA). In addition, he has hypertension and coronary artery disease, which can be associated with RA. After his years of resistance to any medication and his vast improvement with methotrexate, you would think he would be open to one of the newer, more effective drugs, but because of his history of melanoma and antidrug bias, he is passively resistant. Each visit, he smiles and insists he will think about it. He also takes the same approach to his osteoporosis despite having two vertebral fractures. Still he is so charming and such a nice guy it's hard to get angry at him.

Chapter One

Rheumatoid Arthritis (RA)

Fifteen years ago the majority of patients I saw when I opened the door were thin, middle-aged women with varying degrees of deformities of their hands and feet. Their joints were swollen to some degree, and more often than not they limped and had some difficulties with the activities of daily living. I was always struck by their great attitudes. If seen early in the disease's onset, some of the medications we used at the time seemed to have some effect by reducing inflammation, but it seemed inevitably after about five years all patients had deformities. In 2012, the typical patient is a thirty-plus-year-old female who is on one or more medications and has occasional flares but has no deformities and lives a normal life without restrictions.

Rheumatoid arthritis (RA) is probably the most common disease I see in my office. The advances in our understanding of the disease process and therapies have been spectacular over the last ten to fifteen years. They have changed our approach and the disease's prognosis dramatically and made rheumatology much more fun. First of all, RA is a systemic disease. There is a misconception that arthritis is all the same. *Arthritis* literally means "inflammation of the joint," but there are many causes of arthritis and actually different kinds.

The two major categories are inflammatory and noninflammatory. Usually, inflammatory arthritis is systemic, meaning it's caused by inflammatory cells circulating in your bloodstream and causing inflammation in your joints and other areas of your body; whereas noninflammatory arthritis is confined to individual joints. The classic noninflammatory arthritis is osteoarthritis, or degenerative arthritis, which we all develop as we age. Rheumatoid arthritis is a disease, linked to specific gene types, that occurs in approximately one in a hundred people, predominantly female but sometimes males. Not everyone with the gene types develops the disease, but smoking and maybe gingivitis increase the likelihood and severity. Smoking also increases the likelihood and severity of heart and lung disease. There are many factors in the immune system that promote inflammation, and these are the targets of many of the new therapies. Usually, patients will complain of pain, stiffness, and swelling in many joints (especially their fingers), although occasionally they will start with one or few joints. Unlike many other types, this arthritis is usually symmetrical and involves both large and small joints (with a few exceptions). If left untreated, the inflammation can eat away the cartilage and bone in a matter of months or years, leaving the joint deformed and nonfunctional. Patients generally feel fatigued and ill. They may have hours of stiffness in the morning. The inflamed joints are usually swollen and often tender. The swelling is usually synovitis, or inflammation of the lining of the joints, and can feel rubbery to the touch. Inflammation of the hands—especially the metacarpophalangeal joints, or MCPs (the knuckles at the end of the hand)—is classic for rheumatoid arthritis and often helps distinguish it from other causes of arthritis, which either do not involve the hands symmetrically or spare the MCPs. Permanent damage to the joints can occur early in the disease (six months to a year), so it is important to get patients to a rheumatologist early, establish the diagnosis, and start treatment with agents that remit the disease or completely halt its progression. There is convincing data that patients treated earlier and aggressively do better.

The diagnosis is established with a good history and physical, which includes a family history and a good complete joint exam. Lab tests clinch the diagnosis and help monitor activity and rule out other diseases, which can coexist or mimic RA. Most of the autoimmune diseases produce characteristic antibodies to proteins specific to each disease. Anti-CCP (cyclic citrullinated peptide) antibodies are present in 50–75 percent of RA patients but are 90 percent specific for RA; whereas rheumatoid factor is present in about 75–80 percent of RA patients but is less specific. In other words, many other conditions may also be associated with rheumatoid factors, but few are associated with anti-CCP. The presence of anti-CCP also seems to predict a more aggressive disease. Rheumatoid factor and anti-CCP need only be measured once, with a few exceptions. Sedimentation rate (ESR) and C-reactive protein (CRP) are good but nonspecific measurements of inflammation or disease activity. We measure these two factors after each visit to help monitor disease activity and gauge the effectiveness of treatment. Infection or other causes of inflammation may also cause elevations of these factors. Anemia, thrombocytosis (or increased platelets), and high or low white blood cell counts also can reflect active disease and can be used as indicators of inflammation. X-rays, especially of the hands and wrists, are important markers of disease activity and severity and the efficacy of treatment. We look for joint space narrowing or loss of cartilage, erosions of the bones, and bone thinning, or osteopenia, around the joints. Our goal is to prevent any changes or limit them to the ones that are present prior to treatment. Interestingly, radiological changes most correlate with future disability. It is important to monitor patients on a regular basis, at least every three to four months, to look for disease activity or drug toxicity so that we can make adjustments in their medications.

Ten years ago, our ability to control the disease was limited, and our goals were much less ambitious. However, with new medications, especially biologics, we settle for nothing less than complete remission or close to it without drug toxicity. Each visit, we use standardized measures of disease activity that incorporate counts of joint swelling and tenderness, measures of the patient's ability to do daily activities, and sedimentation rates (ESRs) or C'reactive proteins (CRPs). These measures allow us to objectively assess disease activity and effectiveness of treatment. Many of my long-term patients will immediately put their hands in front of me when I enter the room, knowing that I will be squeezing and examining each of their finger joints. These measurements also involve patients filling out questionnaires each visit, and I encounter resistance occasionally. One of my favorite curmudgeonly patients used to insist that he didn't want to do my work for me. However, when I explained that not only did it help me monitor objectively his disease activity but that his insurance was now insisting on these measurements before they would approve his medications, he relented. We also monitor drug toxicity clinically and with labs. Prior to the biologic age, patients developed deformities and became disabled, losing their quality of life. The development of deformities is extremely rare these days, if the patient is diagnosed and treated early.

The inflammation of rheumatoid arthritis may involve many organs. A painful red eye in these patients can be an emergency since inflammation of the sclera or iris can lead to blindness. Sjögren's syndrome, often associated with RA, can cause chronic dry eyes and mouth, leading to visual problems, infections, gingivitis, and loss of teeth. If any of my patients complains of a painful red eye, I send them immediately to an ophthalmologist. I have seen at least two patients develop scleromalacia, or corneal melt, where the white of their eye or cornea just essentially melted down, leading to blindness in days. Iritis, or inflammation of the iris, is more common and can be just as devastating if untreated. Fortunately, these days we can treat most of these cases successfully if we are prompt. So beware of the red eye!

Over the years, we've seen several patients who have developed severe pulmonary fibrosis, or scarring of their lungs, because of inflammation caused by RA. If discovered early, it may be treatable, and it is possible patients who are under good control would never develop this horrible manifestation of their disease. It is important to distinguish it from infectious causes or methotrexate lung (a reaction to this drug we use commonly in RA), which can be similar. In all three cases, misdiagnosis and improper treatment could lead to devastating outcomes, so proper referrals and prompt workups are needed. We recently had a patient on a biologic (a type of medication that targets specific factors in the immune system that are active in RA) and methotrexate (a medication that nonspecifically inhibits certain inflammatory cells) who complained of shortness of breath and had low oxygen saturation despite looking well. A chest X -ray and CAT scan of the lung showed a diffuse interstitial (the space between the cells) inflammation of both lungs. She was hospitalized, and a bronchoscopy revealed a bacterial infection; after antibiotics and withdrawal of methotrexate, she recovered quickly. If we had treated her with steroids or immunosuppressive medications, such as Cytoxan (used in rheumatoid lung), we could have severely worsened her condition. On the other hand, I have a patient who developed severe scarring and inflammation of his lungs before his rheumatoid arthritis was diagnosed. The lung disease was extensively worked up by several specialists, and they concluded that it was due to his RA. He has been treated aggressively, but it's too late, and the only solution is a lung transplant. Earlier aggressive treatment of his RA may have saved his lungs and prolonged his life.

Large pleural effusions or fluid in the lining of the lungs can cause severe shortness of breath. The fluid is inflammatory, just as it is in the joints, and must be distinguished from infection. Patients can also develop rheumatoid nodules in their lungs, just as they do in their skin and other parts of their body. Once again, they rarely occur in patients who are in remission.

The most common location for these nodules is on the extensor surface of the elbows but may occur on the fingers, scalp, buttocks, and other pressure points. The biologics usually make them shrink, but methotrexate may make them grow. Rarely, uncontrolled disease can cause leg ulcers secondary to vasculitis, or inflammation of small blood vessels in the skin. With the new medications, it is rare.

Cardiac involvement is rare but can be severe. Pericardial effusions (fluid between the lining of the heart and the heart), pulmonary hypertension (increased pressure in the artery connecting the heart and lungs), and even heartbeat rhythm abnormalities do occur. Each of these problems can cause either shortness of breath or chest pain and left untreated can lead to respiratory or cardiac failure. They will be discussed in more detail in other sections dealing with different diseases. Also, rheumatoid arthritis is just as much a risk factor for coronary artery disease as is diabetes. The same inflammatory process affecting the bones and cartilage has been found in the coronary arteries of rheumatoid arthritis patients! I often use this cautionary piece of information to convince patients who refuse medication because they "can tolerate the arthritis." Also, if you add smoking to the mix, the risk increases exponentially!

Rheumatoid Arthritis (RA)

Gastrointestinal and genitourinary problems are rare but do occur, although usually secondary to medications. Splenomegaly, or enlarged spleen, does occur and can be associated with low white blood cell count and nodules. Such cases are called *Felty's syndrome* and are rare since we have such effective treatment. Many years ago, before we had good therapies, patients would develop amyloidosis of their intestines, causing them to stop absorbing much of their food and develop diarrhea and profound weight loss. Amyloid is an abnormal protein substance that can infiltrate organs. It will be discussed later and can develop in any uncontrolled inflammatory disease.

Kidney disease is rare in RA but can be caused by many medications, amyloidosis, and overlap with other diseases, such as lupus or Sjögren's. In many cases the first clue will be on blood tests, such as the creatinine (a measure of kidney function), but new onset edema (subcutaneous swelling especially around the ankles) and protein in the urine are red flags.

The most common neurological manifestation is peripheral neuropathy, where the insulation of the nerves in the arms and legs are worn down, and patients can suffer from numbness, tingling, or burning of the involved extremities and lose their internal compass or proprioception. One of the few and rare complications of RA that we rarely see anymore is subluxation, or dislocation of the first two cervical vertebra (the atlas and the axis). Ligaments holding them together can become stretched or torn. Then when the neck is flexed, these two vertebrae dislocate and shear or press on the spinal cord or compromise its blood supply and cause weakness, numbness, and even quadriplegia. When patients complain of neck pain, weakness, or numbness, I always order cervical spine x-rays with flexion and extension views. If there is abnormally large space between the first two vertebrae (the atlas and axis), it is a surgical emergency. That patient must wear a cervical collar until he or she can see a

surgeon. I had one patient who had this disorder and was left untreated. By the time I saw her, she was a quadriplegic and would be
lying on a stretcher each visit. I remember the shock of seeing her
MRI. Her spinal cord had shriveled to about a tenth of the normal
diameter. The image has never left me nor has my memory of the
patient. Cervical spine x-rays should always be ordered with flexion
and extension views!

Treatment

Rather than bore you with all the details and mechanisms of action of all the medications, we will have a riveting chapter at the end
of the book you can reference. I will try to give you the bare bones of
the treatment for each disease and elaborate on these medications
later with some repetition.

The goal in rheumatoid arthritis is to stop the disease cold or
put it in remission. Ideally, that would mean no joint swelling, normal
ESRs and CRPs, very low activity scores, and above all no radiological changes over years. As I mentioned previously, radiological
damage best correlates with disability over time, and for years, researchers have been searching for agents that prevent radiological
damage. These drugs promote remission and are called *remittive
agents*. It's been only over the last decade and a half that studies
have verified that we have such therapy at our disposal, and the
results have been nothing short of astounding. Rheumatoid arthritis
has become one of the easier diseases to manage. Most of the reasons for the success of our treatment are the advances in science.
They help us understand the disease process and how to counteract
it. Simply put, rheumatoid arthritis patients have certain gene types
that predispose them to have this disease, and certain external factors unlock the code. Smoking and possibly gingivitis are two possibilities. Once the code is unlocked, certain factors in the immune

system are released excessively. They stimulate inflammatory cells to multiply in the blood, and these cells infiltrate joints and other organs. Drugs like methotrexate prevent inflammatory cells from multiplying and remit the disease; whereas biologics, such as tumor necrosis factor (TNF) antagonists, affect the inflammatory process a step earlier and inhibit one of the factors that stimulate inflammatory cells. These are long-term agents.

Treatment usually starts with methotrexate, which is increased incrementally in doses over four to six months until full remission is achieved or the patient develops an intolerable adverse effect. If the maximum dose of 30 mg is achieved without remission, we add either a biologic or initiate triple-drug therapy, which includes Plaquenil, Azulfidine, and methotrexate. Occasionally, for very mild cases of RA, we use Plaquenil alone, but it has not proven to be a true remittive drug for RA. Azulfidine alone has remittive qualities, but for some reason British studies tend to suggest that it is more effective than do similar studies in the United States. I find it to be minimally effective even in Brits, but it is extremely inexpensive and worth a try when patients can't afford or take any other drug. Arava, or leflunomide, may be used as an alternative to methotrexate when the latter is not tolerated. Although I will discuss monitoring later, it is important to emphasize that all these medications require monitoring with labs and in the case of Plaquenil eye examinations. I tell patients who can't reach me during the winter and are taking methotrexate or Arava that I need to obtain their liver-function tests and complete blood count every three months, even if I don't see them. I am responsible for their safety. Medication doses can be reduced, or the medication can be discontinued, if there is an abnormality. However, if the problem is detected too late, it may be irreversible. Therefore, I will either discharge the patient or discontinue the medication if the patient can't reliably and regularly undergo testing.

Rudy's Ruminations On **Rheumatology**

What are biologics? They are lasers zeroing in on or inhibiting particular factors that trigger inflammatory and sometimes cancer cells. These factors include circulating proteins called *cytokines*, receptors on inflammatory cells, and even gates on the inflammatory cells themselves that when opened lead to their activation. Biologics include TNF inhibitors or antagonists, such as Enbrel, Humira, Remicade, Simponi, and Cimzia. These drugs are usually prescribed after methotrexate fails or isn't tolerated, but they can also be used first. Remicade and Enbrel were the first biologics introduced for the treatment of RA in 1998. We suddenly had lasers instead of shotguns to treat this disease. Patients rose out of their wheelchairs and remission or complete absence of disease activity, disability, or deformities became realistic expectations. These drugs usually work quickly and are more effective and better tolerated than previous medications. They are all injected under the skin (subcutaneously) except for Remicade. Most recently Simponi can be given intravenously or subcutaneously. Remicade is also the only one of the TNF antagonists that has flexible dosing. I tend to use it in sicker patients, but unfortunately, I am often guided here in the United States by what my patients can afford or more accurately what their insurance will allow. Medicare would only pay for Remicade until recently, so it was the TNF antagonist of choice for all my Medicare patients. (Actemra, Rituxan, and Orencia are non-TNF biologics also covered by Medicare.) Remicade should be paired with methotrexate or Arava to be effective and avoid some of the adverse effects. Remicade and Humira are also effective in patients who have iritis (painful inflammation of the iris leading to a painful red eye and possibly blindness), whereas Enbrel is not; however, it may be safer. They all have different dosing intervals: Enbrel, weekly; Cimzia and Humira, every other week; and Simponi, monthly. These four drugs may be prescribed alone or with methotrexate. Unfortunately, they all have the same risks, especially infection, and testing for TB and hepatitis B needs to be done before starting the medication and then yearly. Vaccinations (nonlive) are important to protect against infection. I won't go into the details of all the risks in this section, but suffice it to say, the first patient I had who rose out of a wheelchair with the help of Remicade died a grisly death soon after because of a severe infection. Over all, these are safe and wonderful drugs for the long term but need close monitoring. Patients look and feel so good that some of them disappear for months or years and have their primary care doctors prescribe the drug without proper monitoring—big mistake! Several years ago, it was frustrating to encounter patients who failed or couldn't tolerate TNF antagonists and all conventional medications because I could not fulfill my promise of partial or complete remission to the patient that I had come to expect. Lo and behold science came to my rescue, and new biologics with different mechanisms became available! They all inhibited a different part of the immune system that was defective in RA. Patients now have many choices. Each has its unique advantage and has a chance of succeeding when the others fail. Most of them are also more effective when paired with methotrexate.

Rituxan is an antibody that inhibits a type of inflammatory cell called *B-lymphocyte*, which is active in RA. It was first used to treat lymphoma, a blood cancer. I find it to be particularly potent and may be given in two six-hour infusions two weeks apart. Patients may respond and remain under control for six to twelve months. The earliest I can reinfuse them is after six months. Patients are often ecstatic with the results, especially after months or years of medication failures and frustration. They will insist there is no need for a repeat infusion until there is. Then it becomes urgent. I have patients who last eight and nine months on one set of infusions and one who lasted a year and a half. Like all the biologics, this medication has some rare but major risks, especially infections and infusion or allergic reactions. It may deplete immunoglobulins or antibodies, and occasionally I will give patients monthly immunoglobulins if they are having recurrent infections. Rituxan has some advantages that make it more attractive than TNF antagonists for some patients. It is used to treat lymphoma, and RA has an increased incidence of lymphoma. It is only given at the most every six months and can last longer. It is effective in some sorts of vasculitis and has shown some promise in Sjögren's and polymyositis. Unlike TNF antagonists it is safe in multiple sclerosis. I have a patient with MS who has RA and Sjögren's, and all three diseases have improved on this agent.

Actemra is an antibody that inhibits interleukin-6 (IL-6), a proinflammatory factor that is reflected in the CRP (one of the principle measures of inflammations). IL-6 is also elevated in obesity and a variety of inflammatory diseases. Actemra is one of the infusions that have been shown to be effective alone and is particularly effective in types of juvenile idiopathic arthritis. It has been effective in a number of patients who have failed other biologics. It has many of the classic adverse reactions, especially risk of infection, but has added risks of raising cholesterol levels and causing liver abnormalities. It should be held when the absolute neutrophil count (a type of white blood cell) is less than two thousand.

Orencia, a selective costimulator modulator, is a protein that blocks two proteins on inflammatory cells that are usually activated during the inflammatory process. It can be administered subcutaneously or intravenously. It has a slow onset but seems to be the safest drug for those prone to infection. I have had some spectacular long-term successes with this drug in difficult patients, although my subjective bias is that it is not as potent as some of the others.

Kineret inhibits interleukin-1 (IL-1), another proinflammatory factor. It is administered subcutaneously daily and is not as potent as the other biologics but is particularly good for certain kinds of juvenile idiopathic (inflammatory) arthritis, especially Still's disease. It also may be the safest biologic because of its short half-life. In other words, it's out of the bloodstream quicker than any of the others. Recently Ilaris, or canakinumab (another IL-1 inhibitor), was approved for treatment of juvenile idiopathic arthritis. It is administered subcutaneously monthly.

A new biologic called Xeljanz, or tofacitinib, is an oral agent that inhibits JAK kinase, the pathway along which the activating signals of certain inflammatory cells travel. It may be used alone or in combination with other remittive medications but not with other biologics. I have had little experience with it yet but have had four or five patients who have had spectacular results after failing or having adverse effects to many of the other biologics. It has many of the same side effects as all biologics, but diarrhea, abnormal liver-function tests, elevated lipid profiles, and low white counts seem to be more prominent. Atypical infections, such as TB and fungus and lymphoma, are also worries. Much to my disappointment and dismay, it is at least as expensive as the injectable biologics, which in my opinion are obscenely overpriced.

All these meds are remittive long-term agents. They are usually more effective when used in combination with methotrexate or Arava and are injected under the skin by the patient or given intravenously at a doctor's office or at an infusion center at a hospital, except for Xeljanz. Some of these medications take a few weeks and others a few months to take effect. We always balance the risks and benefits of each medication to the individual patient before choosing which one is appropriate for him or her. It may take months or sometimes years to find the right combination of medications the patient can tolerate and will be effective. I have had several patients who tolerate very few medications or have contraindications that make it almost impossible to choose an effective regimen that won't hurt them. I have followed a young lady for seven years, since she was sixteen, who has hepatitis B and rheumatoid arthritis. She has no insurance and very little money, despite working three jobs. She can't afford treatment for hepatitis B, and methotrexate, Arava, and all the biologics can't be used in a patient with hepatitis B. Despite trying a combination of Plaquenil, Azulfidine, Imuran, and prednisone, I have watched her hands become more and more deformed. I am saddened and frustrated and hope to get her treatment for her hepatitis B so that we can treat her RA properly. There are a few other patients who develop intolerable side effects to every drug I try. Some patients are fearful of medications and refuse most. These patients are satisfied with medications that just make them comfortable even if their joints become more and more deformed, and they become slowly disabled. Many of them would rather have multiple joint surgeries than take a medication. I try in vain to explain to these patients that RA is a systemic disease and that it is affecting their heart and other organs as well as their joints. However, I never try to force the issue because I have learned that if a patient is sure something bad will happen from taking a medication, it often does!

Oral, IV, or IM (intramuscular) steroids are used as symptomatic treatment, although occasionally they can abort a flare and induce remission while the true remittive agent maintains it. I will often give a patient who is having a flare an intramuscular injection of triamcinolone or betamethasone, a long-acting steroid to quickly reduce inflammation and buy some time until I start a new remittive agent or until the one I am using takes effect. I will also use it during a flare to reset the patient, give some relief, and then reevaluate. I won't consider these injections more than three times a year, to avoid the ill effects of steroids. I rarely use oral prednisone for any prolonged period of time because it is really hard to wean these patients off it and long-term, bad things will happen, especially osteoporosis and infection. Most studies show that the remittive agents have only a small increased incidence of infections unless paired with prednisone; then the incidence increases dramatically. Occasionally I give patients a supply of prednisone as an emergency stash in case of a flare during a trip. Patients who have been on low doses of prednisone for years often show few signs of inflammation but have significant deformities, proving once again that it is not a remittive agent.

Nonsteroidal anti-inflammatory drugs (NSAIDS), such as ibuprofen, Naprosyn, Celebrex, and so forth, treat symptoms and have the extra benefit of being an analgesic for the already damaged joints or those with osteoarthritis. However, they are not remittive agents, and they have many adverse effects I would like to avoid. Therefore, I do not prescribe them as often as I did years ago. See my discussion in the medications chapter for more details.

Up until the late nineties, we had some partial successes in the treatment of RA and many dismal failures. These days we aim for close to 100 percent remission with RA and often achieve it!

Pearls

- RA is an inflammatory arthritis usually involving multiple small and large joints.
- RA is a systemic disease that affects multiple organs, not just the joints.
- If diagnosed and treated early (within six months of onset), it has a much better prognosis.
- Anti-CCP is a very specific antibody for RA. Rheumatoid factor is more sensitive. One antibody can be positive while the other is negative, so initially both should be tested.

- Physicians should be regularly monitoring joint inflammation and activity with joint counts, measures of activities of daily living, ESRs, and/ or CRPs.
- The target should be remission of disease.
- The aim should be rapid escalation of doses of methotrexate within three to six months, and if remission not achieved, add a biologic.
- Triple-drug therapy with methotrexate, Plaquenil, and Azulfidine may be as effective clinically but not radiologically as adding a biologic agent to methotrexate.
- Prognosis is generally very good if treated early and aggressively.
- There are a wide variety of biologic drugs available, and all can be effective but need to be monitored regularly for toxicity, especially infection.
- Only Xeljanz and Actemra have been shown to be effective as monotherapy (without methotrexate). In other words, most medications are more effective when paired with methotrexate or another drug.
- If patient is not responding to most drugs or combinations after three months, consider change of dose or medication.

References

1. Cush, John J., Michael E. Weinblatt, and Arthur Kavanaugh. *Rheumatoid Arthritis: Early Diagnosis and Treatment.*

2. Groekoop-Ruiterman, Y. P., et al. Comparison of Treatment Strategies in Early Rheumatoid Arthritis: A Randomized Trial. *Ann. Int. Med.* 146:40.

3. De Vries-Bouwstra, J. K., et al. Progression of Joint Damage in Early Rheumatoid Arthritis: Association with HLA-DRB1, Rheumatoid Factor, and Anticitrillunated Antibodies in Relation to Different Treatment Strategies. *Arthritis and Rheumatism* 58:1293.

Rheumatoid Arthritis (RA)

4. Grigor, C., et al. Effect of a Treatment Strategy of Tight Control for Rheumatoid Arthritis (the TICORA Study): A Single-Randomized Controlled Trial. *Lancet* 364:263.

5. Choy, E. H., et al. A Two Year Randomized Study of Intramuscular Depot Steroids on Patients with Established Rheumatoid Arthritis Who Have Shown an Incomplete Response to Disease Modifying Antirheumatic Drugs. *Ann. Rheum. Dis.* 64:1288.

6. Russell, A. S., et al. The Role of Anti-Citillunated Cyclic Peptide Antibodies in Predicting Progression of Palindromic Rheumatism to Rheumatoid Arthritis *J Rheumatology* 33:1240.

7. Turreson, C., et al. Extraarticular Disease Manifestations in Rheumatoid Arthritis: Incidence, Trends and Risk Factors over 46 Years. *Ann Rheum Dis* 62:722.

8. Anderson, J. J., G. Wells, A. C. Verhoeven, and D. T. Felson. 2000. "Factors Predicting Response to Treatment in Rheumatoid Arthritis: The Importance of Disease Duration. *Arthritis Rheum* 43:22.

9. Emery, P., F. Breedveld, D. van der Heijde, et al. Two-Year Clinical and Radiographic Results with Combination Etanercept-Methotrexate Therapy versus Monotherapy in Early Rheumatoid Arthritis: A Two-Year, Double-Blind, Randomized Study. *Arthritis Rheum* 62:674.

10. Nam, J. L., K. L. Winthrop, R. F. van Vollenhoven, et al. Current Evidence for the Management of Rheumatoid Arthritis with Biological Disease-Modifying Antirheumatic Drugs: A Systematic Literature Review Informing the EULAR Recommendations for the Management of RA. *Ann Rheum Dis* 69:976.

11. McInnes, I. B., and J. R. O'Dell. State-of-the-Art: Rheumatoid Arthritis. *Ann Rheum Dis* 69:1898.

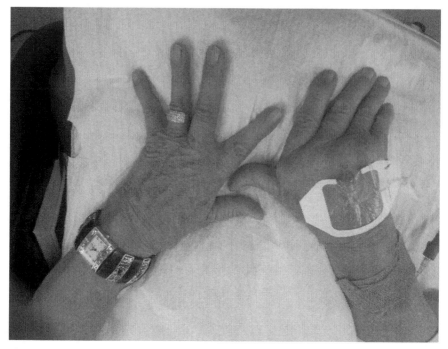

*Advanced rheumatoid
arthritis with deformities*

Chapter Two

Systemic Lupus Erythematosus (Lupus, or SLE)

The Girl with the Butterfly Rash

I made Sandra's diagnosis from across the room when I first met her. She was the stereotypical sex and age and had a classic rash. At the time she was a twenty-year-old African American student who had exceled at her studies but for months had had trouble concentrating and remembering facts. She described extreme fatigue and "brain fog," was generally achy, and had a knife-like chest pain when she took a deep breath. She had a bright red, butterfly-shaped rash on her face, and when she opened her mouth, she had a large, painless ulcer on her hard palate. I thought she had stepped out of a rheumatology textbook chapter on lupus and felt confident I could make a big difference. Sure enough, all her symptoms and signs resolved after a short course of moderate-dose prednisone, and with continued Plaquenil therapy, she is flourishing.

Like most of the diseases we see, it is inflammatory and autoimmune. You might hear the term *collagen vascular disease* because it affects the collagen fibers in blood vessels, but that can be confusing. What does all this mean? I always tell patients that in most of these diseases, their immune system has a defect that unlocks or disinhibits it and allows it to overproduce messengers or signals that stimulate inflammatory cells in their blood, which cause them to multiply and produce many autoantibodies (*auto*, "directed against self"). These renegade cells and antibodies attack organs, joints, and blood vessels, and each of the autoimmune inflammatory diseases have their own unique clinical features depending on the kind of cells and messengers that are released and what part of the body is affected. Lupus is often linked to certain genetic profiles and usually starts in the early twenties, but it can affect infants, children, and the elderly. Like most of our diseases, it is mainly a female disease. It may be hormone related, but we don't really know because there is mixed data. It is one of the classic diseases in rheumatology and has always been considered a great mimicker or chameleon because it has so many guises. Many of its features, such as rashes or even psychoses, can be mistaken for other diseases, such as psoriasis or schizophrenia. The reverse is also true. I have seen "lupus" rashes turn out to be shingles (as I describe below). Although most lupus patients fulfill certain criteria (we rheumatologists love criteria), some have certain classic features, and others have different ones. Also, the disease severity varies from catastrophic and life threatening to mild, not requiring medication. It is the prospect of the former that makes most docs pay extra attention to these patients. Fortunately, unless you work in a tertiary care hospital, the catastrophic patients are rare. In fact, the prognosis of lupus has improved dramatically in the decades since the fifties when survival was short and the diagnosis was considered a death warrant. Many lupus patients during the early years of rheumatology were on high-dose steroids and were disfigured by their disease or their medication. Often, they had some sort of organ failure. It's a different world now, and either we are better at treating this disease, diagnosing it earlier, or dealing with disease that has changed. Overall, patients do well and rarely need steroids, but there are exceptions, and we have to be alert. I tell patients that I am better at putting out little fires than raging ones, so come in early and often. We should watch for red flags in these patients. I find that they all follow their own unique patterns so that if bad flares start with a rash in one patient, they may start with fever and palpitations in another. These patterns tend to repeat themselves.

So who is the classic lupus patient? First, remember this is a systemic disease; it's in the bloodstream, so patients often do not feel well. They are often horribly fatigued, achy, and may even run fevers and lose weight. That's why it can be difficult to distinguish it from infection or even cancer, but there are ways. The pictures of lupus patients you see in textbooks usually include a bright red but-terfly rash on their cheeks, which is raised. This rash is usually sun sensitive, spares the area between the nose and the upper lip, and can be scarring or disfiguring. Lupus is a disease of many kinds of rashes on many locations of the body. Some of the most scarring are called *discoid rashes* and are usually raised and inflammatory. I have seen many patients who have had horrible rashes from head to toe, including their scalp. One older patient had permanent white scars on her trunk by the time I first saw her and did not clear the angry raised blotches on her skin for one year until I found the proper regimen of medications. Another young lady had an extensive rash on her trunk that was leaving whitish scars, which she had been told by a dermatologist was vitiligo. She was soon to be married and was trying to fill in the white spots by tanning. I warned her that tanning might make her rash and scarring worse because lupus patients and their rashes are usually photosensitive (to all light in the ultraviolet spectrum), but I never saw her again. I have had several patients who have developed rashes on Plaquenil, the most commonly used drug for lupus rash. Ironically, it can cause a pretty awful, itchy rash itself if the patient is allergic to it. The Plaquenil rash usually spares the face but not always. If in doubt, I stop the medication, but the allergic reaction can linger for months, so occasionally I consult dermatology and obtain a skin biopsy to sort things out.

Two other unusual kinds of rashes are called *subacute cutaneous lupus* and *lupus profundus*, which can be severe and disfiguring. The former often starts as a small raised lesion and becomes circular with a raised red margin. It can be quite artistically distinctive and also can be caused by a variety of medications. My last case was an eighty-year-old Swedish male who had these circles on his whole trunk. He responded to meds, but as soon as we stopped them, the rash returned. He is now on chronic therapy and is rash-free. Lupus profundus is actually inflammation and atrophy of the subcutaneous fat, so it causes depressions or craters in the skin and subcutaneous area. It usually starts with an inflamed, raised, firm, and painful nodule. Steroid injections into the muscle can cause similar craters by causing fat atrophy, but they are not usually painful. Since these lesions are inflammatory, I have learned to treat them aggressively, often with steroids, and they usually resolve. My last two patients thought that they had some sort of nerve problem leading to muscle atrophy. One had a painful crater in her buttocks, and the other had one at the back of her shoulder. I admit I had my doubts, but a tapering dose of steroids and some adjustment of their maintenance drugs helped resolve this problem. Not all patients have such satisfying results. Again these cutaneous features can be scarring, disfiguring, and distressing (especially to young women) and should be treated aggressively. Remember, lupus can cause many other kinds of rashes, including bullous or blister-like lesions, but be careful because lupus patients who may be immunosuppressed may be susceptible to skin infections, such as shingles or herpes zoster, and treatment for lupus rashes could make these infections worse. Don't treat rashes over the phone because you don't know what you are treating unless you see it. Another common feature of lupus is painless oral or nasal ulcers. Again, don't treat these over the phone because there are many causes of oral ulcers, such as herpes or yeast infections, that may be exacerbated by conventional treatment for lupus. A red flag may be that the ulcers are painful. Rheumatology is a hands-on specialty that is very visual.

It is important to know that patients can have discoid lupus without having systemic lupus. These patients do not have positive antibodies or have low levels and do not have any of the other manifestations of systemic lupus. Of these patients 5 to 10 percent will eventually develop the systemic version. One of the first questions asked by newly diagnosed lupus patients is "What kind of lupus do I have?" It's reassuring to tell them that it's just discoid lupus limited to their skin.

Speaking of hands, Raynaud's phenomenon is fairly common in these patients and is characterized by white, purple, and red color changes of fingers, toes, and even nose in the cold or under stress. Warming measures are all that are usually needed, but occasionally patients may develop digital ulcers and even gangrene. These patients will have cool if not cold fingers, which may be white or dusky during the exam, especially if the room is cold. They may complain of numb and painful hands or feet when coming out of the shower or into any cooling environment. My patients often find it amusing that my hands are colder than theirs or that my nose is purple during the winter. They are comforted and reassured when I tell them that I have Raynaud's, although I have no known underlying disease. I think it makes me more human and perhaps more understanding.

Rudy's Ruminations On **Rheumatology**

We share advice regarding gloves, socks, and warming measures and jokes about Rudy's red nose during Christmas. Raynaud's is usually just a spasm of the small vessels and benign in the vast majority of patients. However, occasionally, it can be the result of vasculitis or inflammation of small or even larger vessels, which can lead to gangrene and loss of limbs. In diseases such as lupus and scleroderma, the inflammation can damage the lining of the blood vessels, leading to permanent damage and narrowing. So, not all Raynaud's is benign.

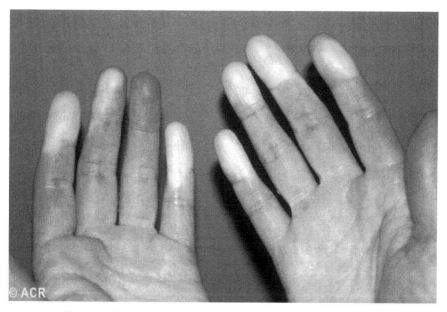

Raynaud's phenomenon—courtesy of ACR image bank

Hair loss, or alopecia, in patches or total can be quite devastating to these often young women. It can be associated with scarring discoid scalp rashes and be permanent. Recently I had a forty year-old lupus patient lift her ponytail and show me that the whole back of her head was bald. We have medications that can treat or prevent the hair loss, such as antimalarials, but ironically they can also cause hair loss. I have had several patients bring me bags of hair to prove this particular point. The hair loss resolves in some cases off these medications. To make it even more confusing, there are several other medications, such as methotrexate, Cytoxan, Imuran, and CellCept, that can cause hair loss. Several unrelated conditions, such as iron deficiency, hypothyroidism, and stress, also cause hair loss. Of course hormones and genetics also may play a part as I discover every time I look in the mirror. Dermatologists often treat alopecia with steroid injections into the scalp with success, but antimalarial medications are the most commonly used medications.

Patients often have joint pain and swelling, especially in the hands. They may have hand deformities called *Jaccoud's arthropathy*, which unlike those in rheumatoid arthritis will disappear if they flatten their hands on a level surface. Although their joints may be very inflamed, they rarely are destroyed as they are in rheumatoid arthritis, but there are exceptions. I have seen a few lupus patients who have a very destructive arthritis. Their finger bones are resorbed and shortened while their joints are destroyed and deformed just like in severe, untreated RA. Joint pain, or arthralgias, without signs of swelling may be the predominant complaint in many patients. Often they are referred with the diagnosis of rheumatoid arthritis, especially since many of the antibody tests for both diagnoses may overlap. A good history and full exam should easily distinguish the two. Most of the time, the joint pain and swelling is polyarticular, or involving many joints, and is symmetrical. If one joint is involved, especially a hip or knee, I look for other causes, such as osteoarthritis or aseptic necrosis. Bone death or aseptic or avascular necrosis may occur in almost any joint in a lupus patient, especially those who have been on high-dose steroids for a long period of time. It means that the circulation to the bone has been compromised, and so the bone dies and eventually collapses, like a dead tree. Unfortunately, these patients tend to have been the sickest and may be fully recovered when the event occurs. One of my favorite patients is a young Vietnamese woman who had a particularly severe case of lupus, which included a stroke at age twenty-one. She was treated with a variety of medications, including a prolonged course of high-dose steroids, to no avail until we tried a "new" medication at the time called *Rituxan*. She had a complete resolution of her signs and symptoms, felt great, and resumed her normal life until one day she limped into my office with a painful hip. An MRI revealed aseptic necrosis of both hips, meaning the bones had died because of poor blood supply caused by prolonged high-dose steroids. She had both hips replaced within the year and resumed her normal life. It's important to distinguish aseptic necrosis as a cause of joint pain from inflammation because aseptic necrosis can lead to collapse of the bone and should not be treated with steroids, for obvious reasons.

Fatigue may be the most common complaint in autoimmune diseases because they are systemic. Lupus is no different. The fatigue may be overwhelming and may have major impact on the patient's personal and work life. Treatment of the underlying disease may resolve the problem, but often the fatigue is multifactorial. Depression, insomnia, sleep apnea, anemia, and hypothyroidism are just some of the factors that need to be considered and addressed. Patients often are not aware of these problems, and I find that subtle detective work and intuition are important. Appropriate lab work and very occasionally sleep studies and psychological analysis by a good therapist who uses psychometric testing can be helpful. I also find it important to have a spouse, sibling, or parent in the exam room to act as an objective witness (a "truth teller") and supplement the patient's memory. Many people will deny depression, and I have had many patients in tears as they are denying it. I also have had patients, especially men, who improve with antidepressants, stop the medications, and only after a return of their symptoms realize that they must have been depressed. Denial is not just a river in Egypt.

Generalized or focal weakness is also common. It may be a function of fatigue, joint pain or dysfunction, or actual muscle involvement. Muscle inflammation, especially in the shoulders, upper arms, thighs, and upper legs, occurs in a small minority of patients and may cause the patients to have difficulty rising from a sitting position, combing their hair, or even walking long distances. Their clinical picture overlaps with another disease I will discuss later—polymyositis. Most of these patients will have abnormal labs such as creatine phosphokinase (CPKs) and aldolases. They may also have abnormal electromyograms, and even muscle biopsies. In my experience muscle involvement in lupus is usually mild and rarely requires extensive workup or treatment. In fact, muscle involvement, like fatigue, often is caused by other factors, such as medications. Plaquenil, or hydroxychloroquine, can cause a weird kind of muscle disease called *vacuolar myopathy*. The definitive diagnosis is based on biopsy. Since many patients with lupus are taking this drug and weakness is common, patients are undiagnosed for years with devastating results. Prednisone and other steroids in higher doses can cause weakness but usually without an elevation of CPKs. Statin drugs, used to treat high cholesterol, are probably the most common cause that I see, often associated with an elevation of CPKs. Hypothyroid is always in the different diagnosis of muscle weakness with an elevated CPK. Sedentary or chronically ill patients may have disuse atrophy of their muscles and be clinically weak. So you can see, rheumatologists need to be good internists and hands-on physicians.

Kidney inflammation and failure are two of the scariest manifestations of lupus. If left untreated, many lupus patients will need dialysis. Treating early and aggressively may prevent the need for dialysis and maintain kidney function. Usually the patients who have kidney disease show activity in other systems. Hypertension, anemia, or edema may be signs of kidney disease, but usually patients are asymptomatic until the disease is advanced. Frequent urinalyses are helpful; they may lead to early treatment and prevent severe kidney damage. Antibodies and other inflammatory factors flood the kidneys and cause inflammation and, if left unchecked, cause increasing damage eventually leading to kidney failure. Occasionally, lupus patients will have diffuse swelling or edema, low albumin in their blood, or very high levels of protein in their urine. The loss of protein in their urine leading to low protein in the blood allows the blood to leak out of blood vessels into the skin, causing edema. Many of these patients have nephrotic syndrome (large amounts of protein in the urine, edema, low albumin or protein, high cholesterol) and can leak fluid into their abdominal and lung cavities. They can be gravely ill. These patients need to be treated aggressively. An effective treatment of 'lupus nephritis or kidney disease has been the Holy Grail for decades. Kidney failure quickly changes the prognosis of lupus from good to poor and certainly affects the quality of life of these typically young women.

In the past, treatments have been only partially effective and have often led to massive weight gain, disfigurement, hair loss, and infertility. No wonder many of these patients were depressed! Fortunately, treatment and outcomes have changed dramatically. I have had the pleasure of watching the science and application evolve with sometimes spectacular results. Two decades ago, many of my patients would disappear from my practice because once their kidneys failed and they were on dialysis, many nephrologists, or kidney doctors, felt their lupus was in remission and they no longer needed rheumatologists. This debatable conclusion is moot now since very few patients treated early and aggressively go into kidney failure. I still use the "little fire" theory, and if I see any sign of activity when examining the patient's urine, I obtain a twenty-four-hour urine collection, check some lupus antibodies and other activity markers, and treat early and aggressively. Many experts advise kidney biopsies in lupus patients with signs of kidney inflammation very early in the disease. The biopsy tissue can reveal the kind and degree of inflammation in the kidney and the degree of fibrosis or scarring. This information can produce an activity and chronicity index, which helps providers choose the appropriate treatment. Obviously, the more scarring and chronicity, the harder it is to reverse kidney dysfunction, and the more activity, the more aggressive the therapy will be required to prevent chronicity and kidney failure. Still, kidney disease can be devastating to lupus patients and should be treated early and aggressively. Blood tests for creatinine and glomerular filtration rates, as well as the urinalyses, should be done regularly, and blood pressures should be monitored closely. Once any of these parameters are abnormal and the patient is not responding to therapy, he or she should be referred to a nephrologist (kidney specialist). However, with the new therapy available, it's been years since I have seen a patient develop irreversible kidney damage unless he or she already had years of severe damage prior to being treated.

Recently, I saw a twenty-nine-year-old woman with lupus and on Plaquenil who developed kidney disease, severe edema, and anemia. She lost her job because she was absent too often, lost her insurance, her husband left her, and the government took away her unemployment benefits. When I saw her, she was extremely pale and had massively swollen legs. We diagnosed nephrotic syndrome (a protein-losing kidney disease that is associated with extreme edema), started her on prednisone and CellCept, and sent her to nephrology. They performed a kidney biopsy and found that she had a particularly bad form of lupus kidney disease (diffuse prolifera-tive nephritis with crescents) with a moderate chronicity and high activity index. We continued her on 40 mg of prednisone and 3 g of CellCept, but I wondered whether we should be even more aggres-sive and treat her with Cytoxan. Although she initially improved, by 2015, her kidney function began deteriorating again much to every-one's dismay. It had been years since I had seen a Lupus patient so resistant to treatment. I took it personally. With the assistance of a kidney doctor, we initiated a six -month trial of intravenous Cytoxan (the medical equivalent of a nuclear bomb) without much success. Her kidney function continued to deteriorate and she developed se-vere headaches, anemia requiring repeated transfusions amd just felt awful. I consulted Bevra Hahn the former chief of rheumatol-ogy at UCLA and one of the world's leading Lupus experts and at her suggestion prescribed Tacrolimus and Rituxan based on some small promising studies. As I write this second edition, the patient is on low dose daily Prednisone and Rituxan every six months. She seems to have stabilized at a kidney function of 30%. I am skeptical that she can avoid dialysis and kidney transplant in the future but stranger things have happened. I have treated several patients who had worse kidney function and have improved and stabilized over two decades but they responded within the first 6 months of treat-ment. The longer it takes, the worse the prognosis. It's been over two years.......

Neurological manifestations of lupus are numerous and also can be very scary. Probably the most common one is headache, which can be quite severe and come in all forms, including migraines. Brain fog or cognitive dysfunction is relatively common and in some rare cases can lead to dementia. I have seen an intelligent lawyer become a disoriented street cleaner in a matter of years. There are some questionably effective treatments, so early detection is important with objective cognitive studies performed by trained psychologists. Sometimes it's hard to distinguish early dementia from depression or the effects of medication. Recently I've been treating a very intelligent, high-functioning lupus patient who insisted her cognitive skills were deteriorating rapidly and begged me to treat her. She did her own research and concluded IV Cytoxan had the most chance of success. I concurred but warned her of the consequences of long-term Cytoxan therapy that include lymphoma and bladder cancer. She had three doses of monthly IV Cytoxan and felt there was a remarkable improvement. Thrilled, I immediately stopped the Cytoxan and maintained her on Benlysta and Quinacrine for 2 years. Unfortunately, she began complaining again of increasing brain fog--losing words and becoming disoriented. A psychological assessment revealed mild cognitive impairment. I tried Prednisone again and a variety of other medications but the patient was beginning to panic because she was losing herself. She felt Cytoxan gave her the best chance for recovery and was willing to take the chance of cancer in future years. After consulting several internationally recognized Lupus specialists, I reluctantly restarted the Cytoxan and at this writing am holding my breath. Oxygen is by my bed.

Seizures of all kind occur and are usually due to brain inflammation. A noninfectious meningitis or encephalitis must be distinguished from infectious causes in these patients whose immune system is often compromised. These patients will often be hospitalized with high fevers, severe headache, vomiting, mental status changes, and even coma. Stroke of the brain or spinal cord can lead to total or partial paralysis, but in some cases, treated aggressively, it is reversible. I already described my twenty-one-year-old Vietnamese patient who had a stroke with speech difficulties and severe right-sided weakness. She had a complete recovery after six months of aggressive treatment. Two years ago, I had a similar experience with a forty-year-old Hispanic woman. Unlike strokes in elderly patients, those in lupus patients may resolve completely—sometimes. I think part of the reason is because the patients are younger and have more plasticity. More recently, I have become aware of PRES syndrome (posterior reversible encephalopathy syndrome), where patients have severe headaches, altered consciousness, visual disturbances, and sometimes seizures. It is often caused by uncontrolled hypertension and rarely by certain immunosuppressive drugs or pregnancy. With prompt treatment and withdrawal of the offending medications, the condition is totally reversible. PRES probably has existed for a long time but only recently has received a lot of press. The longer I study, the more there is to know; but somehow it gets easier. Science I once thought I would never understand has become basic knowledge and has laid the groundwork for much more sophisticated versions. Finally, in lupus, personality changes can occur, and patients can be psychotic. There have been cases of severe paranoia, and untreated patients can be dangerous to themselves or others. I have to admit that since I left Los Angeles, I have rarely seen these extreme cases. It could be that the extreme cases go to the big centers or they are being detected and treated earlier, but again maybe lupus is changing. One of my early and more amusing teachers in rheumatology shared a sad but humorous anecdote with me about one such patient. He admitted an attractive, nice forty-year-old housewife to the rheumatology ward in County Hospital for signs of psychosis and lupus one evening. The next morning during rounds with the rheumatology fellows and residents, she was standing on her bed, pointing her finger at my teacher, and accusing him of infecting her with lupus. I am not sure of the outcome of this encounter, but there have been a few rheumatologists murdered by psychotic, paranoid lupus patients.

Remembering that lupus is an inflammatory disease, it's not hard to imagine its effects on the heart. Pericarditis (inflammation of the covering of the heart) leads to pleurisy, or knife-like chest pain with breathing. It can also lead to pericardial effusion, or fluid accumulating between the pericardium (heart covering: think cellophane wrapping) and the heart. This fluid can prevent the heart from expanding fully and cause shortness of breath, heart failure, or arrest. Inflammation of the heart muscle can lead to heart failure, cardiomyopathy (chronic heart muscle dysfunction or failure), and conduction or rhythm problems. Shortness of breath, syncope, skipped beats, chest pain, and edema can all result. The chest pain is characteristically pleuritic (the knife-like pain with breathing mentioned above). An inflammation of the lung lining may cause a similar pain. I encounter patients several times a year who complain of such pain, and if I'm satisfied that they don't have an infection or a major cardiac problem, I treat them with nonsteroidal anti-inflammatory drugs (NSAIDs); if their symptoms persist, two weeks of 20 mg of prednisone will do the trick. Very rarely, patients can develop noninfectious deposits on their heart valves that flip emboli to the brain. This syndrome is called *Libman-Sachs endocarditis*. Pulmonary hypertension, where the pulmonary artery between the heart and the lung develops high pressures, may be the most insidious manifestation of lupus because patients become increasingly short of breath over time and over a few years become oxygen dependent and eventually die. Often, it is not detected until late in the process and is then irreversible. Yet, I have been impressed by how early detection with a combination of pulmonary function tests, an echocardiogram with Doppler, and finally, right heart catheterization or angiogram by a friendly and competent cardiologist may make a major difference. If the pulmonary pressures are found to be mildly elevated and treatment is initiated early, the process may be stopped in its tracks. So I have become hypervigilant about this disease and have a great working relationship with one of our local cardiologists. We will discuss medications later, but I find it ironic that I am prescribing Viagra-like drugs to these young and middle-aged females who have mild pulmonary hypertension. Finally, lupus or almost any of the systemic inflammatory diseases are risk factors for coronary artery disease. It's important to minimize inflammation and eliminate risk factors, such as smoking, hypertension, and high cholesterol.

Inflammation plays a big part in the lupus lung. Serositis or pleurisy caused by the inflammation of the pleura or the covering of the lungs can cause severe pleuritic chest pain or pleural effusions (fluid between the pleura and the lung), causing shortness of breath, cough, or even respiratory or heart failure. Inflammation of the lungs can cause an acute pneumonitis mimicking an infectious pneumonia. Infection always needs to be ruled out. Remember, these patients are often immunocompromised and can get really weird infections. Chronic low- or high-grade inflammation can lead to scarring and or fibrosis, which can lead to oxygen dependence and severe debility. Treated aggressively and early (my mantra), these processes may be reversed. I think it is important to have an early pulmonary consultation and obtain a biopsy if necessary. If we miss an infection and treat with immunosuppressive therapy, we can do a lot of harm, which violates our Hippocratic Oath. One of the rheumatology emergencies is pulmonary hemorrhage in a lupus patient. They will become critically ill, and 50 percent will die. Patients may cough blood, become acutely short of breath, or even go into respiratory failure. This problem warrants immediate hospitalization, bronchoscopy, and biopsy since diagnosis and aggressive treatment can be lifesaving. The biopsy may show hemosiderin (a remnant form of iron from old, dead red blood cells) in macrophages (a type of white blood cell), which indicates the bleeding has been going on for some time and makes lupus more likely to be the cause. Several years ago, a lupus patient who lived in a city one hour away called me and told me she was coughing blood and acutely short of breath. I told her to go to the emergency room, and I called her primary care physician, urging him to arrange an emergency bronchoscopy. As in many cases with lupus, the treatment for pulmonary hemorrhage could make an infection worse, and since infection is always a possibility, it should be ruled out. The pulmonary doctor on call argued with me regarding the necessity for an urgent bronchoscopy but eventually relented. Within the hour, he called me and sounded almost hysterical about the amount of blood he saw in the patient's lung; because he was not comfortable with the medications we wanted him to order, he transferred the patient to a bigger medical center. The patient is still under my care and doing well today.

The GI (gastrointestinal) system is more frequently involved due to medication side effects, but patients can have mild to moderate liver-function abnormalities, especially during flares. Just like in other systems, general inflammation can cause inflammation of the omentum, the covering of the abdominal cavity, leading to severe abdominal pain that simulates many surgical emergencies, such as appendicitis or an infection. It is the GI equivalent of pericarditis or pleurisy. Inflammatory bowel disease and pancreatitis can occur in a small percentage of patients. I also had one patient who developed a huge spleen—so big I thought she was at risk for spontaneous rupture and death. She recovered nicely from removal of her spleen. Clearly, there are many conditions that cause a big spleen, especially malignancy and infection, but lupus certainly can do it.

Rudy's Ruminations On **Rheumatology**

Various parts of the eyes can be inflamed, such as the sclera (the white of the eye) or iris, and if untreated, it can lead to blindness. Fortunately, these manifestations are treatable and rare. When I am looking for a cause for iritis or scleritis, lupus is usually in the differential. The bottom line is that a red eye in a lupus patient or any chronic inflammatory disease must be taken seriously, with an immediate eye consultation. Recently, I have seen a lupus patient who had very painful eyes and visual blurriness. She was found to have optic neuritis, or inflammation of the optic nerves. It is a fairly uncommon problem in lupus and can be characteristic of multiple sclerosis. The patient's workup for multiple sclerosis was negative, but her measures of lupus activity were very high. We treated her lupus aggressively, with complete resolution of her symptoms. Again our friendly ophthalmologist was a key to making the diagnosis.

Low white and red blood cell and platelet (cells that make blood clot) counts are common because antibodies attach to them and they are either destroyed or sent to the garbage disposal of the body—the spleen. Rarely the counts become so low they are life threatening. Lupus patients seem to tolerate lower counts than the normal population, but they can crash quickly. One of my hardest lupus patients was a young doctor who was also a doctor's wife; she was six months pregnant, was on high-dose prednisone, had a platelet count of nine thousand (normal, one hundred fifty to four hundred fifty thousand), and was bleeding from her nose, vagina, and rectum. Both the mother and baby survived with treatment, but the doctor lost most of his hair. I usually don't worry about platelet counts above thirty thousand unless the patient is bleeding, although hematologists seem to worry around fifteen to twenty thousand. We watch for bruises and petechiae (little red bumps, usually on the legs). Interestingly, most lupus patients will run low white counts when they have active disease (with exceptions), which helps distinguish lupus activity from bacterial infection but not viral. I usually don't worry about white blood cell counts until they are about two thousand, but the key is the neutrophil (a type of white cell) number—it becomes dangerous when it is below fifteen hundred. Patients are then at high risk for infection. It is again rare but worth knowing. Hemolytic anemia means the antibodies are destroying the body's red cells. Again it is rare but very serious. Most of the hematological findings I see are mild but may sometimes indicate disease activity and be helpful in distinguishing lupus from infection.

Pregnancy can be an adventure with lupus. The rules are as follows: If the disease is inactive, kidney functions are normal, and the patient does not have anticardiolipin, beta-2 glycoprotein, phosphatidylserine, anti-SSA or anti-SSB antibodies, or lupus anticoagulant, they are a low-risk pregnancy. Otherwise, they either should not become pregnant or be under the supervision of a high-risk obstetrician. Active disease or severe kidney disease are contraindications to pregnancies because they put the mother at high risk. Anticardiolipin, phosphatidylserine, and beta-2 glycoprotein antibodies and lupus anticoagulant are paradoxically called *circulating anticoagulants*, but they make the blood clot easily, so they can cause the placenta to clot and induce miscarriages. Blood thinners during the pregnancy can be effective. Anti-SSA and anti-SSB antibodies, also called anti-Rho and anti-La antibodies can be associated with complete heart block in the fetus or infant, so you can see that pregnancy can be an adventure. In the last paragraph, I shared one of my most exciting ones with you.

Many of the patients referred to us with the diagnosis of lupus just have a positive ANA (antinuclear antibody) lab test with very few other findings consistent with lupus. The ANA is a very sensitive test for lupus, found in 93 percent of patients, but it is not very specific since only 60 percent of patients with a positive ANA have lupus.

In other words, it's unlikely a patient has lupus if the ANA is negative, but there is a 60 percent chance a patient with a positive ANA has lupus. Medications, infections, thyroid disease, and many other chronic diseases, especially those that are autoimmune, are associated with this antibody. It is a great screening test but does not correlate with activity. Anti-double-stranded DNA antibodies and anti-Smith antibodies are much more specific for lupus, but their accuracy also depends on the lab. Low serum complement (C3, C4, CH50) correlates with disease activity as does elevated ESRs (sedimentation rate) or CRPs (C'reactive protein), but remember that infection, liver disease, and other factors can affect these measurements as well. Bottom line—positive ANA does not equal lupus, and many patients have been incorrectly given that diagnosis based on this test and joint pain. I see many patients who have been handed from physician to physician, carrying the diagnosis of lupus, who really don't have the disease. The flip side of this problem is that some patients may be intermittently negative for these antibodies and asymptomatic on medications. I have made the mistake of discounting the diagnosis made by another physician because of a vague history and no findings. To my chagrin and embarrassment, the diagnosis becomes obvious when the patient stopstaking medication at my request and the symptoms return and so do the positive blood tests.

Treatment or Meds Used in Lupus

(For more information, please refer to the medication chapter.)

Decades ago almost every lupus patient had a round face, was obese, and had arms and legs full of bruises because the only effective treatment for lupus was steroids. High doses treated severe flares, and low doses maintained the patients. Certainly this treatment improved their outcomes dramatically, but it caused new problems and wasn't the panacea envisioned by many. Over the years new science and understanding has led to new therapies and a better prognosis, but a group of older medications that used to be used in malaria is the mainstay of treatment of lupus. Plaquenil, or hydroxychloroquine, is usually the first-line drug for lupus. It is slow acting and often takes up to three months to take effect. It is particularly effective for rashes, fatigue, and oral ulcers and is good for arthritis. Plaquenil seems to have true remittive qualities in lupus. It provides other bonuses, such as lowering blood sugars and reducing the risk of clot with circulating anticoagulants (see the next chapter). Patients may take this drug for years, and it is relatively safe as long as the patient has eye exams on a regular basis. Very rarely it can cause pigment to be deposited in the cornea or retina, but when detected early, there is no impact on vision if the medication is discontinued—so the regular eye exams are vital. I find that the most common side effect is an itchy rash on the trunk that can become quite severe and require months of therapy. Rarely, patients can develop abdominal pain and diarrhea so severe they are hospitalized for extensive workups. Also very occasionally, it can cause a grayish skin tint, muscle weakness, and ringing in the ears. Overall, this drug is very safe if monitored properly. See my section on medications for further details.

If patients cannot tolerate Plaquenil or continue to have a rash or fatigue, I either add or switch to quinacrine. Unlike Plaquenil, eye toxicity or vision is not an issue. It is particularly good for fatigue, but I find it also is good for rash and cognitive problems. It is such an old drug that it is no longer manufactured and has to be compounded at a compounding pharmacy. Inevitably, once a year a pharmacy will call and tell me that it is no longer made, and I have to remind the patient that it needs to be compounded. Patients also should be told that they have a good chance of turning various shades of orange, which is reversible if the medication is discontinued. Most patients actually like the color because it looks like a good suntan. It is also helpful to tell these patients that their eyeballs will remain white, in case they are worried about jaundice. Several years ago one of my elderly lupus patients forgot my warnings about quinacrine and visited her primary care doctor emergently because she was "jaundiced." Her doctor promptly called me, and until she rechecked the patient's eyeballs would not believe that the patient was not jaundiced. She also checked the patient's liver-function tests to be sure and found them to be normal. Nevertheless, the patient was only one of two patients who ever stopped quinacrine because of color changes.

Chloroquine is another antimalarial drug similar to Plaquenil and may even be more toxic to the eyes, so I do not prescribe it, but many rheumatologists do.

NSAIDs (ibuprofen, Naprosyn, etc.) are helpful to treat joint pain and inflammation, but they are not remittive and not to be used in patients with significant kidney dysfunction. Very rarely, they can cause a kind of noninfectious meningitis in lupus patients. Most cases have been associated with ibuprofen, but I have yet to see one.

I still use steroids as first-line drugs for catastrophic or severe organ involvement, especially in hospitalized patients. IV pulses of high-dose steroids for a few days or high doses of oral steroids for a few weeks or months may induce remission; then the steroids are slowly tapered, discontinued, and replaced by another medication. Kidney, pulmonary, hematological, neurological, and even severe dermatological problems can be treated this way. When I was in training at USC, we would see patients in the ICU who were in a coma and had all these systems involved. Often it was a quandary whether to start them on high doses of steroids while there was still a question of infection, knowing that steroids could make them worse. Usually they were placed on both steroids and antibiotics.

Systemic Lupus Erythematosus (Lupus, or SLE)

I use moderate doses of prednisone (20–30 mg) for pleural or pericardial effusions (fluid around the lungs or heart) or pericarditis (inflammation of the sheath surrounding the heart) but only for a few weeks. Mild organ involvement, such as mild muscle disease, may require these doses. Unlike in the early days of steroid use before its long-term toxicity was so well known, I try to use minimal doses of steroids and taper and discontinue as soon as possible. Keep in mind that these patients are usually young women, and long-term steroid use will doom them to obesity, poor tissue healing, diabetes, hypertension, osteoporosis, accelerated atherosclerosis, recurrent infections, and so forth. Occasionally I will try low-dose prednisone (5–10 mg) for a few weeks or longer to treat fatigue, cachexia, or inflammatory arthritis if there is not a benign alternative. Also occasionally, I will prescribe a few weeks of low-dose steroids to patients with fatigue and joint pain to gauge their response. It helps distinguish between fibromyalgia or lupus in patients who have both. More often, I will give such patients an IM shot of 80 mg triamcinolone, a long-acting, more potent steroid that lasts about two weeks.

I rarely treat lupus patients with steroids these days, and when I do, it is for finite periods.

For patients who have inflammatory arthritis or rashes that have not responded to Plaquenil, methotrexate is a good choice. I seem to be using it more and more, but it can cause hair loss, headaches, and oral ulcers, which already may be a problem for these patients. Arava may be an alternative.

CellCept (mycophenolate mofetil) has become my drug of choice for most patients with kidney disease and it is an effective alternative to Plaquenil and methotrexate for many of the manifestations of lupus, including rash, fatigue, and joint pain. It is far safer and better tolerated than Cytoxan, or cyclophosphamide, which was the drug of choice until recently for severe kidney disease and most catastrophic events in lupus. Cytoxan, IV or orally, is still one of the preferred choices for treatment of kidney and severe neurological disease, but after reviewing the studies and years of watching the havoc Cytoxan wreaks, I rarely use it anymore (although I would in extreme cases). Edema, hypertension, and nausea are the adverse effects I most often encounter with CellCept. In contrast, nausea, low blood counts, cancer, infertility, bleeding bladders, and a variety of equally awful side effects are common with the use of Cytoxan. As I mention later, it has been described as the "nuclear bomb" of medications.

Imuran (azathioprine) is still used by many practitioners for patients who have failed Plaquenil and need a drug to maintain their remission as we wean them off steroids. To me, it is a junior Cytoxan with the added "bonus" of the possibility of pancreatitis. I don't like the medication and rarely use it.

Benlysta (belimumab) is the first new medication for lupus in fifty-plus years. It is an antibody directed against B-lymphocytes, which are a type of white blood cell. Interestingly, some of the cells in this lineage produce antibodies, major players in lupus. Administered intravenously monthly, it is effective for most of the manifestations of lupus, but its effectiveness in kidney and neurological disease has not been confirmed. At this point, it is reserved for patients who have failed antimalarial drugs as well as CellCept, methotrexate, or other nonbiologic medications. I have used it in several patients, including some with severe rashes, with good success. It takes up to six weeks to three months to be effective.

Rituxan (rituximab) is another B-cell inhibitor used in rheumatoid arthritis and lymphoma and off-label for Lupus. I have found it to be lifesaving in some cases. For a graphic illustration, see my medication chapter.

Diet

The only diet that has some scientific support or merit in the treatment of Lupus is the Meiterranean diet but see my chapter on complementary and alternative therapies.

Pearls

- Lupus is a multisystem disease.
- It can occur at any age but most often initially in young women (in their twenties).
- Organ involvement (kidney, etc.) requires aggressive treatment.
- Steroids may be required at varied doses but should be used in the short term.
- Positive ANA does not equal lupus.
- Antimalarials, such as Plaquenil, are first-line drugs.
- Methotrexate, CellCept, and Benlysta are good options.
- Cytoxan should be reserved for extreme cases and emergencies, especially involving the kidneys or nervous system.

References

1. Wallace, Daniel J. *The Lupus Book: A Guide for Patients and their Families*.

2. Wallace, Daniel J., and Bevra Hannahs Hahn. *Dubois' Lupus Erythematosus*.

3. Strand, V. New Therapies for Systemic Lupus Erythematosus. *Rheum Dis. Clin. North Am.* 26:34.

4. Wallace, D. J. Antimalarial Agents and Lupus. *Rheum Dis Clin North Am* 20:243.

5. Akhavan, P. S., J. Su, W. Lou, et al. The Early Protective Effect of Hydroxychloroquine on the Risk of Cumulative Damage in Patients with Systemic Lupus Erythematosus." *J Rheumatol* 40:831.

6. Wallace, D. J., W. Stohl, R. A. Furie, et al. A Phase II, Randomized, Double-Blind, Placebo-Controlled, Dose-Ranging Study of Belimumab in Patients with Active Systemic Lupus Erythematosus. *Arthritis Rheum* 61:1168.

7. Tieng, A. T., and E. Peeva. B-cell-Directed Therapies in Systemic Lupus Erythematosus. *Semin Arthritis Rheum* 38:218.

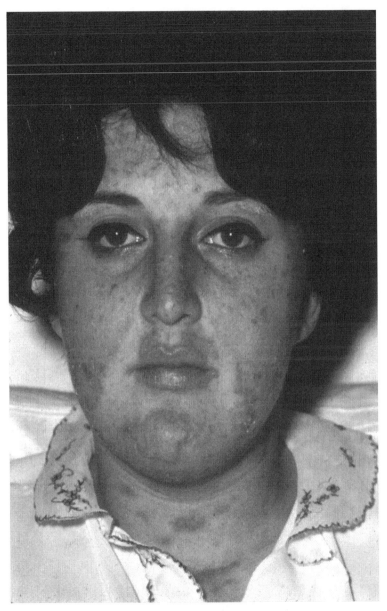

*Lupus with vasculitis, inflammation, and
facial rash—courtesy of ACR image bank*

Chapter Three

Circulating Anticoagulants or Antiphospholipid Antibodies

Three Miscarriages and a Clot

By our first visit, Jackie had had three late-term miscarriages and a blood clot in her leg. Ironically, she was sent to me only because she had Raynaud's phenomenon and a positive ANA. When I examined her, I found that she had a network of dilated blood vessels on her arms and legs and discovered that many of her family members had a history of miscarriages and strokes. Based on all these findings, I suspected that she had an antibody that predisposed her to blood clots, and lo and behold, she had high levels of anticardiolipin antibodies and a lupus anticoagulant. I prescribed a baby aspirin a day for her and have been agonizing over placing her on Coumadin, a potent anticoagulation medication, for life. If the aspirin is not effective, she could have a blot clot to virtually any organ in her body, including her brain or lung. Complicating my decision is her desire for another pregnancy. It would be high risk but could be successful on low-dose heparin (an injectable anticoagulant) and possibly aspirin. Coumadin is contraindicated in pregnancy. And people wonder why I am bald!

Circulating anticoagulants include anticardiolipin antibodies, lupus anticoagulant, and beta-2 glycoprotein antibodies. Paradoxically they make blood clot easily even though they are called "anticoagulants." There are many clotting disorders that predispose patients to blood clots in arteries and veins. They often but not always require a trigger for the clot to occur. Discussion of all these disorders and their diagnostic testing is beyond the scope of this book. However, in the sixties, it was discovered that there was a factor in some patients' blood that made them clot easily. It was called the *lupus anticoagulant* even though it was not just confined to lupus patients. As the years passed, other factors or antibodies were found to have similar properties, and because they had the ability to bind to fatty acids with phosphate molecules, they were called *antiphospholipid antibodies*. They may be associated with lupus, virtually any of the other rheumatologic diseases, or stand alone. They have some genetic links and don't just affect pregnancies. They can cause clots in any blood vessel (vein or artery), most commonly in the deep veins of the legs or arteries of the lungs but virtually anywhere, including the gut, brain, or liver. Results can be devastating. Any patient with recurrent miscarriages or unexplainable blood clots, especially with a family history, should be checked for these antibodies. They must be positive at least twice in a three-month period and at a moderate to high level to be considered valid and warrant treatment. Patients may present with Raynaud's phenomenon—a network of dilated blood vessels on their arms and legs (livedo reticularis)—neurological signs and symptoms, or low platelets. Rarely, they may develop catastrophic antiphospholipid antibody syndrome (CAPS), where they clot off three or more organs in a week or less and become critically ill and require aggressive treatment. Fortunately, the latter scenario is rare and seen in the ICU. I am not sure I have ever seen one. Most cases without a history of major clots may be treated successfully with low-dose aspirin. Once a patient has blood clots, I will treat with him or her with blood thinners, usually Coumadin (warfarin) maintained at a specific anticoagulant level (INR of 2.5–3). As mentioned previously, women with recurrent miscarriages may be treated with a blood thinner called *low molecular weight heparin* and possibly an aspirin. I have successfully treated several lupus pregnancies complicated by these antibodies and a history of miscarriages with this regimen, although I usually send them to a high-risk obstetrician. Patients who have never had a miscarriage but have these antibodies don't necessarily need to be treated unless they have a history of clots. However, they present us with a conundrum regarding whether treating them with low-dose aspirin lowers the risk for future clots. I am not sure we know the answer yet.

I have treated at least two young patients who have had ministrokes. Imaging techniques (MRA and angiogram) have shown signs of clots in the blood vessels of their brains, and both patients have high levels of one of these antibodies. Both are on lifelong Coumadin and have had no recurrences. They are both avid skiers and wear helmets because of their susceptibility to bleed because of their Coumadin.

In conclusion, I screen patients with recurrent miscarriages, arterial occlusive disease, an unexplained stroke, or other unusual arterial or venous thrombotic events for all the antibodies mentioned above, including the lupus anticoagulant. I also search for other conditions or factors that cause hypercoagulable states. These antibodies and conditions are commonly missed, often with tragic repercussions. Treatment can be life and limb saving!

Pearls

- Hypercoagulable states (factors in the blood that make patients clot easily) should be ruled out in patients with recurrent or atypical blood clots or recurrent miscarriages.
- Antiphospholipid antibodies include anticardiolipin antibodies, beta-2 glycoprotein and lupus anticoagulant.
- Other factors that can cause clots include factor 5 Leiden and protein C and S deficiencies.
- If a patient has recurrent or major clots, especially arterial, and has moderate to high titers of antiphospholipid antibodies twice within a three- month interval, the patient should be treated with lifelong Coumadin, with their INR maintained at 2.5–3.
- Pregnancy in a patient with recurrent miscarriages and high to moderate antiphospholipid levels is high risk and may be successfully treated with ASA and low molecular weight heparin.
- So far the new factor X inhibitors or anticoagulants that are being used to replace Coumadin in other venues do not seem to be effective in these patients

References

1. www.rheumatology.org/Practice
(Patient Education—Diseases and Conditions)
2. Levine JS, Branch DW, Rauch J. The antiphospholipid syndrome. N Engl J Med 2002; 346:752.
3. Erkan D, Cervera R, Asherson RA. Catastrophic antiphospholipid syndrome: where do we stand? Arthritis Rheum 2003; 48:3320.

Chapter Four

Gout

Paul's Painful Holiday Cheer

Every year, I used to get a call from Paul during the week after Christmas or New Year's. His foot, knee, or wrist was swollen. It had become a ritual. He was a successful lawyer with a weakness for beer and steak. Unfortunately, he had gout, and despite being well controlled on his medications, his yearly binges precipitated an attack. It had become so ridiculous and predictable that a few years ago I gave him a supply of prednisone and just told him to take it for a few days when he felt the attack coming on. Of course, I preferred he avoid these binges, but he just smiled, nodded, and slapped me on the back when I made the suggestion. Eventually, it became old, and he stopped drinking alcohol. During his first visit, he arrived on crutches with a very painful, swollen foot and swore he would do anything to avoid a recurrence, but it took a few years and several similar visits until his uric acid fell below six on allopurinol and he abstained from beer. His diabetes and hypertension complicated matters but finally came under control. During the first few years of his disease, the attacks came once a year and would last for five days; he responded well to NSAIDs, but the attacks became more frequent and involved more joints until "he got it," except during the holiday season. Eventually, those lapses stopped too. In a strange way, I miss his holiday phone calls, but I can't help but chuckle when he recounts almost nostalgically the agony and ecstasy of his past yearly debaucheries.

First described by the Egyptians in 2640 BC, gout has been called "the disease of kings." I'm sure many royals would have traded their kingdom for relief. Most people think of gout as intermittent podagra: acute arthritis involving the first metatarsophalangeal (MTP) joint of the big toe (where the toe attaches to the foot) caused by hyperuricemia, or high uric acid, and seen mostly in alcoholics. They picture an obese patient with a big bulbous nose sitting in an easy chair with a bandage around a big toe, a large mug of beer in one hand, and a leg of lamb in the other. Although alcohol, especially beer, can cause flares, teatotalers may develop gout too. Obesity, diabetes, and high cholesterol all make gout more likely, but there are many skinny gout patients. Furthermore, only 50 percent of the first attacks involve the big toe, and untreated, in many cases, eventually patients may develop a destructive, deforming inflammatory arthritis involving many joints that can be mistaken for rheumatoid arthritis. A minority of patients' first attack may involve two to four joints and even more rarely more than four joints. So, you see, stereotyping gout patients may be a mistake.

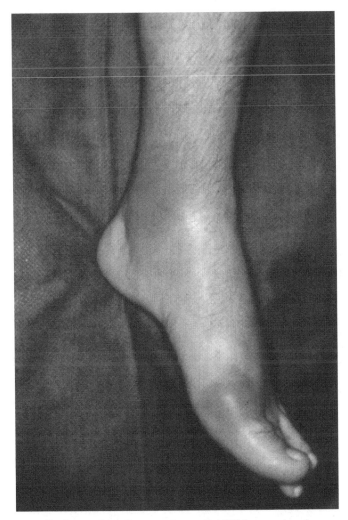

Podagra (gout)—courtesy of ACR image bank

High uric acid can damage joints, kidneys, and even the cardio-vascular system between attacks when patients are asymptomatic. Kidney stones are probably the most painful result of hyperurice-mia (high uric acid in the blood). Women say they are more painful than childbirth. Therefore, gout is a chronic metabolic disease that can cause intermittent acute arthritis attacks that usually involve one joint but eventually can involve many. The arthritis can be chronic and can destroy or damage joints in between attacks. It is not subtle and is extremely painful—the joint is swollen, hot, and red. Patients often enter my office on crutches or even wheelchairs or stretchers. Most will be over the acute attack in twenty-four to forty-eight hours with the proper treatment. The initial attack may even resolve spontaneously in five to seven days. Patients are usually so thrilled after treatment that some of them have entertained me with a jig two days after their initial visit. Gout patients can be very entertaining and satisfying.

Many cells in our skin, GI tract, and respiratory tracts are constantly dying and being replaced by new ones. Uric acid is the byproduct of the metabolism of these dying cells. It is excreted through the kidneys, and a balance is struck between production and excretion maintaining a serum uric acid of around 6 mg/dl. When that balance is disturbed by overproduction (10 percent of gout patients) or underexcretion (90 percent of gout patients), a state of hyperuricemia, or high uric acid, is achieved, making gout more likely. Uric acid is carried from the bloodstream to tissues, and when the serum level rises above 6.5 mg/dl, it has a tendency to combine with sodium and form crystals. The higher the level of uric acid the more likely there will be crystal formation. Crystals may deposit in joints, kidneys, or soft tissue for years, and when they reach a critical level, they precipitate an inflammatory reaction and an acute attack. Large deposits of crystals in soft tissues and joints may form large, hard nodules called *tophi* or form stones in the kidney. The key to prevention is to maintain the uric acid level below 6 mg/dl for life. Interestingly, not everyone with a high uric-acid level will develop gout, and not everyone with arthritis and a high uric acid level have gout. Therefore, we only treat people with confirmed gout attacks and hyperuricemia with uric-acid-lowering drugs. The exceptions are men with uric acids above 12 mg/dl and women with uric acids above 10 mg/dl because the odds are very high they will develop the disease. Many labs will report a normal range of uric acid to be as high as 7–8 mg/dl, but physiologic normal is below 6.5 mg/dl and the target normal should be below 6 mg/dl. Misconceptions about normal ranges of uric acid by primary care physicians just lead to more consults for me. Medications, alcohol, and fructose corn syrup can inhibit the kidney transport of uric acid through the kidneys, increasing serum uric acid. Diet and certain diseases like leukemia can increase its production. Interestingly, estrogen protects premenopausal women from gout unless they are in kidney failure. It usually takes over a decade of high uric acid to accumulate a big enough total body uric acid to develop gout, so it's rare to see a gout patient younger than twenty-five. Still, I recently saw a patient with a strong family history who had his first attack at sixteen. He was from Guam and was one of the 10 percent of patients who overproduced uric acid and probably had an enzyme deficiency (HGPRT) or overactivity (PRPP synthetase). Polynesians, such as Samoans, tend to have genetic defects leading to the worst cases of gout.

Diagnosis of gout should be easy but unfortunately is often bungled. Not every pain or swelling in the first MTP is caused by gout. Degenerative arthritis is much more common and can be quite painful when the joint is overused, such as in running or during long hikes. These patients don't have the dramatic swelling or pain that gout patients do. Psoriatic or rheumatoid arthritis patients may have gout, but more commonly, the swelling in their first MTP is due to their underlying disease. When I was in training (during the Ice Age), we were taught that rheumatoid arthritis and gout did not coexist, but that may have been because high doses of aspirin reduce uric acid (low doses elevate it), and in those days many patients were on this regimen. These days that teaching does not seem to hold true. Nevertheless, if a joint is inflamed in a patient with rheumatoid arthritis, it's probably due to rheumatoid arthritis. Ideally, the best way to diagnose gout definitively is to aspirate an acutely inflamed joint, obtain fluid, and examine it under a polarizing microscope. Gout crystal shedding occurs in the absence of inflammation, so to make the definitive diagnosis of acute gout, it is important to find a urate crystal inside of a white blood cell. Sometimes, we aspirate nodules called *tophi* (singular is *tophus*), which are most common at the elbow but can be on the fingers, knees, feet, or even ears. They contain chalky material full of uric acid crystals. Even a drop of blood from the joints or nodules may yield hundreds of crystals. Their presence indicates that the patient has chronic gout but is not evidence of an acute attack.

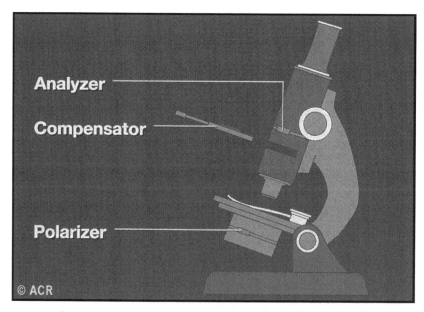

Polarizing Microscope—courtesy of ACR image bank

Gout

Uric acid crystals are large needlelike structures that shine brightly with either blue or yellow colors depending on whether they are lined up vertically or horizontally under a polarizing filter. Few microscopes are fitted with a polarizer. Most hospitals have a separate polarizer they attach to their everyday microscope when needed. I have found them somewhat inadequate over the years in the many hospitals that I have visited as a consultant. Then again, the microscope is only as good as the human using it. Fortunately, one of my first purchases after completion of my fellowship was a polarizing microscope, which has provided me with years of instant gratification and accurate diagnoses. It also is a great teaching tool and entertains my staff because gout crystals are colorful and almost psychedelic. I love sharing the fun with students and staff. The microscope also will help me find calcium pyrophosphate crystals, which shine less brightly, are smaller, rectangular, or bean-shaped, and polarize in a ninety-degree different orientation than uric acid crystals. They are diagnostic of pseudogout, which can simulate gout but most commonly involves the knee or wrist. The number of white blood cells found on the slides helps us to distinguish inflammatory from noninflammatory fluids. However, the number does not always distinguish gout from infectious arthritis since both gout and bacterial infections can cause joint-fluid white blood cell counts to be above one hundred thousand. Tuberculosis, fungi, viruses, Lyme disease, pseudogout, and most gonococcal (gonorrheal) infections can cause joint-fluid white blood cell counts to be between two thousand and fifty thousand, as can gout. Fluid cultures and crystal analysis are keys to distinguishing between gout and infection, and, remember, they can coexist! I love my polarizing microscope. Every rheumatology office should have one, but few offices do, and it's not always possible to aspirate every joint. In those cases, it's OK to use the laws of probability. If the patient is obese, hypertensive, diabetic, has high cholesterol, a high uric acid, and a very inflamed first MTP joint, it's probably gout. If the patient has x -ray changes consistent with recurring or ongoing gout, it makes it more likely, as does a family history, a history of kidney stones, or a history of recurrent attacks. Nodules on the elbows or other body parts that can be aspirated and yield urate crystals also make the diagnosis more probable.

Unfortunately, gout throws us a few curveballs. Uric acid can be normal during an acute attack; it's usually highest two weeks later. Gout inflames joints other than the first MTP during the initial presentation 50 percent of the time. It can also inflame many joints at once or be polyarticular in the minority. In fact, if untreated over many years, it can become chronically polyarticular. Finally, premenopausal women almost never suffer from gout, but a growing number of postmenopausal women do because of the rising incidence of obesity in our society. Ladies, watch your calories! For that matter, guys better do the same.

Treatment of gout is in three stages: managing the acute attack, lowering the uric acid, and maintenance. To treat the acute attack, we use nonsteroidals (NSAIDs) in young patients who have healthy kidneys and livers, and who do not have ulcers, a history of GI bleeds, or bleeding problems or are taking anticoagulants. Many patients, especially older ones, have one of these contraindications. Nevertheless, in many patients they are a good choice. Shorter-acting NSAIDs, such as Motrin, used at higher doses (1,600–3,200 mg daily) are effective and probably less toxic than drugs such as Indocin. Since it is one of the oldest NSAIDs, most of the early studies were done with indocin, so many physicians still think it is the NSAID of choice for gout. It's not true and can be quite toxic in elderly patients. In any case, NSAIDs only work in about 60 percent of cases.

Gout

Another option is colchicine: first 1.2 mg and then 0.6 mg one hour later. It was a popular drug for acute gout attacks for many years. It was dirt cheap and effective in more than half the patients. Years ago, physicians used to tell patients to take it hourly until they developed diarrhea or the attack was aborted. However, a recent study showed that the above-mentioned regimen was equally effective and caused much less cramping, diarrhea, and nausea. Many older gout patients have bad memories of colchicine and refuse to take it. Can you blame them? In addition to diarrhea and abdominal cramps, it occasionally wiped out the white blood cells in the bone marrow, which could be life threatening. In fact, colchicine was sometimes administered intravenously to hospitalized patients, but the incidence of dangerously low white blood cell counts (neutropenia and agranulocytosis) was so high that the medical community stopped using it. Finally, recently because of a wily move by a drug company, colchicine is no longer generic and is extremely expensive. Also, caution must be used in patients with kidney or liver problems. Nevertheless, it is still an option and is also used as a prophylactic drug against acute attack as the uric acid is being lowered to the appropriate level for maintenance. I find steroids injected into the inflamed joint may be the most effective treatment and gives me the option of aspirating first and confirming the diagnosis even if I obtain just a drop of blood. Intramuscular or intravenous steroids are very effective and give very quick relief, although caution must be exercised in diabetics. Oral steroids are also effective but not as instantaneous. I often follow an injection of steroid with two to three days of NSAIDs unless there is a contraindication. Kidney or liver problems are not an issue with steroids. I only prescribe long-term low-dose steroids (usually no more than six months) when NSAIDs or colchicine are contraindicated as prophylaxis while using a uric-lowering agent to lower the uric acid below 6 mg/dl. For some reason, steroids are or were controversial in gout. I remember my favorite teacher during my fellowship scolding me for suggesting their use in a gout patient, and I never could figure out why. He's still around, and I should ask him. There eventually may be an alternative to colchicine or steroids. Some studies indicate that Il-1 inhibitors, such as Ilaris (canakinumab) or Kineret, effectively abort acute attacks, but these medications are not FDA approved for gout and are prohibitively expensive.

Once the acute attack is over, it's time to lower the uric acid below 6 mg/dl unless it is an isolated incident and the patient has no risk factors. I always wait two weeks, so I can measure the uric acid when it's at its apex since it is at its lowest point during the acute attack. Also, any change in the uric acid up or down during an acute attack is going to make the attack worse and may even multiply the number of joints involved. I anticipate the need for prophylaxis against acute attacks during the uric-acid-lowering stage by starting them on NSAIDs, colchicine, or prednisone during the acute attack because as soon as the uric acid starts to drop, the risk of recurrent attacks is high until the uric acid is below 6 mg/dl or the patient is on one of these prophylactic drugs. Recent studies seem to suggest that six months is the ideal duration for prophylaxis, whereas the need for uric-acid-lowering drugs is life-long. Patients will often tell me that uric-acid-lowering drugs were ineffective in the past because they continued to have episodes of gout. Although some patients do not respond to these drugs, the majority have flared because most physicians don't use prophylaxis and surprisingly many start and stop uric-acid-lowering agents even during a flare and don't recognize that gout is a chronic disease and needs chronic therapy. Mess with a patient's uric acid by stopping or starting a uric-acid-lowering drug during an acute flare, and you are asking for trouble and increasing the chance I will get a new consult. The choices of uric-acid-lowering drugs have expand-ed dramatically in the last few years. Before deciding on therapy, I determine whether a patient is an underexcreter or overproducer of uric acid. I obtain a twenty-four-hour urine collection, checking the uric acid level. The majority of patients underexcrete uric acid in the urine, so uricosuric drugs (such as Probenecid), which increase the output of uric acid in the urine, are the drugs of choice in many cases. However, these drugs have their limitations: they are not as effective in patients with kidney disease and should not be used in patients with tophi, uric acid kidney stones, or a high urinary output of uric acid.

The most popular and inexpensive drug that lowers produc-tion of uric acid is allopurinol. It is inexpensive and effective in most cases. I use it in doses between 100 and 800 mg; some physicians use higher doses, but most never use doses that exceed 300 mg daily, leading to inadequate control of uric acid and recurrent attacks of gout. The medication needs some adjustment in kidney disease, but rheumatologists are a little less timid about increasing doses even in patients with impaired kidney disease. Allopurinol strikes fear in many physicians because of a small but significant incidence of Stevens-Johnson syndrome associated with it. Once you have seen a patient with it, you never want to see one again. It is an allergic reaction that starts with a rash and quickly turns into a blister-like eruption on the body, oral cavity, GI and GU tract, and even the eyes. These lesions weep large amounts of fluid, and patients can go into shock. The blisters and subsequent scars on the eyes can lead to blindness. I have seen two cases, and they both died. It's a horrible, hideous death. Fortunately, it is rare, and if patients on allopurinol tell me they have a rash, I tell them to stop it immediately.

Recently, we have the first three new drugs introduced for the treatment of gout in over forty years—Uloric Krystexxa and Lesinurad.

Uloric is similar to allopurinol in that it inhibits similar pathways (xanthine oxidase) but is structurally a different drug and has a few different actions, so it doesn't cross-react with allopurinol and can be used in patients who have had allergic reactions. It is safer in patients with mild to moderate kidney disease and seems to be more effective. Cost and newness make this the drug of second or third choice. Maybe when it is generic and has a longer track record, it may surpass allopurinol.

Krystexxa is a biweekly intravenous drug that works on a completely different pathway converting uric acid to allantoin, a benign compound. Birds and other nonmammals have an enzyme similar to this drug (uricase) that does it naturally. The drug lowers the uric acid quickly and dramatically, but there is a significant incidence of scary infusion or allergic reactions; the drug is expensive and has to be given every two weeks. For those patients with a large load of uric acid who are resistant to the other agents regardless of their kidney function, it is a good choice and a breakthrough. I have little experience with it thus far but have had great success with one dialysis patient. Two other patients could not tolerate the drug, and one other failed treatment. Still, there have been reports of spectacular success and complete resolution of tophi.

Leisenurad (Zurampic) is a drug approved by the FDA in 2015. It helps the kidney excrete uric acid by by inhibiting the function of transportation proteins involved in the reabsorption of uric acid. Leisenurad is prescribed in combination with Allopurinol or Uloric (xanthine oxidase inhibitors). When prescribed alone kidney failure is more common. I have yet to prescribe it but allegedly it should enhance the effect of these drugs for difficult cases.

Diet can affect uric acid and lower it by about 0.5–1.5 mg/dl, which is unlikely to be sufficient. Alcohol, especially beer, will precipitate attacks and make it difficult to treat gout in the long run. Four ounces of wine is the exception. One of my first gout patients in Oregon was a Hispanic male about my age who hobbled into my office on crutches. I treated his acute attack, and he was better by the next day. I counseled him about his diet, especially his "cerveza" (or beer) and started him on allopurinol along with colchicine since he had a very high uric acid level and a huge uric acid load in his urine. Several months later he returned in a wheelchair with an attack involving several joints. He swore he was taking all his medications, but after repeated denials, he admitted he was drinking beer. Again I treated his acute attack successfully and counseled him about beer. Three months later, he arrived to my office on a stretcher, and we went through the same routine with the same confession and counseling. It took two more visits until he finally got it. Fourteen years have passed without beer or attacks, and when I asked him recently if he ever drank beer, his response was: "Are you crazy? Do you know how much gout hurts?"

Food high in purines, like red meat, seafood, and organ meat (such as liver or kidneys), will increase uric acid as will tomatoes. Products high in fructose corn syrup, such as soft drinks, will also do it. Vitamin C, coffee (caffeinated and decaffeinated), and cherry juice will reduce uric acid. A diet high in dairy products is probably best for gout patients.

Certain medications, such as diuretics or water pills, can increase uric acid but need not be avoided if the uric-acid-lowering drugs are adjusted accordingly. Low-dose aspirin impairs urate excretion, but 81–325 mg daily has negligible effect, and it is more important to continue it in patients with vascular disease. Certain medications used in organ transplants (cyclosporine and tacrolimus) can cause rapid onset of hyperuricemia and gout. Other medications, such as Arava, losartan, and fenofibrate, can decrease uric acid slightly.

Pearls

- Gout is a metabolic disease caused by elevated blood levels of uric acid.
- Gout is a chronic disease with intermittent flares.
- Joint destruction may occur in between flares.
- Initial attack is in the big toe 50 percent of the time but may occur in other joints and affect multiple joints.
- Untreated, gout may cause chronic polyarticular (more than five joints) inflammatory arthritis.
- Acute attacks may be treated with NSAIDs, colchicine, or oral, intramuscular, intra-articular, or oral steroids, or rarely an IL-1 inhibitor.
- Once an acute attack is resolved, a patient should be treated with a uric-acid-lowering drug with a target uric acid level of 6 mg/dl or below for life.
- Never reduce uric acid during an acute attack, or the inflammation will get worse, and the number of joints affected will increase!
- While lowering uric acid, add a prophylactic drug, such as an NSAID, prednisone, or colchicine, for the first six months, or the patients will have continued flares.
- Diet changes will only reduce uric acid 0.5–1.5 mg/dl.
- Diagnosis of acute gout is ideally made by aspirating a joint, examining the fluid under a polarizing microscope, and finding negatively birefringent intracellular crystals

References

1. www.rheumatology.org/Practice
(Patient Education—Diseases and Conditions)
(On this website, see ACR 2012 guidelines for management of gout or Google them.)

2. Terkeltaub, R., J. S. Sundy, H. R. Schumacher, et al. The Interleukin 1 Inhibitor Rilonacept in Treatment of Chronic Gouty Arthritis: Results of a Placebo-Controlled, Monosequence Crossover, Non-randomised, Single-Blind Pilot Study. *Ann Rheum Dis* 68:1613.

3. Choi, H. K., K. Atkinson, E. W. Karlson, et al. "Purine-Rich Foods, Dairy and Protein Intake, and the Risk of Gout in Men." *N Engl J Med* 350:1093.

4. Choi, H. K., W. Willett, and G. Curhan. Coffee Consumption and Risk of Incident Gout in Men: A Prospective Study. *Arthritis Rheum* 56:2049.

5. Dalbeth, N., and D. O. Haskard. Pathophysiology of Crystal-Induced Arthritis. In *Crystal-Induced Arthropathies*, edited by R. L. Wortmann, H. R. Schumacher, Jr., M. A. Becker, and L. M. Ryan, 239. New York: Taylor & Francis.

6. Becker, M. A., and M. Jolly. Hyperuricemia and Associated Diseases. *Rheum Dis Clin North Am* 32:275.

7. Becker, M. A., and M. Jolly. Clinical Gout and the Pathogenesis of Hyperuricemia. In *Arthritis and Allied Conditions*, 15th edition, edited by W. J. Koopman and L. W. Moreland, 2303. Philadelphia: Lippincott, Williams & Wilkins.

8. Choi, H. K., and G. Curhan. 2Soft Drinks, Fructose Consumption, and the Risk of Gout in Men: Prospective Cohort Study. *BMJ* 336:309.

9. Choi, H. K., W. Willett, and G. Curhan. Fructose-Rich Beverages and Risk of Gout in Women. *JAMA* 304:2270.

10. Zhang, Y., T. Neogi, C. Chen, et al. Cherry Consumption and Decreased Risk of Recurrent Gout Attacks. *Arthritis Rheum* 64:4004.

11. Borstad, G. C., L. R. Bryant, M. P. Abel, et al. Colchicine for Prophylaxis of Acute Flares When Initiating Allopurinol for Chronic Gouty Arthritis. *J Rheumatol* 31:2429.

12. Stamp, L. K., J. L. O'Donnell, M. Zhang, et al. Using Allopurinol above the Dose Based on Creatinine Clearance is Effective and

Safe in Patients with Chronic Gout, Including Those with Renal Impairment. *Arthritis Rheum* 63:412.

13 Khanna, D., P. P. Khanna, J. D. Fitzgerald, et al. 2012 American College of Rheumatology Guidelines for Management of Gout: Part 2: Therapy and Antiinflammatory Prophylaxis of Acute Gouty Arthritis. *Arthritis Care Res* (Hoboken) 64:1447.

14. Sundy, J. S., M. A. Becker, H. S. Baraf, et al. Reduction of Plasma Urate Levels following Treatment with Multiple Doses of Pegloticase (Polyethylene Glycol-conjugated Uricase) in Patients with Treatment-Failure Gout: Results of a Phase II Randomized Study. *Arthritis Rheum* 58:2882.

16. Becker, M. A., H. R. Schumacher, L. R. Espinoza, et al. The Urate-Lowering Efficacy and Safety of Febuxostat in the Treatment of the Hyperuricemia of Gout: The CONFIRMS Trial. *Arthritis Res Ther* 12:R63.

17. Schumacher, Jr., H. R., M. A. Becker, R. L. Wortmann, et al. Effects of Febuxostat versus Allopurinol and Placebo in Reducing Serum Urate in Subjects with Hyperuricemia and Gout: A 28-Week, Phase III, Randomized, Double-Blind, Parallel-Group Trial. *Arthritis Rheum* 59:1540.

18. Becker, M. A., H. R. Schumacher, Jr., R. L. Wortmann, et al. Febuxostat Compared with Allopurinol in Patients with Hyperuricemia and Gout. *N Engl J Med* 353:2450.

19. Shoji, A., H. Yamanaka, and N. Kamatani. A Retrospective Study of the Relationship between Serum Urate Level and Recurrent Attacks of Gouty Arthritis: Evidence for Reduction of Recurrent Gouty Arthritis with Antihyperuricemic Therapy. *Arthritis Rheum* 51:321.

20. Neogi, T. 2011. Clinical Practice: Gout. *N Engl J Med* 364:443.

21. Khanna, D., J. D. Fitzgerald, P. P. Khanna, et al. 2012 American College of Rheumatology Guidelines for Management of Gout. Part

1: Systematic Nonpharmacologic and Pharmacologic Therapeutic Approaches to Hyperuricemia. *Arthritis Care Res* (Hoboken) 64:1431.

22. Saag K, Fitz-Patrick, Kopicko, et al; Leisenurad, a selective uric acid reabsorption inhibitor in combination with Allopurinol: Results from a phase 3 study in gout patients having an inadequate response to standard of care (clear 1). Ann. Rheum Dis. 2015, June; 74 (sup. 2): 540. Abstract. Fr 10320. Doi: 10.136/Ann. Rheum Dis.—2015. Eular. 3273.

23. Bardiaa T, Keenan R, Khanna P, et al. Leisenurad, a selective uric acid reabsorption inhibitor in combination with Allopurinol: Results from a phase 3 study in gout patients having an inadequate response to standard of care (clear 2). Ann. Rheum Dis. 2015, June; 74 (sup. 2): 545. Abstract Fr 10333. Doi: 10.1136/ Ann. Rheum Disease—2015— Eular. 1238

Chapter Five

Pseudogout

Joanna's Knee

I always seemed to see Joanna after a hospitalization for fever and a swollen knee. She was seventy, with steely gray eyes and a wry smile. Joanna had a few medical problems, but each hospitalization would inevitably end with the same scenario. After many knee aspirations and negative cultures for infection, it was determined that she probably had crystal-induced arthritis—either gout or pseudogout. Despite knee-fluid white blood cell counts of twenty to thirty thousand, no crystals were ever found until her third episode. I aspirated her knee and in the fluid found rhomboid-shaped crystals that were weakly positively birefringent (remember, gout is negatively birefringent) under a polarizing microscope and changed from blue to yellow depending on whether they were horizontal or perpendicular to the microscope field. These crystals were contained inside white blood cells. I established the diagnosis of pseudogout and injected her knee with triamcinolone for the third time in twelve months. I then started her on colchicine (0.6 mg daily) as prophylaxis, but she not only continued to have recurrences but they started to involve her wrists. She failed NSAIDs, Plaquenil, and methotrexate but stabilized on 5 mg of prednisone, 0.6 mg of colchicine daily, and two total knee arthroplasties. Recently she tested positive for hyperparathyroidism, a glandular problem that causes high blood calcium and may be associated with pseudogout. She is now eighty and reluctant to have any new procedures, but let's see what the endocrinologist proposes. I suspect Joanna will greet any suggestion with a smile and resign herself to a life on prednisone.

Pseudogout usually involves an older age group (average seventy-two years). It is caused by calcium pyrophosphate crystals precipitating out into the connective tissues, especially joints and cartilage. It is an inflammatory arthritis that can easily be mistaken for gout but usually involves the knees or wrists and has characteristic findings under polarizing microscopy as described above. Because the crystals are small and only light up faintly, they are often missed. Attacks are usually acute, intermittent, inflammatory, and self-limited and involve one or a few joints. The joint-fluid white blood cell count is usually between twenty and thirty thousand but may be higher or lower. Most cases are idiopathic, but some may be associated with joint trauma, hyperparathyroidism, hemochromatosis, familial chondrocalcinosis, hypomagnesemia (low magnesium), hypophosphatasia (a rare bone disease), and Gittelman's syndrome (kidney disease resulting in low potassium and magnesium). There are many other loose associations, such as hypothyroid disease, diabetes, Wilson's disease, and acromegaly. I suspect pseudogout in patients with classic osteoarthritis who suddenly develop an inflammatory arthritis.

I usually treat acute attacks by aspirating the joint, confirming the diagnosis, if there is fluid, and then injecting the joint with triamcinolone. Occasionally I will try NSAIDs but find they are rarely effective, as are oral steroids. If the attacks are frequent, I will try NSAIDs or colchicine as prophylaxis and occasionally low-dose steroids. There is some evidence that interleukin-1 (IL-1) inhibitors, such as Kineret or Ilaris, may be effective.

Calcium pyrophosphate crystals are formed when there are elevated levels of calcium or pyrophosphate in cartilage. Enzyme overactivity or deficiency in local cartilage may account for the excess and cause crystal precipitation. Systemic metabolic abnormalities, such as hyperparathyroidism, are other possible causes. Once the crystals precipitate out into the joint or soft tissue, they induce an inflammatory response similar to gout involving many of the same players, including interleukin-1. The arthritis can be very destructive, similar to gout, but may present in many forms. Crystal deposition may also be asymptomatic and incidentally found on X-rays, especially in knee or wrist cartilage. This finding is called *chondrocalcinosis*. In patients whose clinical picture is suggestive of pseudogout and every other test, including joint-fluid analysis, is negative, radiological chondrocalcinosis may be helpful in making the diagnosis, although not definitive.

Calcium pyrophosphate disease may take a few other forms. It may mimic rheumatoid arthritis and cause a chronic polyarticular disease with swollen finger joints and even fever and elevated white blood cell count. However, x-rays resemble an aggressive form of osteoarthritis rather than rheumatoid arthritis, and there may be evidence of chondrocalcinosis, especially in the wrist. I have treated May, a delightful English lady with snow-white hair, for ten years for the presumptive diagnosis of RA. She failed methotrexate, Arava, Plaquenil, Rituxan, and a variety of TNF antagonists, and I felt something was not right, so I decided to reevaluate. Her proximal interphalangeal joints (the knuckles in the middle of the fingers) had bony swelling, and her x-rays looked like an aggressive form of osteoarthritis, with cysts and bone spurs. Her shoulder joint had been totally destroyed and had multiple areas of calcification. I decided that she probably had a form of calcium phosphate disease and treated her with Actemra (an IL-6 inhibitor) with initially great success, although lately I'm not so sure. As mentioned previously, there is some evidence that IL-1 inhibitors, like Kineret or Ilaris (canakinumab), may be effective in this form of calcium pyrophosphate disease as well. At this point in her disease, May's arthritis also resembled another form of calcium pyrophosphate disease—pseudo-osteoarthritis. These patients seem to have an aggressive form of osteoarthritis involving the hands, wrists, elbows, shoulders, and/or knees but have evidence of calcium pyrophosphate either on x- ray or in their joint fluid. They should probably be treated like recurrent pseudogout, with the same regimen.

Finally, there is a form of calcium pyrophosphate disease called *pseudoneuropathic arthritis* that is extremely disruptive and destructive and resembles the type of joint destruction seen in diabetes and other diseases where there has been disruption of nerve signaling to the joint. These joints are called *Charcot's* or *neuropathic*.

Pearls

- Pseudogout is an inflammatory arthritis often mistaken for gout, septic arthritis, and sometimes rheumatoid arthritis or degenerative arthritis.
- It usually causes episodic and explosive attacks involving a wrist or knee (monoarticular) but may involve other joints and be polyarticular (more the four joints).
- It may be chronic and cause joint destruction resembling rheumatoid arthritis or erosive osteoarthritis.
- It may be associated with metabolic diseases, such as hyperparathyroidism or hemochromatosis.
- A diagnosis can be definitively made by aspiration of joint and examination of fluid under polarizing microscope (finding intracellular, positively birefringent crystals).

- Infection must be ruled out!
- A radiological finding of calcium in the cartilage of the offending joint is suggestive of diagnosis but not definitive.
- The best treatment for an acute attack is aspiration and injection of the joint with steroids when one or two joints are involved.
- NSAIDs or oral steroids are sometimes helpful.
- Literature suggests that IL-1 inhibitors are effective, but they are not approved by the FDA.
- Long-term prophylaxis is difficult, but colchicine, low-dose prednisone, or IL-1 inhibitors may be helpful.

References

1. www.uptodate.com

2. McCarty, D. J. Calcium Pyrophosphate Dihydrate Crystal Deposition Disease—1975, supplement. *Arthritis Rheum* 19 (S3): S275.

3. Rosenthal, A. K., L. M. Ryan, and D. J. McCarty. Calcium Pyrophosphate Crystal Deposition Disease, Pseudogout, and Articular Chondrocalcinosis. In *Arthritis and Allied Conditions*, 15th edition, edited by W. J. Koopman and L. W. Moreland LW, 2373. Philadelphia: Lippincott Williams & Wilkins.

4. Zhang, W., M. Doherty, T. Bardin, et al. 2011. "European League Against Rheumatism Recommendations for Calcium Pyrophosphate Deposition: Part I: Terminology and Diagnosis." *Ann Rheum Dis* 70:563.

5. Zhang, W., M. Doherty, E. Pascual, et al. EULAR Recommendations for Calcium Pyrophosphate Deposition. Part II: Management. *Ann Rheum Dis* 70:571.

6. Alvarellos, A., and I. Spilberg. Colchicine Prophylaxis in Pseudogout. *J Rheumatol* 13:804.

Chapter Six

Septic Arthritis

Aaron's Near Fatal Choice

Aaron was one of the scariest patients I have ever seen. He was a forty-year-old anesthesiologist buddy of mine and a hardcore skier and tennis player. I saw him the first time for a mildly swollen finger, which I thought was due to osteoarthritis. He had some mild eczema on his hand, and I injected one of his knuckles, trying to avoid the rash. A few days later, he returned to my office with a big swollen knuckle, a high fever, and lightheadedness. He looked like he was about to pass out. One look at him and I knew he had an infected joint, and the infection had spread to his bloodstream. I insisted that he be admitted to the hospital, but he refused because he had plans to go skiing with his son. He threatened to leave my office, but after he almost passed out and his wife, with tears streaming down her face, begged him to listen, he relented. He was hospitalized and found to have staph in his blood and joint. He recovered completely after having the joint opened and drained and receiving two weeks of IV antibiotics. It was a lesson in more ways than one.

Rudy's Ruminations On **Rheumatology**

One of the axioms of rheumatology is as follows: inflammatory monoarticular (one joint) arthritis is an infection until proven otherwise. In other words, an undiagnosed patient with one red-hot joint, with or without fever, needs to have that joint aspirated and cultured for infection immediately. Even if the patient has an underlying disease, such as gout, one lone, hot joint should raise suspicion in certain settings. Patients may have coexistent gout or RA and infection, although it is rare. I remember a toothless, elderly gout patient with a great smile and a long history of prednisone therapy who was hospitalized for some sort of surgery and developed a hot, swollen right knee. After aspirating pus-like material and almost injecting it with steroids, I sent the fluid for culture, and lo and behold, the patient had both active gout and a staph infection! He was treated successfully with antibiotics and nonsteroidals. I could have done some major damage had I injected the steroids. Certainly a gout patient who develops a big swollen toe or an RA patient who develops a swollen finger is unlikely to have an infection, but you never know. If in doubt, aspirate the joint. I feel I can save many patients hospitalizations, if I see them in the office, aspirate the joint, and examine the synovial fluid under the polarizing microscope. Gout and pseudogout are probably more common than infection.

Septic arthritis usually refers to bacterial infections. The vast majority of these are caused by *Staph aureus*. These patients are usually very sick with fever, fatigue, and weakness. Staph is usually seeded to the bloodstream from an open wound on the skin (such as in our patient), from an artificial joint, or from an infected heart valve. Usually one joint is involved, but occasionally there may be two or more, especially when the patient has been seeding the bloodstream from an infectious source such as an infected heart valve. The joint-fluid white blood cell count may be from fifty to more than one hundred thousand but often the latter. These patients need to be hospitalized and treated immediately with at least two weeks of IV antibiotics followed by two weeks of oral antibiotics. Serial aspirations should be performed in the hospital to determine the effect of the antibiotics and to make sure there is adequate drainage of the very toxic infected fluid. If in doubt, an orthopedic surgeon should place a drain in the joint; otherwise the joint could be totally and permanently destroyed. Untreated, patients may die. When a septic joint is suspected, it needs to be aspirated immediately and sent for cultures. At the same time, blood cultures (usually three) should be obtained.

The next most common bacterial cause of septic arthritis is gonorrhea. If it is suspected, especially in a young person or patients who engage in high-risk activity, always culture the patient's urethra, cervix, rectum, and throat because joint fluid is often sterile and not helpful. Also, these cultures need to be done at the bedside and placed on a certain medium called *Thayer-Martin agar* or *chocolate agar*. They should be transported immediately at body temperature to the lab. When I was a rheumatology fellow, we would transport these covered plates containing the cultures under our armpits or in our pants. It sounds and felt ridiculous, but you did what you had to do. Many gonococcal arthritis patients have small, grouped pustules or blisters (vesicles) on a reddish base on their skin. The most common joints involved are the knee and wrist, and once again the infection usually involves only one joint, but two or more are not uncommon. The joints are hot, red, swollen, and painful and associated with fever. The joint-fluid white blood cell counts may be between ten thousand and fifty thousand and can be deceiving. The patients need to be hospitalized and treated with IV antibiotics (ceftriaxone 1 g IV or IM every twenty-four hours) for at least seven days. Their sexual partners should be treated as well.

Other bacterial causes of arthritis are much less common. Organisms that originate from the gut (gram-negative rods) can get into the bloodstream and joints after an infection of the appendix, gallbladder, or intestine. Also intravenous drug abusers may introduce strange organisms into the bloodstreams via dirty needles. These patients are usually extremely ill and need immediate hospitalization with all the investigations outlined in the paragraph on staph infection. The treatment with IV antibiotics is usually for four weeks, depending on the organism.

To be honest I haven't treated a bacterial or septic arthritis case for years. It rarely appears in an office practice. I hesitated to include it in this book, but my friend and colleague Larry insisted that it was important to make everyone aware of its existence. With the advent of hospitalists, it's rare for rheumatologists to be consulted on these patients. However, now that we are using biologics and more and more immunosuppressive therapies, I guess it's important to be aware that we might see more septic arthritis, with unusual organisms. So far, that has not proven to be the case, but I should mention that tuberculosis and a variety of fungi may infect joints in immunosuppressed patients. The onset of the infection is much more insidious, subtle, and chronic. Patients may not seem sick at all or just chronically ill. Joint white blood cell counts tend to be lower than in bacterial infections. If TB is suspected, aspiration of the joint should be performed with appropriate cultures and staining of the fluid. Cultures can take up to four weeks to grow, so in the meantime, skin and serological tests should be performed on the patient and a chest x-ray ordered. If I have a patient with one chronically inflamed joint and I have no explanation for it and cultures are negative, I will order a biopsy of the synovial lining of the joint, especially if I have a high index of suspicion of infection. If the patient eventually tests positive for TB or fungus, I consult my favorite infectious disease specialist, Ruth.

Septic Arthritis

Before leaving this topic, I think I need to mention rheumatic fever, usually seen in an acute care setting. This disease is most common in five- to fifteen-year-olds. It always follows a group A streptococcal bacterial pharyngitis (sore throat) and commonly causes fever and arthritis. However, it's not clear that toxins from the bacteria cause the arthritis or whether it is a genetically programmed autoimmune response to the infection. In fact, there is an entity-caused poststreptoccocal reactive arthritis, which is an autoimmune reaction to the bacteria (see my section on reactive arthritis). In any case, any child or adult who develops fever and arthritis following a sore throat should be investigated for recent streptococcal infection with a throat swab and blood tests (ASO titers or streptolysin assay). An EKG and sometimes an echocardiogram should be ordered, and the patient should be examined for nodules and rashes. Of course as in many rheumatic diseases, there are certain criteria (*Jones criteria*) that need to be met to confirm the diagnosis. The five major criteria are migratory arthritis usually involving large joints, carditis (congestive heart failure or third-degree heart block) or valvulitis (inflammation of heart valves), erythema marginatum (a faint rash), central nervous system involvement especially chorea, a movement disorder), and subcutaneous nodules. Minor criteria include elevated ESRs or CRPs, fever, prolonged PR interval on EKG, and arthralgias. Evidence of a recent strep infection and two major and minor criteria are necessary to make the diagnosis. Treatment should start with complete eradication of the infection, usually with penicillin for seven to eleven days; then aspirin (80–100 mg/kg daily in children or 4–8 g daily for adults) should be started until all symptoms have resolved. If the patient has carditis or has had a previous episode of rheumatic fever, he or she should be treated with antibiotics for life. Don't forget to swab all sore throats associated with fever, and treat strep infections aggressively!

Pearls

- Inflammatory monoarticular arthritis (one joint) is septic (bacterial) arthritis until proven otherwise.
- Septic arthritis is a medical emergency and should be diagnosed and treated immediately.
- The affected joint should be aspirated, and the fluid should be sent for appropriate cultures.
- If gonorrhea is suspected, aspirate the joint, swab the cervix, urethra, and rectum, transport the material at body temperature, and culture in chocolate agar medium.
- Staph is the most common cause of bacterial arthritis.
- Look for the source of the bacteria (blood cultures, artificial joint, or heart valve).
- Initial treatment is almost always IV antibiotics, and duration varies with organism.
  If rheumatic fever is suspected, note the following:
  - Indications include sore throat followed by fever, arthritis, and/or rash in a younger person.
  - Review the Jones criteria.
  - Rule out carditis (heart involvement).
  - Treat with anti-inflammatory drugs for several weeks following a short course of antibiotics.
  - If there is heart involvement, long-term antibiotics (lifelong?) are often required.
  - Monitor temperature, ESRs, and CRPs.

References

1. www.uptodate.com
2. Goldenberg, D. L. Septic Arthritis and Other Infections of Rheumatologic Significance. *Rheum Dis Clin North Am* 17:149.

3. Goldenberg, D. L., and J. I. Reed. Bacterial Arthritis. *N Engl J Med* 312:764.

4. Mikhail, I. S., and G. S. Alarcón. Nongonococcal Bacterial Arthritis. *Rheum Dis Clin North Am* 19:311.

5.6. "Jones Criteria (Revised) for Guidance in the Diagnosis of Rheumatic Fever." *Circulation* 32:664.

7. Ferrieri, P. Jones Criteria Working Group: Proceedings of the Jones Criteria Workshop. *Circulation* 106:2521.

8. Arnold, M. H., and A. Tyndall. Poststreptococcal Reactive Arthritis. *Ann Rheum Dis* 48:686.

9. Mackie, S. L, and A. Keat. Poststreptococcal Reactive Arthritis: What Is It and How Do We Know? *Rheumatology* (Oxford) 43:949.

10. Gerber, M. A., R. S. Baltimore, C. B. Eaton, et al. Prevention of Rheumatic Fever and Diagnosis and Treatment of Acute Streptococcal Pharyngitis: A Scientific Statement from the American Heart Association Rheumatic Fever, Endocarditis, and Kawasaki Disease Committee of the Council on Cardiovascular Disease in the Young, the Interdisciplinary Council on Functional Genomics and Translational Biology, and the Interdisciplinary Council on Quality of Care and Outcomes Research: endorsed by the American Academy of Pediatrics. *Circulation* 119:1541.

11. Cilliers, A. M. "Rheumatic Fever and Its Management." *BMJ* 333:1153.

Chapter Seven

Viral Arthritis

Young Parents and Schoolteachers Beware!

When I saw Susie for the first time, her occupation made me suspect the eventual diagnosis immediately. She had been a very energetic preschool teacher and mother of two young kids until two months prior to the visit. At that time, she developed a rash, severe fatigue, and swollen, painful hands. The rash resolved in a few days, but the other symptoms persisted. She was a short, thin woman with freckles, a warm smile, and black hair tied in a ponytail. Although she had a vivacious air, she seemed exhausted, and her MCP and PIP joints of her hands were all swollen and tender. She looked like a typical RA patient, but because she was a preschool teacher and had had a transient rash, I suspected parvovirus. It commonly causes a febrile illness with a rash in young children but often can cause arthritis in adults. Symptoms can last for months and may be associated with positive ANAs and rheumatoid factors. Sure enough, Susie had a low-level rheumatoid factor but high levels of both parvovirus IGG and IGM antibodies. The IGG was indicative of a previous infection, but IGM indicated acuteness. IGM is needed to make the diagnosis. Her hand x-rays were unremarkable. When I next saw Susie and interpreted her lab results for her, I reassured her that I thought she had parvovirus, with the outside chance of RA. I prescribed NSAIDs, and within two months her symptoms had resolved, and the rheumatoid factor had disappeared. She has remained asymptomatic for three years.

Viral arthritis can be deceiving. It can simulate RA, be rich in antibodies, and last for days or years. There are many viruses that cause arthritis, but the two I see most often are hepatitis C and parvovirus. Most viruses are associated with fever and other viral symptoms and are usually self-limited. They may be polyarticular, involving many joints, or oligoarticular involving a few joints. Often the joint symptoms are migratory, moving from joint to joint over a matter of days or weeks. Joint fluids may be noninflammatory or moderately inflammatory, rarely causing joint white blood cell counts in the range of septic arthritis (over one hundred thousand). Sed rates and CRPs may be very elevated. Most viral arthritis will resolve in weeks, but hepatitis C, parvovirus, and HIV can last much longer. Rubella and Alphaviruses are also commonly seen viral causes of arthritis, but there are many more. I test for parvovirus, hepatitis C, or HIV when patients have risk factors such as IV drug abuse, tattoos, blood transfusions, high-risk sexual encounters, or exposure to small children. I routinely ask these questions during our first consultation. Unfortunately, rheumatoid factors and ANAs are common in these patients, although anti-CCP is absent. These antibodies usually resolve with the illness. X-rays are helpful because they are usually normal, and if there are changes, then RA is much more likely.

Parvovirus usually resolves in a few months. It is key to remember that many people have been exposed to the virus and will have IGG antibodies, but they are not helpful unless accompanied by IGM antibodies to the virus, which indicates that the infection is acute. I order both. Usually I treat these patients with NSAIDs but occasionally need to prescribe low-dose prednisone or even Plaquenil. Most cases resolve in months, but there are occasional recurrences, and I have had a few cases where the ANAs never disappear, and I suspect these patients had underlying lupus or a lupus-like disease all along. Since many of these patients have a rash and arthritis at the outset, discovering a positive ANA leads many a learned physician to conclude that these patients have lupus. Can you blame them?

Hepatitis C can be frustrating, deceiving, stealthy, and life altering. When I first moved to Ashland, I became aware of a group of patients who had either fibromyalgia or an RA type of inflammatory arthritis associated with some liver abnormalities. I soon discovered that many of these patients had recently gotten tattoos and had contracted hepatitis C. After careful questioning, I felt fairly confident that most of these patients were not IV drug abusers and the source of the virus was the tattoo. I assumed the artist was using dirty needles, but one particularly angry patient disabused me of this assumption. She discovered that the local artists were using fresh needles but not changing their ink. Patients developed an immune reaction to the virus months or even many years after their exposure. I treated one patient who was seventy, didn't have a tattoo, and swore she had injected heroin only once in the sixties. She denied any symptoms until the early two thousands and had only mildly elevated liver-function tests. Many of these patients, as mentioned above, may have high levels of rheumatoid factors and ANAs but not anti-CCPs unless they have coexistent RA. In fact, many of my referrals of patients with hepatitis C have been for supposed RA with a positive rheumatoid factor. The key distinguishing factors are their x-rays (no erosions) and lack of anti-CCP.

Rudy's Ruminations On **Rheumatology**

Occasionally, I see patients who have coexistent RA and hepatitis C. I have followed such a patient for ten years. When I first saw her, she was a thirty-five-year-old single mom of three boys and had severe inflammatory arthritis involving most of her joints, especially her hands. I found her to have a positive anti-CCP, a positive rheumatoid factor, an abnormal x -ray of her hands, and a large viral load of hepatitis C. She failed Plaquenil and Azulfidine, and developed finger deformities and a higher viral load on prednisone. Since I wanted to avoid drugs that were toxic to the liver, methotrexate and Arava were out of the question, so I prescribed Enbrel. Several studies indicated it was safe and effective in hepatitis C. Indeed it was effective, but her viral load increased, and she developed a bad pneumonia. For years after her infection, I was reluctant to treat her with a biologic, so I treated her semisuccessfully with Imuran. However, she developed more and more deformities and eventually breast cancer. Her cancer was treated successfully, and last year we decided to try Enbrel again and watch her viral levels. Misfortune seemed to follow this nice single mom, because she developed lung cancer just as she quit smoking, and I have not seen her since. Most gastroenterologists are reluctant to treat hepatitis C in patients with lupus or RA because the medications (especially interferon) can make the arthritis worse. I have one brave patient with severe RA who underwent six months of difficult treatment for her hepatitis C and was cured. I was then free to use any medication for her RA since her liver seemed undamaged. She is doing well on methotrexate and, despite many damaged joints, is relatively pain and inflammation free.

Patients who have hepatitis C alone may have a constellation of rheumatologic problems, including arthritis, fibromyalgia, or vasculitis. It is important to test these patients for cryoglobulins (described later in the book), which are abnormal proteins or immunoglobulins that precipitate out in the cold and can cause arthritis and vascular problems. They may be associated with hepatitis C and must be stored at body temperature before being tested. Also the routine test for hepatitis C is an antibody that just indicates exposure but not active disease, so to make the diagnosis, I order hepatitis PCR or viral load, which will tell me how much virus the patient has on board. To develop the autoimmune problems, patients don't need to have extremely high loads, and since there is effective treatment for many hepatitis C patients, I recommend their gastroenterologists treat them if they have the type of hepatitis C that will respond. However, many of these patients will have only minor liver damage, and the GI docs are reluctant to treat them. I have tried to explain to them that the viral load and degree of liver damage does not always correlate with their rheumatologic symptoms, but they still refuse to treat. But, the newer oral regimens for hepatitis C just introduced in 2014 have changed their attitudes somewhat. Admittedly, not every successful treatment abolishes the symptoms, especially if the patient has fibromyalgia. The arthritis of hepatitis C can last for years and I have had varied success with Plaquenil, NSAIDs, and prednisone. When I use prednisone, I watch the viral load. If the patients have high cryoglobulins, they can develop a severe vasculitis-like illness (see the section on cryoglobulins and vasculitis), and they may need to be treated with steroids, Rituxan, and Riboviran (an antiviral agent).

It's common for patients with new onset arthritis to ask to be tested for viruses other than HIV or hepatitis C because they want to have something self-limited, not chronic. Some spend months in denial when I give them a diagnosis of RA or lupus. One of the other diagnoses patients are sure that I missed is Lyme disease because they think it is curable.

Pearls

- Viruses can cause a variety of rheumatological problems, including inflammatory arthritis, fibromyalgia, and vasculitis.
- Most viruses cause self-limited problems, but some can cause conditions that last for six months to a year, and others, for a lifetime.
- The arthritis associated with viruses is usually migratory and low-grade inflammatory.
- Many viruses are associated with positive ANAs, RFs, and a variety of other antibodies and don't mean that the patient has lupus or RA
- Take a good history!
- Young mothers or preschool teachers with acute onset of arthralgias or arthritis should be tested for parvovirus.
- Patients with tattoos, a history of blood transfusion, or IV drug abuse, and arthritis and arthralgias should be tested for hepatitis B and C (and HIV?).
- Hepatitis C is a an antibody-rich disease, and patients may test positive for RA or lupus (RF, ANA) but should not be positive for anti-CCP or have erosions on x-rays unless they truly have RA.
- Patient may have minimal damage to liver and still have severe autoimmune or rheumatological problems if they have a significant hepatitis C viral load.
- Viral arthritis or arthralgias in most cases are self-limited.
- HIV has multiple rheumatological manifestations.

References

1. www.uptodate.com

2. Naides, S. J., and T. J. Schnitzer. Viral Arthritis. In *Textbook of Rheumatology*, edited by W. N. Kelley, E. D. Harris, R. C. Budd, et al. Philadelphia: WB Saunders.

3. Cacoub, P., T. Poynard, P. Ghillani, et al. Extrahepatic Manifestations of Chronic Hepatitis C: MULTIVIRC Group: Multidepartment Virus C. *Arthritis Rheum* 42:2204.

4. Rosner, I., M. Rozenbaum, E. Toubi, et al. The Case for Hepatitis C Arthritis. *Semin Arthritis Rheum* 33:375.

5. Nesher, G., T. G. Osborn, and T. L. Moore. Parvovirus Infection Mimicking Systemic Lupus Erythematosus. *Semin Arthritis Rheum* 24:297.

6. Naides, S. J. Rheumatic Manifestations of Parvovirus B19 Infection. *Rheum Dis Clin North Am* 24:375.

7. Chantler, J. K., A. J. Tingle, and R. E. Petty. Persistent Rubella Virus Infection Associated with Chronic Arthritis in Children. *N Engl J Med* 313:1117.

8. Ford, D. K., D. M. da Roza, G. D. Reid, et al. Synovial Mononuclear Cell Responses to Rubella Antigen in Rheumatoid Arthritis and Unexplained Persistent Knee Arthritis. *J Rheumatol* 9:420.

9. Calabrese, L. H., and S. J. Naides. Viral Arthritis. *Infect Dis Clin North Am* 19:963.

10. Calabrese, L. H., E. Kirchner, and R. Shrestha. Rheumatic Complications of Human Immunodeficiency Virus Infection in the Era of Highly Active Antiretroviral Therapy: Emergence of a New Syndrome of Immune Reconstitution and Changing Patterns of Disease. *Semin Arthritis Rheum* 35:166.

Chapter Eight

Lyme Disease

Ticks, Joints, and Misconceptions

Phillip and his daughter Spring usually would visit me together. They had similar stories. A few years ago, they were bitten by ticks and developed a rash. They tested positive for Lyme disease and were treated appropriately with oral antibiotics for a month. However, months after they finished treatment, they developed diffuse joint pain with occasional swelling of their joints. Their primary care doctor and a local infectious disease doctor reassured them after some testing that they did not have a recurrence of their Lyme disease, nor did they have "chronic Lyme disease." However, they found a website located in another state that disputed the findings of the Center of Disease Control and the American College of Rheumatology and claimed that chronic Lyme disease is a real entity. By the time I first saw them, they had been on various antibiotics continuously for two years and had all kinds of bowel issues and continued joint pain. Interestingly, the father had clear-cut fibromyalgia, and the daughter had recurrent large effusions (fluid) in both knees. I would routinely aspirate 200–300 cc of fluid out of both knees and inject them with steroids every four months. They were both HLA-B27 positive, and I thought that Spring and possibly Phillip had reactive arthritis, which was an immunological reaction to the Lyme disease infection or organism. I explained to both of them that they were no longer infected and did not need antibiotics but needed an immunosuppressive agent, such as methotrexate, or a TNF antagonist. I did not want to continue aspirating and injecting her knees, and she did not respond to NSAIDs. However, both father and daughter chose to believe that they had chronic Lyme disease, went back on antibiotics, and disappeared from my practice.

A sizable number of patients with joint or muscle pains are sure they have Lyme disease and demand testing. They are skeptical when I tell them that their tests are negative and, if they have been diagnosed and treated in the past and still have symptoms, are convinced they still need antibiotics. I am not sure how many true cases I have seen, but I do know there are a lot of misconceptions about the disease, and the "chronic Lyme disease" believers cling to their beliefs with almost religious fervor. Lyme disease is an infection caused by an unusual organism called a *spirochete* (*Borrelia burgdorferi*), borne by deer ticks and transmitted to humans. It causes a target-like rash called *erythema chronicum migrans* (ECM) early in the disease, associated with fatigue, joint pain, and sometimes fever. In the second stage of the disease, when the infection has spread through the bloodstream, patients can develop multiple ECM skin lesions and neurological and/or cardiac problems. Finally, in the late stages of the disease, patients can develop arthritis involving a few large joints and rare neurologic symptoms. Diagnosis is actually straightforward but becomes a point of controversy among the Lyme disease zealots, making them very difficult patients. The initial test should be an ELISA blood test (a test that uses antibodies and color changes to identify a substance) and should be reserved for patients living in endemic areas that have a history of tick bite or are at high risk and have one of the systemic symptoms associated with Lyme disease, such as arthritis, meningitis, or carditis. I do not test patients with nonspecific complaints, such as fatigue or joint pain, or those who have not been to endemic areas. Those who have been to those areas and have ECM, I would treat without testing. There is a significant incidence of false-positive ELISA tests, so they should be followed by Western blot tests. These tests are composed of IGM and IGG antibodies and since arthritis occurs only in the late (third) stage of disease, they are only significant if IGG antibodies are positive since they reflect relect later disease. The confusion occurs with the misconception of high-incidence false-negative tests, which occur in the first two to four weeks of infection when the patient has ECM but very rarely in late disease when the patient has arthritis. So patients who have had joint symptoms for months and have negative tests do not have Lyme disease. The other very frustrating point of controversy, illustrated in my two patients above, is "chronic Lyme disease." It does not exist! There are a group of doctors and support groups who advocate treating these patients with years of antibiotics despite lack of scientific evidence that once Lyme disease is treated with two to three months of antibiotics any active infection persists. There is a post-Lyme disease syndrome, which can last up to six months and often involves joint pain, brain fog, and fatigue and usually subsides spontaneously or with symptomatic treatment. Fibromyalgia is not chronic Lyme disease. Occasionally, patients, such as Spring, will develop inflammatory arthritis months after treatment. They are thought to have reactive arthritis (see section below), which is an autoimmune inflammatory response to the infection and needs to be treated with anti-inflammatory and/or immunosuppressive drugs. Despite adequate research and guidelines from the Center for Disease Control, many people choose to believe the outliers and call "chronic Lyme disease" deniers, such as me, "Lyme illiterate doctors." I find these doctors and groups irresponsible, dangerous, and self-serving, but that's just one man's opinion, and they probably say the same about me. Oh well...

Since I am generally treating patients with arthritis, which is a later manifestation, I generally prescribe doxycycline 100 mg twice a day for one month or amoxicillin 500 mg three times a day for one month. However, if they have neurologic disease or recurrent arthritis despite adequate oral antibiotics, I refer them to my favorite infectious disease consultant, Ruth, who would probably treat them with ceftriaxone two grams IV for twenty-eight days.

Oregon is one of the endemic areas for Lyme disease, and I do test for it in high-risk patients, but because of the controversy and zealotry surrounding the disease, I refer any ambiguous patients to Ruth and try to avoid patients who are disciples of "literate Lyme doctors" or advocacy groups.

Pearls

- False-negative Lyme tests occur in the first two to four weeks after a tick bite.
- Arthritis occurs in the late stages of Lyme disease, so a negative test means the patient does not have Lyme disease.
- There is no such thing as chronic Lyme disease, but noninfectious reactive arthritis or diffuse muscle or joint pain can occur after the infection is eradicated. It should not be treated with antibiotics.

References

1. www.uptodate.com
2. Steere, A. C. Lyme Disease. *N Engl J Med* 345:115.
3. Feder, Jr., H. M., B. J. Johnson, S. O'Connell, et al. A Critical Appraisal of 'Chronic Lyme Disease'. *N Engl J Med* 357:1422

4. Steere, A. C. Reinfection versus Relapse in Lyme Disease. *N Engl J Med* 367:1950.

5. Steere, A. C., R. T. Schoen, and E. Taylor. The Clinical Evolution of Lyme Arthritis. *Ann Intern Med* 107:725.

6. Dinerman, H., and A. C. Steere. Lyme Disease Associated with Fibromyalgia. *Ann Intern Med* 117:281.

7. Steere, A. C., G. J. Hutchinson, D. W. Rahn, et al. Treatment of the Early Manifestations of Lyme Disease. *Ann Intern Med* 99:22.

8. Massarotti, E. M., S. W. Luger, D. W. Rahn, et al. Treatment of Early Lyme Disease. *Am J Med* 92:396.

9. Shadick, N. A., C. B. Phillips, O. Sangha, et al. Musculoskeletal and Neurologic Outcomes in Patients with Previously Treated Lyme Disease. *Ann Intern Med* 131:919.

10. Steere, A. C. Diagnosis and Treatment of Lyme Arthritis. *Med Clin North Am* 81:179.

Chapter Nine

Fibromyalgia or Central Pain Syndrome

The Princess and the Pea

Michele has come a long way. When I first saw her, she was a pretty young lady of thirty who was on several narcotics, an anti-depressant, and a muscle relaxant. She carried the diagnoses of possible lupus, depression, and fibromyalgia and was trying to hold her life together as a single mother with two kids and a job as a three-quarter-time office manager in a medical practice. Her major complaints were overwhelming fatigue, muscle and joint pain, and brain fog. She also had some bizarre neurological and GI complaints with diffuse numbness and constipation alternating with diarrhea. She snored, and her boyfriend swore she stopped breathing during the night. I cringed when I read the inventory of her symptoms on our questionnaire because virtually every box in every system was checked. Also when I examined her, she was tender to the touch from head to toe. However, after I ruled out lupus and saw that she had a good grip on her depression, I encouraged her to wean off her narcotics and slowly build up her aerobic exercise over months to thirty minutes a day and take hot baths during pain flares. To my surprise, with the help of her primary care physician, she was weaned off all her narcotics and was going to the gym before work daily. She also used a CPAP machine (a form of pressurized oxygen) for newfound sleep apnea. Today, she informs me she has weaned off her antidepressant medication, and her energy level is at an all-time high while her pain level is the lowest in years. I am ecstatic! She made my day.

For years, like most physicians, when I saw a fibromyalgia patient's name on my schedule, I would wince and swallow hard before taking the long walk to the room. Inevitably, when I reviewed the written questionnaire each patient filled out every visit, there would be a rambling narrative in the space allotted for comments and questions. The checkboxes for the review of recent symptoms were all checked with notations made in the margins. When I showed the questionnaire to office personnel in passing, they would smile and say, "Fibromyalgia—sorry." With the recent advances in technology and better understanding of the cause of this condition and some successful, well-conducted drug studies, our attitude has changed… sort of. At least we seem to have more success with these patients, and they are more satisfied. Over the years there has been a great deal of misinformation circulated about fibromyalgia, so at times my first task is to sort out fact and fiction for these patients. I tell them that fibromyalgia is a condition where people develop diffuse aches and pains associated with fatigue, sleeping abnormalities, sometimes sleep apnea, restless legs, brain fog, subjective numbness, chemical hypersensitivity, and irritable bowel syndrome. Patients have tender points on both sides of the body and above and below the waist. The rest of the physical and laboratory exam should be normal unless the patient has a coexisting condition or an incorrect diagnosis.

Fibromyalgia or Central Pain Syndrome

Functional MRIs have shown that the pain pathways leading to and from the brain are accelerated, and the sensory parts of the brain have a much lower threshold due to certain chemical imbalances. In plain language, the part of the brain that processes sensory input and output is out of balance, and the volume of everything is turned up. One of my patients described herself as "The Princess and the Pea." This description is spot on and usually elicits nods and smiles from patients and their family when I share it with them. Women are the majority of these patients, and many will complain that their husbands can't even touch or hug them because they are so tender. I think that one of the cornerstones of treatment is patient education, and a reassuring explanation can go a long way in initiating the healing process. We used to rigidly adhere to a specified number of tender points to make the diagnosis, but now if the patient has the proper clinical profile and four-quadrant tender points, the diagnosis is pretty certain. I avoid pressure on many tender points during the exam since the pain caused by pressure can linger for hours and is magnified. I have had patients tell me that one of these exams can force them to bed for days. This condition is truly an amplification syndrome—perceived pain and fatigue and virtually any sensory input is amplified, including sound and light. These patients amplify their caregivers' stress and anxiety with their myriad of complaints and their hypersensitivity. Their complaints can be bizarre and include numbness and vibratory sensations. This condition can coexist with many other chronic pain conditions, such as rheumatoid arthritis, chronic back pain, or lupus. In fact, chronic pain caused by these conditions may change the brain chemistry and precipitate fibromyalgia. There is some evidence that long-term use of narcotics may at least exacerbate if not cause fibromyalgia. Interestingly, depression may simulate fibromyalgia and have a similar brain chemistry profile. Depressed patients, like their fibromyalgia counterparts, may dim all the lights and turn down the volume on their TV or stereo. I tell these patients that if they were a stereo, their volume would be on twelve, while the rest of ours is on four. Fortunately, studies show that only 33 percent of fibromyalgia patients are depressed, but when they are, it is a difficult combination and should be treated jointly. In fact, any comorbid condition should be ferreted out and treated. Otherwise, you are doomed to failure. Most patients are fairly easily treated and are happy to have been diagnosed, but those with severe psychological problems or substance dependence can be a major challenge. I find those who enter my office in a wheelchair and claim complete disability without any comorbid diagnosis inevitably have psychological issues or have another diagnosis that's been missed. The American College of Rheumatology recommends against giving these patients long-term disability because studies suggest that those who continue to work do much better. They also recommend against long-term narcotic since they are ineffective in this disease and may cause more harm than good. I find that many of these patients are taking a large number of prescribed medications, including narcotics and antidepressants.

The most effective treatment well supported by good studies is aerobic exercise approximately thirty minutes a day. Unfortunately, many of the patients are deconditioned and feel too fatigued to exercise. They will claim that even ten minutes of exercise creates so much pain that they are bedbound for days. They may also have another condition, such as a bad knee or hip that makes it difficult. I find that "go slow and low" is a good approach. In other words, start with five or ten minutes of the aerobic activity they find easiest and most enjoyable, and slowly increase time and intensity over months. Soaking in a bath, shower, or hot tub after each activity may alleviate the pain and encourage them to try again the next day. In fact, hot tub soaks or hot baths probably provide the best short-term relief of any modality in fibromyalgia. I often tell patients who are having a flare that a hot soak is more effective than most medications. Other nonpharmacological modalities that have been shown in studies to have some short-term effectiveness include acupuncture and light, but not deep, massage. Cognitive behavioral therapy (a form of psychotherapy) has been shown to have long-lasting benefits and may be particularly effective in depressed patients or ones with other psychological issues.

There are three FDA-approved medications for fibromyalgia—Lyrica, Cymbalta, and Savella. I find them to be effective in about 60 percent of patients if they can tolerate or afford them. Patients have usually read about them or seen their commercials and request them. They all can reduce pain and fatigue and in some patients work like magic and allow them to start exercising and resume a normal life. Lyrica may be the most effective for insomnia and pain; Savella, for fatigue; and Cymbalta, for depression.

Lyrica blocks calcium channels in the brain and therefore slows down the pain pathways, which are in hyperdrive in fibromyalgia. The most common side effects are fluid retention, fatigue, dizziness, loss of balance, tremor, and the most bothersome fluid weight gain. I have had at least two patients who have suffered from amnesia from this drug. I try to avoid using it in patients who are obese or have a tendency to retain fluid.

Cymbalta and Savella are serotonin norepinephrine receptor inhibitors (SNRIs). Cymbalta increases serotonin more than norepinephrine and the reverse is true for Savella. Since norepinephrine is an adrenaline-like substance, one can imagine that taking these drugs is like an adrenaline rush—Savella more so than Cymbalta. There is a norepinephrine and serotonin imbalance in fibromyalgia in at least some patients. (Other chemical imbalances have been noted as well.) Therefore, theoretically these drugs should help some patients. These imbalances are also found in depressed and chronic pain patients as well. Cymbalta is FDA approved for depression and chronic pain, and Savella is approved in the United Kingdom for depression. The medications work magically in some patients, especially those who have an element of depression. They are expensive (as is Lyrica) and have some worrisome side effects. Cymbalta can cause headaches, fatigue, sweats, dry mouth, nausea, and constipation. Savella may increase the heart rate or blood pressure and cause palpitations and also can cause tremor, nausea, dizziness, sweats, and difficulty urinating, which can be particularly problematic in older men. I try to avoid Savella in patients with any kind of heart or blood pressure problem. I have also had many older women tell me that they feel they are going through menopause again, with night sweats and hot flashes, with both of these drugs. All three of these medications need to be weaned off slowly and not abruptly discontinued. In quite a few cases, patients can use these medications as bridge therapy to a healthy lifestyle, with exercise, and eventually be medication free.

There are a variety of medications that are not FDA approved but have some efficacy in fibromyalgia. They include tricyclic antidepressants (amitriptyline, imipramine, desipramine, and nortriptyline), which are usually used as sleep aids but in some patients at high doses can alleviate many of their symptoms. Unfortunately, most patients can't tolerate the higher doses. They can cause dizziness, fatigue, voracious appetites (with weight gain), compulsive gambling, and very dry mouth. Nevertheless, they can be very effective in some patients and are very inexpensive. Early in my career, they were really the only drugs available that had any effect. I did see one woman go on a gambling spree and one gain fifty pounds in a several-month period after taking one of these drugs. I rarely use these medications as anything more than sleep aids these days. They can be particularly toxic in elderly patients and increase dementia, dizziness, and the risk of falling. They increase norepinephrine and serotonin so must be used with caution with SNRIs or SSRIs (selective serotonin uptake inhibitors) since they can cause serotonin syndrome, which can be quite nasty—even fatal—and also can increase blood pressure and the heart rate. Just think of norepinephrine as adrenaline, and you can imagine what it could do in high doses to someone with a shaky cardiovascular system. Tricyclics also have an anticholinergic or atropine-like affect. What does that mean? I was taught that these patients become mad as a hatter, red as a beet, and dry as a bone. I know these drugs sound nasty, but in the right setting and the right patient, they are very helpful for central pain, including fibromyalgia.

Another medication that may be helpful in some patients is Neurontin, or gabapentin. It has a somewhat similar mechanism of action as Lyrica but is not identical. There are some studies supporting its effectiveness at doses of 1,800 mg daily, but the results have been lukewarm. Since it is inexpensive and fairly well tolerated (with similar side effects as Lyrica), it's worth a try. Recently, a study showed that it may be effective as a sleep aid in these patients at doses of 600 mg nightly.

Tramadol is another medication that some studies have shown to be effective, and that would make sense since it has some SNRI effects, so it is similar to Cymbalta and Savella but less potent. It is also a partial opiate agonist, so it is a narcotic despite some misconceptions to the contrary. In some respects, it is a very dangerous drug because practitioners who are unaware that it increases norepinephrine and serotonin will mix it with a SNRI or SSRI and increase the possibility of toxicity. I saw a pregnant young lady who was taking an SSRI, tramadol, and Elavil (all not good in pregnancy) and had a grand mal seizure, a known side effect of tramadol. She may have also had serotonin syndrome on this combination. Patients are often under the false impression that tramadol is not an opiate and not addicting. As mentioned before, long-term narcotics can cause hyperalgesia syndrome, which lowers the pain threshold in central pain patients and in the long run increases their pain. I try to stay away from this drug if I can and only occasionally give it for a short term, but that can be difficult.

Cyclobenzaprine is a muscle relaxant that has been useful in the insomnia associated with fibromyalgia. There have been some small studies supporting it, and it is inexpensive, but I have been receiving more and more "Dear Doctor" letters warning of its toxicity in elderly people.

As far as I know, there are no good studies on the long-term effects of any diet on central pain, but avoiding alcohol, nicotine, caffeine, or anything that can disturb sleep or increase brain fog is just common sense. Since central pain syndrome, or fibromyalgia, is not an inflammatory process, anti-inflammatory supplements would not be useful. There are many supplements that have been promoted as effective in fibromyalgia but without any long-term, controlled, double-blinded studies supporting them. Placebo works in 30 percent of people, and I tell patients that if a website or person is selling a product or it's expensive, they shouldn't buy it if it hasn't been prescribed. Also testimonials (especially by celebrities) that haven't been backed up by good studies do not confirm a product's effectiveness.

Recently, there have been some studies that indicate that there are some small fiber nerve abnormalities in the skin of Fibromyalgia patients. These findings cast some doubt on the brain chemistry or central pain model I have outlined. More than likely it will all be related in some way. The wheels of research and medicine keep turning!

Pearls

- Fibromyalgia is a condition associated with diffuse aches and pains, tender points above and below the waist, fatigue, brain fog, and sleeping abnormalities.
- It is considered a central pain syndrome. In other words, there is an abnormality or chemical imbalance in the parts of the brain that process sensory input and output so that sensory pathways are amplified.
- Patients are essentially "Princesses or Princes and the Pea."
- A minority of patients are depressed.
- There is a genetic link, so check family history.
- There is a high incidence of sleep apnea; therefore, sleep studies are helpful.
- The best long-term treatment is a slow buildup of aerobic exercise.
- The best short-term treatments are hot baths or hot tubs.
- Cymbalta, Lyrica, Savella, Neurontin, and tricyclics are sometimes helpful but not always needed.
- Treat any coexisting problem, such as a bad back, inflammatory process (RA etc.) or depression.
- Narcotics may make it worse, so avoid them.
- Most patients improve.
- It should not be a source of disability.

References

1. Clauw, Daniel J., and Daniel J. Wallace. *Fibromyalgia: The Essential Clinician's Guide*.

2. www.rheumatology.org/Practice
(Patient Education—Diseases and Conditions)

3. Yunus, M. B. Fibromyalgia and Overlapping Disorders: The Unifying Concept of Central Sensitivity Syndromes. *Semin Arthritis Rheum* 36:339.

4. Wolfe, F., D. J. Clauw, M. A. Fitzcharles, et al. The American College of Rheumatology Preliminary Diagnostic Criteria for Fibromyalgia and Measurement of Symptom Severity. *Arthritis Care Res* (Hoboken) 62:600.

5. Buskila, D., and P. Sarzi-Puttini. Biology and Therapy of Fibromyalgia: Genetic Aspects of Fibromyalgia Syndrome. *Arthritis Res Ther* 8:218.

6. Arnold, L. M., J. I. Hudson, E. V. Hess, et al. Family Study of Fibromyalgia. *Arthritis Rheum* 50:944.

7. Jensen, K. B., E. Kosek, F. Petzke, et al. Evidence of Dysfunctional Pain Inhibition in Fibromyalgia Reflected in rACC during Provoked Pain. *Pain* 144:95.

8. Emad, Y., Y. Ragab, F. Zeinhom, et al. Hippocampus Dysfunction May Explain Symptoms of Fibromyalgia Syndrome: A Study with Single-Voxel Magnetic Resonance Spectroscopy. *J Rheumatol* 35:1371.

9. Mork, PJ., and T. I. Nilsen. Sleep Problems and Risk of Fibromyalgia: Longitudinal Data on an Adult Female Population in Norway. *Arthritis Rheum* 64:281.

10. Hassett, A. L., and R. N. Gevirtz. Nonpharmacologic Treatment for Fibromyalgia: Patient Education, Cognitive-Behavioral Therapy, Relaxation Techniques, and Complementary and Alternative Medicine. *Rheum Dis Clin North Am* 35:393.

11. Boomershine, C. S., and L. J. Crofford. A Symptom-Based Approach to Pharmacologic Management of Fibromyalgia. *Nat Rev Rheumatol* 5:191.

12. Schmidt-Wilcke, T., and D. J. Clauw. Fibromyalgia: From Pathophysiology to Therapy. *Nat Rev Rheumatol* 7:518.

13. Arnold, L. M., D. L. Goldenberg, S. B. Stanford, et al. Gabapentin in the Treatment of Fibromyalgia: A Randomized, Double-Blind, Placebo-Controlled, Multicenter Trial. *Arthritis Rheum* 56:1336.

14. Crofford, L. J., M. C. Rowbotham, P. J. Mease, et al. Pregabalin for the Treatment of Fibromyalgia Syndrome: Results of a Randomized, Double-Blind, Placebo-Controlled Trial. *Arthritis Rheum* 52:1264.

15. Branco, J. C., P. Cherin, A. Montagne, et al. 2011. "Long-Term Therapeutic Response to Milnacipran Treatment for Fibromyalgia: A European 1-Year Extension Study Following a 3-Month Study." *J Rheumatol* 38:1403.

16. Arnold, L. M., R. M. Gendreau, R. H. Palmer, et al. Efficacy and Safety of Milnacipran 100 mg/day in Patients with Fibromyalgia: Results of a Randomized, Double-Blind, Placebo-Controlled Trial. *Arthritis Rheum* 62:2745.

17. Painter, J. T., and L. J. Crofford. Chronic Opioid Use in Fibromyalgia Syndrome: A Clinical Review. *Journal of Clinical Rheumatology* 19 (2): 72–77.

18. Crofford, L. J. 2012. *Nat. Rev Rheumatology* 6, no. 4: 191–97.

Chapter Ten

Systemic Sclerosis or Scleroderma

The Boy in the Leather Mask
(Not a Laughing Matter)

When I walked into the room a few months ago, I encountered a twenty-seven-year-old man whose skin tightness drew his face into a mask of perpetual amazement or pain. It drew his lips into a tight frown and prevented his mouth from opening more than two finger breadths. His hands were claws, with his fingers permanently clenched in a flexed position, and he had an open sore on the knuckle of his right baby finger. His leather-tight arms and legs and matted trunk sent shivers up my spine. When he related to me that he was unable to walk any distance without shortness of breath and that he had to stay close to a toilet because of the unpredictability of his bowels, it confirmed my worst suspicions that this patient had the most malignant form of a difficult disease.

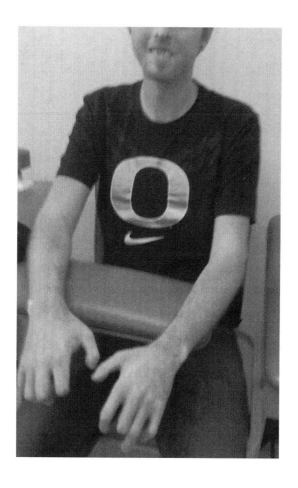

I have a special place in my heart for scleroderma. It was the subject of my research during my training at USC, and recently my scleroderma patients have formed a wonderful support group that is both therapeutic and educational. It is a sometimes frustrating disease, but slowly we are making breakthroughs in therapy. To understand scleroderma, it's best to describe in simple terms its pathophysiology, or what is going on microscopically to cause these physical changes. Scleroderma is another disease where the immune system is overproducing certain factors that are stimulating inflammatory cells and causing them to multiply and circulate systemically. In this case, they cause inflammation in small blood vessels (arterioles) in multiple organs (the skin, lungs, kidneys, heart, GI tract, etc.) leading to spasm and narrowing. Therefore, there is reduced circulation and function, leading to scarring and sometimes severe organ damage and shut down. Raynaud's phenomenon in this disease is particularly malignant because of the blood vessel narrowing and can lead to gangrene and loss of fingers or limbs. The scarring in the lungs can lead to extreme respiratory difficulties and failure.

There are two basic forms of scleroderma—diffuse or limited. Limited is the most common kind and has a much better prognosis. *Scleroderma* means "hardening or thickening of the skin" and may be limited to the skin only. In fact, morphea is a form of scleroderma that is limited to the skin, without internal organ involvement. Systemic sclerosis involves the skin and internal organs, but we tend to use the term interchangeably with *scleroderma*. In limited scleroderma, the skin changes involve only the hands, feet, and distal forearms, legs below the knees, and sometimes the face and neck. Diffuse scleroderma involves the whole body, including the trunk. It is usually explosive and has severe kidney and lung involvement much more frequently than the limited form, although pulmonary hypertension (increased pressures in the artery going from the heart to the lungs) is more frequent in the limited form in the absence of interstitial lung disease. In both forms patients go through three stages of skin change—edematous, fibrotic, and then atrophic. Initially they complain of just severe swelling, not the pitting kind but sort of a brawny texture. Several months or years later, the skin goes through the fibrotic stage and becomes almost like leather. It causes patients to lose all lines in their skin and develop flexion contractures of their joints, especially fingers. Patients sometimes find a silver lining in the changes because their skin, especially their face, loses all lines and wrinkles, making them appear younger. During my research days, I remember one forty- to forty-five-year-old female patient who would proudly remove her shirt, unsolicited, to show off her flawless, tight breasts. Unfortunately, they were just a reflection of the disease process.

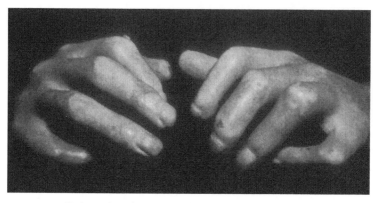

Scleroderma, acrosclerosis, sclerodactyly, hyperpigmentation—courtesy of ACR image bank

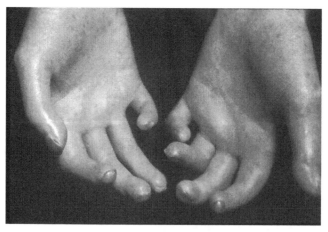

Scleroderma with acrosclerosis, sclerodactyly, resorption—courtesy of ACR image bank

Systemic Sclerosis or Scleroderma

The scariest and most lethal but fortunately rare manifestation is called *renal crisis*, which occurs much more frequently in the diffuse form. Patients develop a sudden, astronomical rise in their blood pressure, and their kidneys shut down permanently. Unless they are treated right away, they can die suddenly; otherwise, they can survive on dialysis, antihypertensives, and in some cases kidney transplants. I remember talking to one of my diffuse scleroderma patients while he was sitting up in bed in the hospital, and suddenly he became drowsy and less and less responsive. His blood pressure readings were so high I thought I was misreading them. Within minutes he was dead, despite every effort to revive him. His death could have been prevented if we had monitored his blood pressure closely and at the first sign of elevation had put him on a certain family of antihypertensive drugs called *ACE inhibitors*. These medications revolutionized the treatment of scleroderma renal failure and changed it from an almost uniformly fatal disease. Good blood pressure control is a key to preventing kidney failure or death in these patients because most of them will initially have moderate elevations and then have sudden dangerous rises in pressure. Captopril, the first available ACE (angiotensin converting enzyme) inhibitor, has a rapid onset so that it is ideal for treating these sudden changes. Newer drugs from the same family are equally effective.

We now tell diffuse scleroderma patients with certain specific antibodies (ant-RNA polymerase 3) to buy home blood pressure monitors and at the first sign of elevation to call their doctor. ACE inhibitors should always be included in any blood pressure regimen in scleroderma. So, renal crisis with malignant hypertension need not be fatal if treated in the hospital immediately. Most of these patients will lose kidney function, although a minority may recover it after some time on dialysis. They can develop flash pulmonary edema (fluid in the lungs), encephalopathy, strokes, seizures, or microangiopathic hemolytic anemia (the red blood cells are destroyed or sheared by factors in the blood vessels). When autopsy is performed, the small blood vessels in their kidneys will have specific changes, called "onion skinning," with a lot of scarring. Fortunately, only 15–20 percent of diffuse scleroderma patients will develop this lethal problem, and it is very rare in limited scleroderma. Blood pressure monitoring and treatment are essential in scleroderma! I also perform semiregular urinalyses on all scleroderma patients to look for protein or any changes that reflect kidney problems. I regularly check for any changes in creatinine and GFR on their blood tests, which may be an indicator of bad things to come. Finally, it is important to avoid vigorous use of diuretics in these patients as well as drugs like cyclosporine because they may precipitate a renal crisis. I was always taught that high-dose prednisone (more than 20 mg) is also a risk, but recently that fact is being questioned. Nevertheless, I rarely prescribe more than 10 mg of prednisone in scleroderma patients, particularly those with the diffuse form.

I hope I'm not scaring everyone by starting with the toughest and potentially fatal manifestations of this disease, but scleroderma is not to be taken lightly. We have made major strides in treating many of the individual organ systems involved, but diffuse scleroderma remains one of our toughest clinical nuts to crack therapeutically. I have learned that these days if you treat scleroderma early and aggressively, especially in the limited subset, you can preserve quality of life and make a huge impact on survival. The number one cause of scleroderma-related death is interstitial lung disease (ILD). It usually is an indolent, low-grade process, which is slowly progressive, leading to increasing shortness of breath over years. Chest x-rays are insensitive early measures of this process. Pulmonary function tests and CAT scans of the lung are helpful but are again relatively insensitive measures of early activity. In most limited scleroderma patients and many diffuse cases, it's probably not a big deal since the ILD is so low grade and slowly progressive that it may take twenty to thirty years to affect quality of life. However, in a minority of patients, the lung disease is a rapidly progressive disease that leads to the need for oxygen therapy and disability and death in months or a year. Research in scleroderma lung has been mainly targeted at detecting early changes in the lungs of these patients. When I was in training, discovering exactly what those early changes were and how to detect them were the Holy Grail. At the time (the early to mideighties), bronchial lavage, which entailed bronchoscopy (or putting a tube down into the patient's lungs and washing out some of the inflammatory cells and then analyzing them), was popular and promising. This procedure requires a competent pulmonologist and pathologist and is not without risk. It does not seem to be as popular these days but is still used in research and at major centers. It may be due to the lack of expertise and comfort with the procedure that it is not done in smaller centers. Fortunately, I have not seen an explosive case of scleroderma lung in years, but we now have some relatively effective treatment early in the disease-- Cytoxan and Cellcept Recently, a large multicenter controlled study indicated that Cellcept is an effective treatment and in my mind, a much safer alternative to Cytoxan. There is some anecdotal evidnce that Rituxan may also be effective. It has been particularly effective in a few of my patients with inflammatory arthritis and may have even softened their skin. I await some large placebo control studies.

Finally, 15–20 percent of limited scleroderma patients and a lower percentage of diffuse patients will develop pulmonary hypertension, where the pressure in the artery between the lung and the heart is elevated and oxygen saturation slowly diminishes. Patients become increasingly short of breath, disabled, and oxygen dependent. In the past, I would watch helplessly as these patients would slowly and miserably fade away before my eyes. Several therapies are now available to avert the inevitable deterioration if initiated early in the disease. PDE5 (cyclic GMP phosphodiesterase type 5) inhibitors (such as sildenafil [Revatio]), endothelin receptor antagonists (such as bosentan), and calcium channel blockers (such as nifedipine [Procardia]) or a combination of all three can have an enormous effectiveness if used early in the disease. Therefore, early and frequent testing even if the patient is asymptomatic is a must. Pulmonary function tests (PFTS) with a DLCO and echocardiograms with Doppler can gauge pulmonary artery pressures to some degree, but a right heart catheterization is the gold standard. I tend to order PFTS and echocardiograms yearly and have my favorite cardiologist do an initial catheterization and a repeat only if the other tests are showing some changes. By the time the patients are symptomatic, they are in trouble. The new medications tend to be much less effective later in the disease. It's important to note that in the absence of severe ILD, pulmonary hypertension is more common in limited scleroderma, as I have mentioned previously.

Heart disease is the next most common cause of death in scleroderma. Other than pulmonary hypertension, I rarely see unusual cardiac events related to the disease, but some of the more devastating ones include restrictive cardiomyopathy, in which the heart is restricted from expanding, and conduction defects and arrhythmias, all of which can be treated but can be deadly. It's good to have a friendly, knowledgeable, and competent cardiologist readily available. Occasionally I see pericardial effusions or pericarditis in these patients, but they are mild. The pericardium is the lining that surrounds the heart, and sometimes it can get inflamed, and fluid can accumulate between the lining and the heart, impeding its expansion or causing chest pain. Of course patients can develop coronary artery disease unrelated to scleroderma, but strangely, they can have heart attacks with normal angiograms because scleroderma is a disease of the small blood vessels, which may not be detected with angiography. Rhythm problems, heart blocks, or conduction abnormalities found on electrocardiogram can be ominous and hard to treat but are usually benign. Again, I rarely deal with unusual cardiac events in scleroderma patients but am always glad to have a smart and friendly cardiologist readily available and don't hesitate to consult one.

Gastrointestinal problems are common in scleroderma. Most stem from motility problems (GI tract smooth muscle dysfunction). The small vessels in the gut from the esophagus down to the anus are narrowed, causing damage to small nerves, which initiate motility by causing the contraction of smooth muscle in the GI tract. The most common target is the esophagus so that patients complain of difficulty swallowing and acid reflux. Years ago, patients would inevitably develop esophageal strictures because acid would reflux up from the stomach chronically and cause inflammation and eventually narrowing of the esophagus. Gastroenterologists were constantly dilating these patients' esophagi—an unpleasant procedure fraught with the devastating potential of rupture. However, over the last few decades, with the development and daily use of proton pump inhibitors, such as omeprazole (Prilosec), pantoprazole (Protonix), rabeprazole (Aciphex), dexlansoprazole (Dexilant), esomeprazole (Nexium), or lansoprazole (Prevacid), I rarely see these complications. It's important to emphasize to patients the daily use of these medications because in most other cases, they are used for only a finite period of time. Recently, there has been concern about osteoporosis with long-term use of these drugs because of poor calcium absorption, and I am especially vigilant about bone densities and appropriate treatment and prophylaxis for these patients. Nevertheless, patients and pharmacists are constantly questioning me about the risk-benefit ratio of long-term treatment. The next most common complaint is abdominal bloating, pain, and alternating constipation and diarrhea caused by poor intestinal motility and either bacterial overgrowth or malabsorption. These problems can lead to malnutrition and extreme weight loss, occasionally requiring parenteral (IV) feeding. I often use erythromycin in these patients (alternating two weeks on and two weeks off) because of its promotility and antibacterial qualities, but other physicians prefer clarithromycin, ketoconazole, fluconazole, metronidazole, rifaximin, ciprofloxacin, or doxycycline. Promotility agents, such as Reglan (or metoclopramide) and cisapride, have had mixed success in these patients but also can have some serious neurological side effects. It may be worthwhile to check these patients for malabsorption and have a good GI workup, but I would find a gastroenterologist who has had special training in scleroderma or a lot of experience. Good coordination with GI doctors is essential. However, patients well versed in their disease complain that they are more familiar with potential problems and treatment than most gastroenterologists. Our very strong local scleroderma support group has been very verbal about this problem.

Most GI problems I find easy to treat, but a condition called *intestinal pseudo-obstruction* can be difficult to diagnose and devastating. Because of a complete loss of motility in the intestine, nothing moves and patients develop intense abdominal pain and a very tense, painful abdomen. To the uneducated physician's eye in the emergency room or office, the patient has a mechanical obstruction and should have immediate surgery or a barium enema—the wrong and possibly fatal things to do. With the right testing and analysis, a nasogastropharyngeal tube, and bowel rest, disaster can be averted. Again, this condition is rare but needs to be recognized and treated immediately. In the last year, I have had several scleroderma patients have sudden drops in their hemoglobin or red blood cell count. Every one of them was found to have dilated blood vessels in their stomach or colon that were easily cauterized by a gastroenterologist. Today, I saw a limited scleroderma patient who has severe pulmonary hypertension, inflammatory arthritis, and a face full of telangiectasia (dilated blood vessels). She has had several GI bleeds and cauterizations of dilated blood vessels in her colon. I tend to think the number of telangiectasia on her face correlates with the number in her GI tract, and they should serve as a red flag. Most recently, a similar patient bled from telangiectasia in her eye—that's a new one!

The only liver involvement I worry about is primary biliary cirrhosis (PBC), most commonly associated with specific antibodies (anticentromere and antimitochondrial antibody) seen in limited scleroderma. Bile becomes static in the biliary tract with increasing fibrosis or scarring of the bile ducts, leading to the worst-case scenario of liver cirrhosis. Patients may complain of intense itching, and their liver functions, especially their alkaline phosphatase and bilirubin, may start rising quite dramatically. Liver biopsy can be definitive. Like all other problems in scleroderma, if it is recognized early, with the right antibody and liver-function tests, there is treatment. Patients may have mild liver-function abnormalities on their lab tests for years before anyone recognizes the possibility of PBC. Ursodiol may slow the progression. Cholestyramine, colestipol, or rifampin may help lessen the associated itching. Adequate vitamin D and calcium supplementation may treat or prevent the osteoporosis or osteomalacia (thin brittle bones due to Vitamin D deficiency) complication. Finally, liver transplantation may be lifesaving in rare occasions.

OK, I think I have covered most of the organ-related problems caused by scleroderma and painted a less bleak picture than I would have even five years ago, if patients are treated early and aggressively. Still, I want to discuss the daily, more mundane problems I typically encounter with these patients. Usually, their first complaint will be swollen hands and/or swollen feet. The skin is indurated and loses all its creases and markings. Fingers with such swelling are said to have sclerodactyly. They are often dusky and cool, showing evidence of Raynaud's phenomenon in which fingers, toes, and even full extremities will undergo tricolor changes of white, purple, and red when exposed to cold or stress. These color changes are reversible with warming measures and sometimes medications, except in rare cases of severe vasculitis or vasculopathy, where inflammation or scarring obstruct the small vessels, and the effected fingertip or extremity infarcts or dies and will fall off. More frequently, patients develop little painful ulcers on their fingertips, which can become infected and cause gangrene and loss of the finger or even hand or foot. I tell patients that pain they encounter with lesions is the equivalent of having a heart attack or angina of their finger because of the compromised blood supply and loss of oxygen to that area. We treat this problem very aggressively with blood-vessel-dilating drugs (most reliably nifedipine), oral antibiotics, and topical antiseptics, such as hydrogen peroxide or betadine. However, in severe cases patients may require intravenous drugs, such as prostacyclin, or some of the newer, expensive oral drugs, such as sildenafil. Even rarer, patients may require vascular surgery or even amputation, which is fraught with risk because poor blood supply leads to poor healing. Patients with gangrene or severe ulceration may demarcate an area on their limb or fingers or toes between healthy and dead tissue, and the unhealthy portion will autoamputate, or fall off, over weeks or months. It sounds worse than it actually appears. During that period, adequate pain control, wound care, infection control, and vasodilation (dilating the surrounding blood vessels) with medications are essential. It is also important to counsel smokers that smoking decreases blood flow to the fingers and will probably doom them to loss of digits in addition to lung damage and so forth.

Systemic Sclerosis or Scleroderma

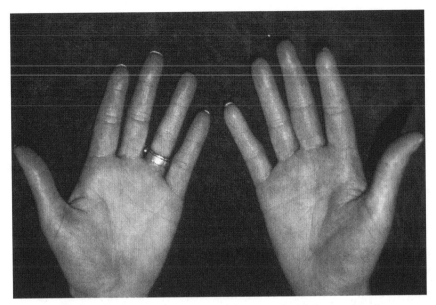

Raynaud's Phenomenon—courtesy of ACR image bank

Winter is a bad season because of the cold, but air conditioning during the summer can be difficult. Remember, most patients can reverse Raynaud's with just warming measures, and if they can't, I know we're dealing with something more. I tell patients to have gloves for every occasion and remember to warm their core. Not every patient who has Raynaud's has scleroderma. It is associated with lupus and many other diseases and may be present without any known underlying disease. In fact, as I have mentioned before, I have Raynaud's phenomenon, and it affects my fingers, toes, and nose much to the delight and sometimes amusement of my patients. The skin changes in scleroderma can be disfiguring, painful, and debilitating. Before I leave Raynaud's and the topic of poor circulation in scleroderma, it's important to mention that erectile dysfunction is common in males. Not surprisingly, sildenafil (Viagra) may be effective therapy.

Rudy's Ruminations On **Rheumatology**

The tendons in the arms or legs may be inflamed or even compressed, so patients develop painful rubs. They also can develop inflammation of their joints and even complete resorption of bones in their hands, forearms, or feet. Medications such as methotrexate or nonsteroidals may be helpful. Recently, Remicade, Rituxan and Actemra have shown some promise. The skin can develop areas of hyper- or hypopigmentation and dilated blood vessels, called *telangiectasia*. Finally, one of the most difficult cutaneous problems is called *calcinosis*, where calcium deposits appear under the skin and at times are bone deep. These deposits may be large and multiple and drain. They can be miniscule little painful bumps on the finger that open and drain toothpaste-like material. Although there have been many reports of successful therapies, none have been shown to be consistently effective. When you ask scleroderma specialists about therapies for calcinosis, they roll their eyes and either change the subject or list all the therapies that have been tried with mixed success. I have tried many of them. Anecdotally, I had some success with diltiazem, a blood pressure medicine which that has had mixed results in studies. Coumadin, bisphosphonates, and colchicine all have their supporters but are questionable. In summary, scleroderma can be a scary disease that needs to be taken seriously and treated early and aggressively. There has been some major progress in treating individual manifestations. Patients need to consult rheumatologists early and often. The majority of scleroderma patients has the limited form and with proper monitoring lives long, productive, good-quality lives. However, diffuse scleroderma still has a grave prognosis and a very rapid progression, so I usually refer these patients to major scleroderma centers, such as UCLA. There has been some spectacular success in some cases treated with stem cell transplants, but it is a high-risk procedure. Then again, diffuse scleroderma is a high-risk disease! Finally, there are always new studies and hope.

Pearls

- *Scleroderma* means "hardening or thickening of the skin."
- It is a systemic disease causing inflammation of small blood vessels (arterioles) in the skin and multiple organs, leading to scarring, narrowing, poor blood flow, and dysfunction.
- There are multiple forms, but the two major ones are limited and diffuse.
- Skin changes in diffuse involve the whole body and can be disfiguring.
- Skin changes in limited involve the face, hands, feet, and distal forearms and legs.
- The diffuse form has a poor prognosis and should be treated aggressively and quickly (stem cell transplant?).
- The limited form has an indolent course and can be quite manageable but very debilitating unless treated promptly and aggressively.
- There is no proven remittive agent, but individual manifestations may be treated successfully.
- Home blood pressure monitors are a must, especially in diffuse scleroderma.
- Any sudden change in kidney function or blood pressure should be immediately addressed.
- ACE inhibitors are keys to blood pressure control and prevention of renal crisis.
- Renal crisis can be fatal but is reversible if treated immediately.
- Closely monitor blood pressure and kidney, lung, and cardiac function.
- Check for pulmonary hypertension yearly with echocardiograms, pulmonary-function tests, and, if indicated, right heart catheterizations.

- Aggressive treatment of mild or early pulmonary hypertension can be successful and lifesaving. When it becomes moderate or severe, it's too late.
- Treat Raynaud's with warming measures, calcium channel blockers, and other blood vessel dilators.
- Skin ulcers should be treated with vasodilators and hydrogen peroxide or betadine soaks mixed with warm water. Short-term analgesics may be necessary.
- Infected ulcers should be treated aggressively with oral antibiotics and hydrogen peroxide or betadine soaks.
- Most patients should be on lifelong proton inhibitors (Prilosec, etc.) for GERD.
- Most GI problems are due to motility dysfunction.
- Intermittent (two weeks on, two weeks off) treatment with antibiotics (my favorite is erythromycin) may be helpful.
- Eat small, frequent meals.
- Beware of biliary cirrhosis! Check alkaline phosphatase on blood tests and antimitochondrial antibody.
- If patient has aggressive interstitial lung disease, Cytoxan and maybe CellCept may be the only chance at reversing or halting the process.
- Most scleroderma patients will live long, productive lives but should have frequent visits with rheumatologists and close relationships with a gastroenterologist, cardiologist, and pulmonologist.

References

1. www.rheumatology.org/Practice
(Patient Education—Diseases and Conditions)
2. LeRoy, E. C., C. Black, R. Fleischmajer R, et al. Scleroderma (Systemic Sclerosis): Classification, Subsets and Pathogenesis. *J Rheumatol* 15:202.

3 Janosik, D. L., T. G. Osborn, T. L. Moore, et al. Heart Disease in Systemic Sclerosis. *Semin Arthritis Rheum* 19:191.

4. Doré, A., M. Lucas, D. Ivanco, et al. Significance of Palpable Tendon Friction Rubs in Early Diffuse Cutaneous Systemic Sclerosis. *Arthritis Care Res* (Hoboken) 65:1385.

5. Walker, U. A., A. Tyndall, and R. Ruszat. Erectile Dysfunction in Systemic Sclerosis. *Ann Rheum Dis* 68:1083.

6. Derk, C. T., L. I. Sakkas, M. Rasheed, et al. Autoantibodies in Patients with Systemic Sclerosis and Cancer: A Case-Control Study. *J Rheumatol* 30:1994.

7. Black, C. M. Scleroderma—Clinical Aspects. *J Intern Med* 234:115.

8. Akesson, A., and F. A. Wollheim. Organ Manifestations in 100 Patients with Progressive Systemic Sclerosis: A Comparison between the CREST Syndrome and Diffuse Scleroderma. *Br J Rheumatol* 28:281.

9. Ferri, C., G. Valentini, F. Cozzi, et al. Systemic Sclerosis: Demographic, Clinical, and Serologic Features and Survival in 1,012 Italian Patients. *Medicine* (Baltimore) 81:139.

10. Alton, E., and M. Turner-Warwick. Lung Involvement in Scleroderma. In *Systemic Sclerosis (Scleroderma)*, edited by C. M. Black and M. I. V. Jayson, xx–xx. Chichester, UK: Wiley.

11. Steen, V. D., D. L. Powell, and T. A. Medsger, Jr. Clinical Correlations and Prognosis Based on Serum Autoantibodies in Patients with Systemic Sclerosis. *Arthritis Rheum* 31:196.

12. Steen, V. D. Systemic Sclerosis. In *The Lung in Rheumatic Diseases*, G. Zimmerman, 279. New York: Marcel Dekker.

13. Kowal-Bielecka, O., K. Kowal, K. B. Highland, and R. M. Silver. Bronchoalveolar Lavage Fluid in Scleroderma Interstitial Lung Disease: Technical Aspects and Clinical Correlations: Review of the Literature. *Semin Arthritis Rheum* 40:73.

14. Tashkin, D. P., R. Elashoff, P. J. Clements, et al. Cyclophosphamide versus Placebo in Scleroderma Lung Disease. *N Engl J Med* 354:2655.

15. Battle, R. W., M. A. Davitt, S. M. Cooper, et al. Prevalence of Pulmonary Hypertension in Limited and Diffuse Scleroderma. *Chest* 110:1515.

16. Steen, V. Advancements in Diagnosis of Pulmonary Arterial Hypertension in Scleroderma. *Arthritis Rheum* 52:3698.

17. Mukerjee, D., D. St. George, C. Knight, et al. Echocardiography and Pulmonary Function as Screening Tests for Pulmonary Arterial Hypertension in Systemic Sclerosis. *Rheumatology* (Oxford) 43:461.

18. Steen, V. D., and T. A. Medsger, Jr. Epidemiology and Natural History of Systemic Sclerosis. *Rheum Dis Clin North Am* 16:1.

19. LeRoy, E. C., and T. A. Medsger, Jr. Criteria for the Classification of Early Systemic Sclerosis. *J Rheumatol* 28:1573.

20. Wigley, F. M. Clinical Practice: Raynaud's Phenomenon. *N Engl J Med* 347:1001.

21. Herrick, A. Diagnosis and Management of Scleroderma Peripheral Vascular Disease. *Rheum Dis Clin North Am* 34:89.

22. Thoua, N. M., C. Bunce, G. Brough, et al. Assessment of Gastrointestinal Symptoms in Patients with Systemic Sclerosis in a UK Tertiary Referral Centre. *Rheumatology* (Oxford) 49:1770.

23. Steen, V. D., and T. A. Medsger, Jr. Severe Organ Involvement in Systemic Sclerosis with Diffuse Scleroderma. *Arthritis Rheum* 43:2437.

24. Silver, R. M. Clinical Aspects of Systemic Sclerosis (Scleroderma), supplement. *Ann Rheum Dis* 50 (4): S854.

25. Sjogren, R. W. Gastrointestinal Motility Disorders in Scleroderma. *Arthritis Rheum* 37:1265.

26. Denton, C. P., and V. H. Ong. Targeted Therapies for Systemic Sclerosis. *Nat Rev Rheumatol* 9:451.

7. Palmieri, G. M., J. I. Sebes, J. A. Aelion, et al. Treatment of Calcinosis with Diltiazem. *Arthritis Rheum* 38:1646.

28. Korn, J. H., M. Mayes, M. Matucci-Cerinic, et al. Digital Ulcers in Systemic Sclerosis: Prevention by Treatment with Bosentan, an Oral Endothelin Receptor Antagonist. *Arthritis Rheum* 50:3985.

29. Avouac, J., P. J. Clements, D. Khanna, et al. Articular Involvement in Systemic Sclerosis. *Rheumatology* (Oxford) 51:1347.

30. Elhai, M., M. Meunier, M. Matucci-Cerinic, et al. Outcomes of Patients with Systemic Sclerosis-Associated Polyarthritis and Myopathy Treated with Tocilizumab or Abatacept: A EUSTAR Observational Study. *Ann Rheum Dis* 72:1217.

32. Omair, M. A., V. Phumethum, and S. R. Johnson. Long-Term Safety and Effectiveness of Tumour Necrosis Factor Inhibitors in Systemic Sclerosis Patients with Inflammatory Arthritis. *Clin Exp Rheumatol* 30:S55.

Chapter Eleven

Eosinophilic Fasciitis (EF), or Shulman's Syndrome

The Athlete with Orange-Peel Skin

Richard is an athletic forty-year-old man who complained of pain and swelling of his lower legs when I first saw him. He was a runner and cyclist and had been inactive for weeks. When I examined his legs, they had a tight, orange-peel quality to them and were very tender. They were similar but not quite what you would find in scleroderma. Also in contrast to scleroderma patients, he had no other skin or internal organ involvement. His labs were only remarkable for a large amount of eosinophils, which are a kind of white blood cell most frequently associated with allergies and parasitic infections. I suspected eosinophilic fasciitis, and a biopsy from a leg confirmed the diagnosis. A six-month course of prednisone resolved the problem completely. Today, he sits in the room in his running shorts, beaming. He just completed his first marathon in years. I feel great.

Rudy's Ruminations On **Rheumatology**

There is a whole group of scleroderma-like illnesses. I won't mention all of them, but the one I have seen the most (four to five cases) is eosinophilic fasciitis. It starts with symmetrical, nonpitting swelling of extremities, which may evolve into an orange-peel, or "peau d'orange," type of texture. It usually spares the hands and feet and is ANA negative, unlike scleroderma. Muscle pain, weakness, and sometimes arthritis or neuropathies can occur, but the most characteristic feature is an increased number of eosinophils in the blood count or in biopsies of the skin, which need to be full thickness, including the fascia and muscle. The patients typically have overexerted themselves and may be athletes or manual laborers. Usually prednisone, starting at 1 mg/kg and tapering over months, is quite effective, but occasionally some of the usual suspects, such as methotrexate or Plaquenil or even Remicade, may be used in resistant cases.

A group of similar syndromes involving more muscle pain and internal organ involvement began to appear in 1989. Toxic oil syndrome was thought to be due to contaminated rapeseed oil in Spain and eosinophilia-myalgia syndrome was due to contaminated tryptophan (a sleep supplement) in the United States. They could be quite disabling and were the subject of class-action suits. Lawyers have often tried to involve themselves in the life of many of my patients, whether it was for disability claims or class-action suits. Although some of them have been helpful and had good intentions, many of them have just been opportunistic. I try to avoid these cases.

Another scleroderma-like illness is nephrogenic systemic fibrosis, seen in dialysis or kidney-failure patients who undergo an MRI exam with gadolinium dye. It is similar to EF, but it involves the hands and feet rather than the arms and legs; it is not associated with eosinophils and does not respond to steroids. Avoid gadolinium in kidney-failure patients!

Pearls

- Eosinophilic fasciitis causes nonpitting swelling of the arms and legs and spares the hands and feet.
- It is usually seen in very active people—manual laborers or athletes.
- Weakness, numbness, and muscle pain are features.
- Diagnosis is clinched by a high eosinophil (a kind of white blood cell) count in the blood when a full-thickness skin biopsy (must include the fascia and muscle) is performed.
- The mainstay of treatment is prednisone, with methotrexate, Plaquenil, and Remicade reserved for resistant cases.
- Nephrogenic systemic fibrosis is similar to eosinophilic fasciitis but involves the hands and feet; it is not associated with an elevated eosinophil count and is resistant to steroids.
- It almost exclusively occurs in patients with kidney failure who receive gadolinium dye for MRIs.
- Do not use gadolinium in kidney-failure patients!

References

1. www.rheumatology.org/Practice
(Patient Education—Diseases and Conditions)
2. Lakhanpal, S., W. W. Ginsburg, C. J. Michet, et al. Eosinophilic Fasciitis: Clinical Spectrum and Therapeutic Response in 52 Cases. *Semin Arthritis Rheum* 17:221.
3. Varga, J., R. Griffin, J. H. Newman, and S. A. Jimenez. Eosinophilic Fasciitis Is Clinically Distinguishable from the Eosinophilia-Myalgia Syndrome and Is Not Associated with L-tryptophan Use. *J Rheumatol* 18:259.
4. Allen, J. A., A. Peterson, R. Sufit, et al. Post-epidemic Eosinophilia-Myalgia Syndrome Associated with L-tryptophan. *Arthritis Rheum* 63:3633.

5. Alonso-Ruiz, A., A. C. Zea-Mendoza, J. M. Salazar-Vallinas, et al. Toxic Oil Syndrome: A Syndrome with Features Overlapping Those of Various Forms of Scleroderma. *Semin Arthritis Rheum* 15:200.

6. Kaufman, L. D., and L. B. Krupp. Eosinophilia-Myalgia Syndrome, Toxic-Oil Syndrome, and Diffuse Fasciitis with Eosinophilia. *Curr Opin Rheumatol* 7:560.

7. Lebeaux, D., C. Francès, S. Barete, et al. Eosinophilic Fasciitis (Shulman Disease): New Insights into the Therapeutic Management from a Series of 34 Patients. *Rheumatology* (Oxford) 51:557.

8. Khanna, D., H. Agrawal, and P. J. Clements. Infliximab May Be Effective in the Treatment of Steroid-Resistant Eosinophilic Fasciitis: Report of Three Cases. *Rheumatology* (Oxford) 49:1184.

9. Galan, A., S. E. Cowper, and R. Bucala. Nephrogenic Systemic Fibrosis (Nephrogenic Fibrosing Dermopathy). *Curr Opin Rheumatol* 18:614.

10. Mendoza, F. A., C. M. Artlett, N. Sandorfi, et al. Description of 12 Cases of Nephrogenic Fibrosing Dermopathy and Review of the Literature. *Semin Arthritis Rheum* 35:238.

Chapter Twelve

Undifferentiated, Overlap, or Mixed Connective Tissue Disease

The Girl with a Little Bit of Everything

Effie was fifty when I first saw her and had swollen hands, severe Raynaud's, dry eyes and dry mouth, and an intermittent rash on her chest. She also has had occasional fatigue, weakness, and signs of muscle inflammation. Her blood work revealed some nonspecific abnormal antibodies. I could not make a definitive diagnosis of lupus, RA, Sjögren's, or polymyositis, although she had features of each of these diseases. I always wonder whether eventually one of these diseases will declare itself, but it is unlikely. At this visit, she is flaring with significant, painful hand swelling and some chest pain. She has been on Plaquenil with good results but has been under stress lately because of tension at home. I am going to give her an intramuscular injection of triamcinolone and counsel her regarding stress management, and if she is no better by next visit, we will consider treating her with methotrexate.

Some patients defy categorization; they have features from many of the above diseases but don't fit any specific disease. They may have features of lupus, Sjögren's, RA, scleroderma, or polymyositis in any combination. I find that patients want a specific label and are skeptical and disappointed when I tell them they have a "combo" disease. Many of these patients will eventually develop a specific disease over time, but some won't. I tend to find most of these patients have a better prognosis and are treated with many of the same medications we use in the specific diseases depending on their features. Mixed connective disease actually is a specific disease described about thirty years ago to differentiate it from lupus because it had its own specific set of antibodies (anti-RNP), and patients rarely developed kidney disease. Its features include swollen hands, Raynaud's, muscle disease, arthritis, fatigue, and occasionally trigeminal neuralgia, fevers, and meningitis. I try to reassure patients that they have a treatable autoimmune disease, and if they need to use a label, tell people they have a lupus-like disease.

Pearls

- Mixed connective disease (MCTD) has features of lupus, polymyositis, scleroderma, Sjögren's, and/or RA and is associated with anti-RNP antibodies.
- Undifferentiated connective disease has many of these features but no anti-RNP antibodies.
- MCTD patients often have swollen hands and Raynaud's and seldom kidney disease.
- Treatment is similar to lupus and RA.

References

www.rheumatology.org/Practice (Patient Education—Diseases and Conditions)

1. Cervera, R., M. A. Khamashta, and G. R. Hughes. 'Overlap' Syndromes. *Ann Rheum Dis* 49:947.

2. Doria, A., M. Mosca, P. F. Gambari, and S. Bombardieri. Defining Unclassifiable Connective Tissue Diseases: Incomplete, Undifferentiated, or Both? *J Rheumatol* 32:213.

3. LeRoy, E. C., H. R. Maricq, and M. B. Kahaleh. Undifferentiated Connective Tissue Syndromes. *Arthritis Rheum* 23:341.

4. Alarcón, G. S., G. V. Williams, J. Z. Singer, et al. Early Undifferentiated Connective Tissue Disease. I. Early Clinical Manifestation in a Large Cohort of Patients with Undifferentiated Connective Tissue Diseases Compared with Cohorts of Well Established Connective Tissue Disease. *J Rheumatol* 18:1332.

5. Bennett, R. M. Overlap Syndromes. In *Textbook of Rheumatology*, 8th edition, 1381. Philadelphia: WB Saunders Co.

6. Sharp, G. C., W. S. Irvin, E. M. Tan, et al. Mixed Connective Tissue Disease—An Apparently Distinct Rheumatic Disease Syndrome Associated with a Specific Antibody to an Extractable Nuclear Antigen (ENA). *Am J Med* 52:148.

7. Piirainen, H. I. Patients with Arthritis and anti-U1-RNP Antibodies: A 10-Year Follow-Up. *Br J Rheumatol* 29:345.

8. Sharp, G. C. Therapy and Prognosis of MCTD. In *Mixed Connective Tissue Disease and Antinuclear Antibodies*, edited by R. Kasukawa and G. Sharp, 315. Amsterdam: Excerpta Medica.

9. Pope, J. E. Other Manifestations of Mixed Connective Tissue Disease. *Rheum Dis Clin North Am* 31:519.

Chapter Thirteen

Seronegative Spondyloarthritis

Too Young to Have Back Pain

During my first several visits with Rob, a twenty-five-year-old car salesman with a shy smile and stocky build, he was usually standing and moving around to alleviate his back pain. He was initially sent to me by an ophthalmologist because of recurrent iritis, a very painful red eye, which often can be associated with a variety of rheumatologic diseases I treat. I noticed the patient's discomfort immediately and discovered he'd had back pain for the last two years. On further inquiry, I found that his father and one brother had developed back pain at a similar age. His exam had been normal except for a slight reduction in his ability to bend and some tenderness at his buttocks. His labs revealed a mildly elevated ESR and a genetic marker associated with ankylosing spondylitis. X-rays revealed narrowing and a little bit of blurring of his sacroiliac joints—clinching the diagnosis. After one year of Humira and an NSAID, he is asymptomatic and able to stand for long periods in the showroom talking to customers. He has not had an episode of iritis since starting the Humira. When I enter the room these days, he is usually sitting comfortably and talking on his cellphone.

Rudy's Ruminations On **Rheumatology**

In the same room, the week previously I saw a thin seventy-year-old patient with a droopy moustache who has a long history of neck and low back problems. His neck was fused in a permanently flexed position, and he couldn't straighten his back to an upright position. He recently was diagnosed with Crohn's disease, or inflammatory bowel disease. Since being on Humira for the last six months, he still can't stand straight, but he has less pain and diarrhea.

Seronegative means patients with these diseases test negative for rheumatoid arthritis. *Spondyloarthritis* means that they have an inflammatory arthritis that typically involves the axial skeleton or spine (but not always). The four major diseases associated with this category are ankylosing spondylitis, psoriatic arthritis, reactive arthritis, and inflammatory bowel disease. The prototype is ankylosing spondylitis. Most patients with this disease will start having symptoms in their teens or early twenties. Unlike most of the other rheumatologic diseases, there is at least equal distribution between males and females. They will most often complain of stiffness and pain in their lower back radiating into both buttocks. It wakes them from a sound sleep. It is worse in the morning, may be associated with hours of morning stiffness, and usually responds at least partially to NSAIDs. The pain is usually not positional and gets better with exercise. It may be associated with neck, midback, or chest wall pain. This particular kind of back pain is classified as inflammatory and should make health providers suspicious of a seronegative spondyloarthritis, especially ankylosing spondylitis. It should be distinguished from mechanical back pain, which we all develop at one time or another. Usually this pain is worse with prolonged standing or sitting and exercise and worsens as the day progresses. Many ankylosing spondylitis patients have a family history of back pain. They may have sacroiliitis, or inflammation of their sacroiliac joints (joints in the back of the pelvis under both buttocks), which may be visible on x- ray, CT scan, or MRI. Some have a history of iritis, which is a particularly serious and painful red eye. Others have psoriasis or inflammatory bowel disease, and many will test positive for HLA-B27, a histocompatibility gene also seen in a small proportion of the normal population—it is not used to make the diagnosis, just to increase probability. In fact, the majority of people with this gene will not develop any of these diseases. Approximately 6 percent of Caucasians will have this gene, and incidence is higher in other races.

Patients may also present to the office with huge swelling of a knee or a severely painful hip. If a young patient is referred to the office with one or two swollen knees and the fluid is inflammatory (meaning there are more than three thousand white blood cells and often between twenty and one hundred thousand), then chances are they have one of these diseases. Interestingly, they often have an amazing amount of fluid in their knees—I've withdrawn 4,000–5,000 cc (or six to seven 60 cc syringes full) out of one knee. Ankylosing spondylitis patients may develop increasing stiffness and deformities of their backs and necks unless treated. Their x- rays can show beautiful, pristine disc spaces but may have bony bridges between the vertebra with calcification of the ligaments in front and behind the vertebra. Eventually the spine can totally fuse, and therefore some wise person coined the term "bamboo spine." If left untreated, these patients can fuse at a ninety-degree angle, unable to straighten or look up. Their neck may also be fused in permanent flexion, leading to significant disability. We, therefore, send patients to physical therapy to teach them to maintain good posture and protect their joints so that if they did fuse, it would be in an upright position. It was our only recourse years ago, but with new medications, we may be able to reduce the pain and prevent the fusion. NSAIDs may inhibit the extra bone formation, and TNF antagonists (Remicade, Enbrel, Cimzia, Humira, and Simponi) will reduce the inflammation, pain, and possibly the fusion. Azulfidine is useful in some patients, and methotrexate is effective in patients who peripheral joint involvement exclusively (not sacroiliitis). Secukinumab (Cosentryx), an IL-17A inhibitor, has been shown to be effective in early studies but is not FDA approved for Ankylosing Spondylitis as yet.

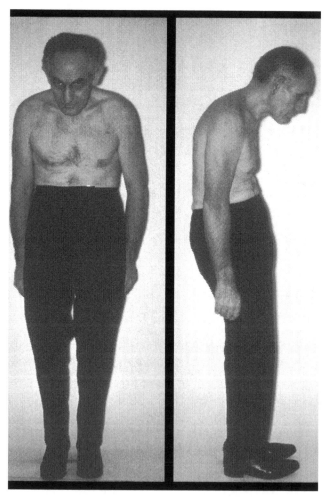

Ankylosing Spondylitis—ACR image bank

Pearls

- Inflammatory back pain in ankylosing spondylitis is usually worse in the morning, better with exercise, and responds at least partially to NSAIDs; it is associated with hours of morning stiffness.
- Check HLA-B27 (genetic histocompatibility marker), x-rays, or MRI of SI joints.
- Rule out history of iritis, psoriasis, or inflammatory bowel disease.
- Its usual age of onset is in the teens and twenties.
- It can cause unusually large knee effusions.
- Bilateral sacroiliitis is associated with ankylosing spondylitis and inflammatory bowel disease; unilateral, with psoriatic and reactive arthritis.
- NSAIDs may prevent fusion of the spine.
- TNF antagonists are effective for inflammation in the spine and SI joints, peripheral joints, and for iritis.
- Methotrexate and possibly Azulfidine are effective for peripheral joint disease but not axial skeleton or SI joints.

Reactive Arthritis

Two Indiscretions and I Get This?

I consulted on Josh for the first time several months ago. He was a suave, athletic fifty-year-old professor of linguistics with a silver mane and moustache who went through a nasty divorce twenty years ago and enjoyed a year of sexual promiscuity until he developed a chlamydial infection in his urethra. It was treated, but shortly thereafter, he developed recurrent massive swelling of his knees that needed to be aspirated and injected with steroids three times in one year. Eventually, a rheumatologist found that he was HLA-B27 positive and made the diagnosis of reactive arthritis. He treated Josh with methotrexate successfully for five years until he moved to a different state and stopped the medication. He remained asymptomatic and pursued his passions of skiing and cycling until a month before seeing me, when he developed severe swelling of his right hand and massive effusions of both knees. I aspirated both knees and injected them with steroids. The joint fluid was moderately inflamed, and the patient's ESR and CRP were extremely elevated. I then prescribed NSAIDs, but his hand remained swollen. Eventually, I restarted the methotrexate, and he showed major improvement.

Reactive arthritis is an inflammatory arthritis that follows an infection. Salmonella, shigella, streptococcus, chlamydia, and campylobacter are some of the organisms implicated. The immune system already activated goes haywire and produces systemic inflammation, attacking joints and sometimes the eyes, urethra, oral mucosa, and skin. Years ago it was called *Reiter's syndrome* and was characterized by arthritis, conjunctivitis or iritis, urethritis (inflammation of the urethra), and sometimes oral ulcers, a swollen penis or labia (circinate balanitis), and a scaly rash on the palms and soles (keratodermia blennorrhagica). Most patients had only the arthritis, so they decided to rename it just *reactive arthritis*, although many of these patients still have the other characteristics. They also may have sacroiliitis (often one-sided) and have a good chance of being positive for HLA-B27. They can present with a swollen knee, but sometimes they may start with hip or back pain or even conjunctivitis or iritis. We used to think that this was an intermittent or even one-time disease, which still can occur, but more often the inflammation is chronic and can cause destruction of joints. All members of this family of arthritis are incestuous and share some features. The treatment is essentially the same as for ankylosing spondylitis, although since this disease affects predominantly peripheral joints (not the spine) methotrexate and NSAIDs are the most commonly used medications.

Pearls

- It is usually an autoimmune reaction to an infection and is noninfectious.
- It may be intermittent or chronic.
- It often involves inflammation of just one sacroiliac joint.
- Rash, iritis, and urethritis are common associations.
- It usually involves large joints, such as the knees.
- It can cause unusually large inflammatory knee swelling or effusions.
- Treatment is essentially the same as for ankylosing spondylitis.

References

1. www.rheumatology.org/Practice
2. Zeidler, H., and B. Amor. The Assessment in Spondyloarthritis International Society (ASAS) Classification Criteria for Peripheral Spondyloarthritis and for Spondyloarthritis in General: The Spondyloarthritis Concept in Progress. *Ann Rheum Dis* 70:1.

3. Healy, P. J., and P. S. Helliwell. Classification of the Spondyloar-thropathies. *Curr Opin Rheumatol* 17:395.

4. Rudwaleit, M., D. van der Heijde, R. Landewé, et al. The Assessment of Spondyloarthritis International Society Classification Criteria for Peripheral Spondyloarthritis and for Spondyloarthritis in General. *Ann Rheum Dis* 70:25.

5. Rosenbaum, J. T. Characterization of Uveitis Associated with Spondyloarthritis. *J Rheumatol* 16:792.

6. Rudwaleit, M., D. van der Heijde, R. Landewé, et al. The Development of Assessment of SpondyloArthritis International Society Classification Criteria for Axial Spondyloarthritis (Part II): Validation and Final Selection. *Ann Rheum Dis* 68:777.

7. Sieper, J., J. Lenaerts, J. Wollenhaupt, et al. Efficacy and Safety of Infliximab plus Naproxen versus Naproxen Alone in Patients with Early, Active Axial Spondyloarthritis: Results from the Double-Blind, Placebo-Controlled INFAST Study, Part 1. *Ann Rheum Dis* 73:101.

8. Sieper, J., D. van der Heijde, M. Dougados, et al. Efficacy and Safety of Adalimumab in Patients with Non-radiographic Axial Spondyloarthritis: Results of a Randomised Placebo-Controlled Trial (ABILITY-1). *Ann Rheum Dis* 72:815.

9. Song, I. H., A. Weiß, K. G. Hermann, et al. Similar Response Rates in Patients with Ankylosing Spondylitis and Non-radiographic Axial Spondyloarthritis after 1 Year of Treatment with Etanercept: Results from the ESTHER Trial. *Ann Rheum Dis* 72:823.

10. Dougados, M., D. van der Heijde, J. Sieper, et al. Clinical and Imaging Efficacy of Etanercept in Early Non-radiographic Axial Spondyloarthritis: A 12-Week, Randomized, Double-Blinded, Placebo-Controlled Trial, supplement. *Ann Rheum Dis* 72:S87.

11. Landewe, R. B. M., M. Rudwaleit, D. van der Heijde, et al. Effect of Certolizumab Pegol on Signs and Symptoms of Ankylosing

Spondylitis and Non-radiographic Axial Spondylarthritis: 24 Week Results of a Double Blind Randomized Placebo-Controlled Phase 3 Axial Spondyloarthritis Study. *Arthritis Rheum* 64:S336.

12. Braun, J., R. van den Berg, X. Baraliakos, et al. 2010 Update of the ASAS/EULAR Recommendations for the Management of Ankylosing Spondylitis. *Ann Rheum Dis* 70:896.

13. Zochling, J., D. van der Heijde, Burgos-Vargas, et al. ASAS/EULAR Recommendations for the Management of Ankylosing Spondylitis. *Ann Rheum Dis* 65:442.

14. Smolen, J. S., J. Braun, M. Dougados, et al. Treating Spondyloarthritis, Including Ankylosing Spondylitis and Psoriatic Arthritis, to Target: Recommendations of an International Task Force. *Ann Rheum Dis* 73:6.

15. Passalent, L. A., L. J. Soever, F. D. O'Shea, and R. D. Inman. Exercise in Ankylosing Spondylitis: Discrepancies between Recommendations and Reality. *J Rheumatol* 37:835.

16. Sidiropoulos, P. I., G. Hatemi, I. H. Song, et al. Evidence-Based Recommendations for the Management of Ankylosing Spondylitis: Systematic Literature Search of the 3E Initiative in Rheumatology Involving a Broad Panel of Experts and Practising Rheumatologists. *Rheumatology* (Oxford) 47:355.

17. Wanders, A., D. van der Heijde, R. Landewé, et al. Nonsteroidal Antiinflammatory Drugs Reduce Radiographic Progression in Patients with Ankylosing Spondylitis: A Randomized Clinical Trial. *Arthritis Rheum* 52:1756.

18. Baraliakos, X., J. Brandt, J. Listing, et al. Outcome of Patients with Active Ankylosing Spondylitis after Two Years of Therapy with Etanercept: Clinical and Magnetic Resonance Imaging Data. *Arthritis Rheum* 53:856.

19. van der Heijde, D., M. H. Schiff, J. Sieper, et al. Adalimumab Effectiveness for the Treatment of Ankylosing Spondylitis Is

Maintained for up to 2 Years: Long-Term Results from the ATLAS Trial. *Ann Rheum Dis* 68:922.

20. Braun, J., X. Baraliakos, J. Listing, et al. Persistent Clinical Efficacy and Safety of Anti-tumour Necrosis Factor Alpha Therapy with Infliximab in Patients with Ankylosing Spondylitis over 5 Years: Evidence for Different Types of Response. *Ann Rheum Dis* 67:340.

21. Braun, J., X. Baraliakos, J. Listing, and J. Sieper. Decreased Incidence of Anterior Uveitis in Patients with Ankylosing Spondylitis Treated with the Anti-tumor Necrosis Factor Agents Infliximab and Etanercept." *Arthritis Rheum* 52:2447.

22. van der Heijde, D., J. Sieper, W. P. Maksymowych, et al.2010 Update of the International ASAS Recommendations for the Use of Anti-TNF Agents in Patients with Axial Spondyloarthritis. *Ann Rheum Dis* 70:905.

23. Van der Heijde, D., R. Landewé, X. Baraliakos, et al. Radiographic Findings Following Two Years of Infliximab Therapy in Patients with Ankylosing Spondylitis. *Arthritis Rheum* 58:3063.

24. Baraliakos, X., H. Haibel H, J. Listing, et al. Continuous Long-Term Anti-TNF Therapy Does Not Lead to an Increase in the Rate of New Bone Formation over 8 Years in Patients with Ankylosing Spondylitis. *Ann Rheum Dis*4; 73:710.

25. van der Heijde, D., R. Landewé, S. Einstein, et al. Radiographic Progression of Ankylosing Spondylitis after up to Two Years of Treatment with Etanercept. *Arthritis Rheum* 58:1324.

26. Braun, J., G. Kingsley, D. van der Heijde D, and J. Sieper. On the Difficulties of Establishing a Consensus on the Definition of and Diagnostic Investigations for Reactive Arthritis: Results and Discussion of a Questionnaire Prepared for the 4th International Workshop on Reactive Arthritis, Berlin, Germany, July 3–6, 1999. *J Rheumatol* 27:2185.

27. Morris, D., and R. D. Inman. Reactive Arthritis: Developments and Challenges in Diagnosis and Treatment. *Curr Rheumatol Rep* 14:390.

28. Carter, J. D., and A. P. Hudson. Reactive Arthritis: Clinical Aspects and Medical Management. *Rheum Dis Clin North Am* 35:21.

29. Baeten, D, Sieper J., et al. Secukinamab, an Interleukin-17A Inhibitor, in Ankylosing Spondylitis. NEJM 2015. 373:26 p.2534-2547

Psoriatic Arthritis

The Rash, the Joint Pain, and the Jail Sentence

Ben, one of my favorite patients, came to me as a twelve-year-old Hispanic boy who could not walk because of knee, hip, and heel pain. I could not find any signs of joint swelling, but he was tender over tendon insertions and had a very high sedimentation rate (measure of inflammation). I thought he had enthesitis (inflammation of tendons and ligament insertions) but couldn't find any causes. He was very overweight and tall for his age and had a very easygoing demeanor, so it was easy to dismiss the severity of his problem. He responded partially to NSAIDs and could not tolerate methotrexate and Arava. However, two years later, when he started missing school, arriving in a wheelchair, and suddenly developed psoriasis from hell, covering his whole body, I became more aggressive and tried Humira with good success. He developed hematuria (blood in his urine), and I immediately stopped the drug. For the last two years, he's done great on Remicade. However, tragedy has struck. At age eighteen, he's in jail facing some serious charges, and I don't know what will become of him. I didn't see this coming.

Psoriatic arthritis occurs in 4–30 percent of psoriasis patients and rarely can precede the skin changes, which make it very confusing. I recently saw a patient who had been followed by a retired colleague of mine for years. The patient had a subtle inflammatory arthritis, which did not quite fit any diagnosis, and all lab tests and x-rays were normal. During her second visit with me, she showed me a rash on her elbows that was classic psoriasis. The diagnosis of psoriatic arthritis became a good possibility, although not definitive. Psoriatic arthritis can appear in many forms and have many associations, such as obesity and metabolic problems. The first form involves the distal joints of the hand called the *distal inter-phalangeal*, or dip, joints. They become swollen, painful, and red. Rheumatoid arthritis usually spares these joints, but osteoarthritis usually involves them, though there is much less inflammation. The second form is polyarticular (involving many joints) and looks identical to rheumatoid arthritis except patients usually but not always test negative for rheumatoid factor and anti-CCCP, and there can be some radiological differences such as new bone formation around the joints and sclerosis (darkening) of the bone around the joints rather than the osteopenia, or lightening, seen in rheumatoid and other inflammatory arthritides. This form of arthritis can be mistaken for a rare form of gout. The third form is called *oligoarticular* and involves a few large joints, such as the hips or knees. The fourth is called *arthritis mutilans* and is, as it sounds, "mutilating." Bone can be totally resorbed so that fingers can become floppy shortened bags of skin. X-rays are remarkable—with bones either partially or completely disappearing. It is a form of arthritis I dread to see because it is so destructive, aggressive, and disabling. The final form involves the spine and resembles other members of this family, such as ankylosing spondylitis or reactive arthritis, but just like reactive arthritis, it usually involves one sacroiliac joint. Unique associations with psoriatic arthritis include enthesitis or enthesopathy, which involves inflammation of insertions of tendons or ligaments, such as the Achilles tendon, and may be associated with extra bone formation or spurring. This finding can be seen in all member of the spondyloarthritis family. In pediatrics, it is considered a separate form or category of psoriatic arthritis. Dactylitis, or a sausage-like inflammation of a toe or finger, is another rare manifestation of psoriasis but can be seen in reactive arthritis or sarcoidosis. Iritis or inflammatory bowel disease are other associations. Treatment of psoriatic arthritis starts with NSAIDs when patients have just arthralgias or joint pain without physical or radiological findings. Otherwise, we use methotrexate, Arava, and occasionally Azulfidine or cyclosporine. Most physicians use exclusively methotrexate as a first-line drug because it treats the skin so well, but dermatologists tend to think that methotrexate causes more liver problems in psoriasis patients than it does in rheumatoid patients and are reluctant to use it. Some studies indicate it is not that effective in the arthritis, although I have seen some good results. I do use more Arava in these patients and sometimes add cyclosporine with good success. TNF antagonists are fast becoming the gold standard in psoriatic arthritis, but their expense and risks make them secondary choices except when the disease mainly involves the axial skeleton or the tendons—none of the other medications are effective. Although they all seem equally effective in joint disease, they have varying success in controlling the skin disease. Simponi seems to be the most effective, followed by Humira, Remicade, and then Enbrel.

There are some frustrating cases where patients have either failed or have a contraindication to TNF antagonists. Recently however, two new therapies have been approved for treatment of psoriasis and psoriatic arthritis. Stelara, or ustekinumab, is a biologic that inhibits two proteins, called *interleukin-17* (IL-17) and *IL-23*. The studies have shown impressive results. I have three patients doing well on it but find that the 90 mg. dose is much more effective than 45 mg. even in smaller patients. It has much of the same potential side-effect profile as other biologics.

One other biologic, secukinamab or Cosentryx, an IL-17 antaganonist has been approved for skin disease but studies seem to indicate it may be effective in both the skin and joint disease. I am just about to prescribe it for the first time.

Another recently FDA-approved oral medication, called *apremilast* (a phosphodiesterase 4 inhibitor), is showing great promise, although its effects on joint disease are not as impressive as that seen as a result of biologic treatment. Because it is not a biologic, it does not increase the risk of serious infections, such as TB, and unlike methotrexate or Arava, it does not affect the liver. So it may be ideal for orphan patients who can't find a drug to fit them. However, one of my patients on Apremilast became psychotically depressed (a known side effect) and two others developed severe diarrhea and discontinued the medication. Still, three others have had remarkable relief from both their severe skin and joint problems. Other physicians have reported great success with psoriatic enthesitis. Unfortunately, all these new medications are very expensive but with the right person doing your negotiations and good documentation, they are worth a try. Good luck!

Pearls

- Psoriatic arthritis occurs in 4–30 percent of psoriasis patients.
- The most reliable predictor of its occurrence in these patients is the presence of pitting in the finger- or toenails.
- Psoriatic arthritis may cause enthesitis, or inflammation of tendon or ligament insertions.
- Dactylitis, or a sausage-like digit, is a rare manifestation also seen in sarcoidosis or reactive arthritis.
- The arthritis may precede the rash in a minority of patients.
- Sacroiliitis is often unilateral.
- There are many forms of psoriatic arthritis.
- Unlike RA, psoriatic arthritis often involves distal interphalangeal joints DIPs) of the hands.
- X-rays may show new bone formation around the joints and sclerosis, rather than the osteopenia around the joints seen in RA.
- In one form of psoriatic arthritis (mutilans), bones can be completely resorbed.

- Psoriasis and psoriatic arthritis are often associated with metabolic problems, such as obesity.
- Some question the efficacy of methotrexate, but it is still used for skin and joint disease.
- Arava may be a better choice.
- TNF antagonists are effective in many for both the skin and joint disease but less so for skin in my experience.
- Stelara and Otezla (apremilast) are new and promising medications for the skin and joints.

Inflammatory Bowel Disease

Tightly Wound but Loosely Bound

Inflammatory bowel disease—that is, Crohn's disease or ulcerative colitis—is the last member of the family. Usually the arthritis appears during flares or active periods of the bowel disease. It is almost identical to ankylosing spondylitis, with inflammation of large joints, both sacroiliac joints, and the axial skeleton. Crohn's disease usually is associated with pauciarticular (few joints) arthritis, which is acute and correlates with flares, whereas ulcerative colitis causes polyarticular (more than or equal to five joints) arthritis, which is chronic and independent of flares. Alternatively, patients may just have arthralgias and may have iritis or even psoriasis. Usually treatment of the underlying bowel disease will take care of the symptoms. TNF antagonists, methotrexate, or steroids are all used in this disease. I try to keep a close relationship with their gastroenterologists since we have to coordinate care. I have seen many patients over the years that were diagnosed with ankylosing spondylitis and years later with inflammatory bowel disease. I order some specialized antibodies, ASCA (Crohn's) and ANCA (ulcerative colitis), and often a gastroenterology consultation in any patient with a seronegative spondyloarthritis who complains of chronic diarrhea or abdominal pain. Recently, GI experts seem to think that the antibodies are unreliable, and a stool test, called a *calprotectin test*, or a GI consult alone may be more effective.

Some of these patients may be very difficult to manage until their GI problems are resolved. I have a fifty-year-old male accountant with Crohn's disease who has maximized doses of Remicade and now Cimzia but continues to have severe back and hip pain and bloody diarrhea. He is a fun, great guy but is a tightly wound accountant who loves karate and other kamikaze sports and is constantly injuring himself. Sometimes it's hard to distinguish between his injuries and the disease process. He knows stress and anxiety exacerbate his diseases and has mellowed significantly, but he can't change his personality. The Crohn's and his arthritis go hand in hand: when one is quiescent, so is the other. His gastroenterologist and I have to find a way to control his Crohn's disease.

Pearls

- The arthritis simulates ankylosing spondylitis, including symmetrical sacroiliitis.
- It usually correlates with bowel disease activity in Crohn's disease.
- Patients who have had a colectomy can still have active arthritis.
- The arthritis and sacroiliitis may precede the bowel disease, so any seronegative spondyloarthritis patient with bowel symptoms should have a thorough GI workup.
- A fecal calprotectin test may be helpful in ruling out inflammatory bowel disease.
- Treat the underlying bowel disease, and you may use much the same meds used in ankylosing spondylitis.

References

1. www.rheumatology.org/Practice
(Patient Education—Diseases and Conditions)
2. Gladman, D. D. Current Concepts in Psoriatic Arthritis. *Curr Opin Rheumatol* 14:361.
3. Alamanos, Y., P. V. Voulgari, and A. A. Drosos. Incidence and Prevalence of Psoriatic Arthritis: A Systematic Review. *J Rheumatol* 35:1354.
4. Haddad, A., and V. Chandran. Arthritis Mutilans. *Curr Rheumatol Rep* 15:321.
5. Gisondi, P., I. Tinazzi, G. El-Dalati, et al. Lower Limb Enthesopathy in Patients with Psoriasis without Clinical Signs of Arthropathy: A Hospital-Based Case-Control Study. *Ann Rheum Dis* 67:26.

6. Chandran, V., C. T. Schentag, and D. D. Gladman. Sensitivity and Specificity of the CASPAR Criteria for Psoriatic Arthritis in a Family Medicine Clinic Setting. *J Rheumatol* 35:2069.

7. Ritchlin, C. T., A. Kavanaugh, D. D. Gladman, et al. Treatment Recommendations for Psoriatic Arthritis. *Ann Rheum Dis* 68:1387.

8. Bogliolo, L., C. Alpini, R. Caporali, et al. Antibodies to Cyclic Citrullinated Peptides in Psoriatic Arthritis. *J Rheumatol* 32:511.

9. Mease, P. J., A. J. Kivitz, F. X. Burch, et al. Continued Inhibition of Radiographic Progression in Patients with Psoriatic Arthritis Following 2 Years of Treatment with Etanercept. *J Rheumatol* 33:712.

10. Salvarani, C., F. Cantini, I. Olivieri, et al. Efficacy of Infliximab in Resistant Psoriatic Arthritis. *Arthritis Rheum* 49:541.

11. Genovese, M. C., P. J. Mease, G. T. Thomson, et al. Safety and Efficacy of Adalimumab in Treatment of Patients with Psoriatic Arthritis Who Had Failed Disease Modifying Antirheumatic Drug Therapy. *J Rheumatol* 34:1040.

12. Goulabchand, R., G. Mouterde, T. Barnetche, et al. Effect of Tumour Necrosis Factor Blockers on Radiographic Progression of Psoriatic Arthritis: A Systematic Review and Meta-analysis of Randomised Controlled Trials. *Ann Rheum Dis* 73:414.

13. Ritchlin, C., A. B. Gottlieb, I. B. McInnes, et al. Ustekinumab in Active Psoriatic Arthritis Including Patients Previously Treated with Anti-TNF Agents: Results of a Phase 3, Multicenter, Double-Blind, Placebo-Controlled Study. *Arthritis Rheum* 64:S1080.

14. Inman, R. D. Arthritis and Enteritis—An Interface of Protean Manifestations. *J Rheumatol* 14:406.

15. Weiner, S. R., J. Clarke, N. Taggart, and P. D. Utsinger. Rheumatic Manifestations of Inflammatory Bowel Disease. *Semin Arthritis Rheum* 20:353.

16. Smale, S., R. S. Natt, T. R. Orchard, et al. Inflammatory Bowel Disease and Spondylarthropathy. *Arthritis Rheum* 44:2728.

17. Generini, S., R. Giacomelli, R. Fedi, et al. Infliximab in Spondyloarthropathy Associated with Crohn's Disease: An Open Study on the Efficacy of Inducing and Maintaining Remission of Musculoskeletal and Gut Manifestations. *Ann Rheum Dis* 63:1664.

18. Marzo-Ortega, H., D. McGonagle, P. O'Connor, and P. Emery. Efficacy of Etanercept for Treatment of Crohn's Related Spondyloarthritis but Not Colitis. *Ann Rheum Dis* 62:74.

19. Langley RG, Elewki BE, Lebwohl . et al ecukinumab in Plaque Psoriasis-results of two phase 3 trials. N. Eng. J. Med. 2014; 371:326

Chapter Fourteen

Polymyositis, Dermatomyositis, and Other Muscle Diseases

So Weak, So Young, So Scared

Two of my most frightening but satisfying cases in the last several years have had one of these diseases. The first was a thirty-five-year-old woman literally led into the office by her parents, holding each of her arms. She hadn't eaten in weeks and was emaciated. She had trouble swallowing, maintaining a sitting position, rising from a seat, washing or combing her hair, dressing herself, and walking independently. She had seen several doctors who thought she might have cancer or a neurological problem. Finally, a bright neurologist checked her CPK (creatine phosphokinase) and found it to be 7,600 (normal in most labs is below 170). Elevated CPK reflects either muscle breakdown or inflammation. The neurologist performed an EMG (electromyogram) of her quadriceps, which indicated severe muscle abnormalities. He then very astutely suspected that this patient had polymyositis, which is another autoimmune systemic inflammatory disease that predominantly affects the proximal muscles, especially the shoulders and hips. This patient's esophagus could not contract well because the muscles in its upper part were inflamed. Therefore, she had trouble swallowing liquids and solids and was at risk of aspirating her food and developing pneumonia or even respiratory arrest. In fact someone so severely and universally affected was at risk of respiratory failure on the basis of inflamed and weakened respiratory muscles. These patients left untreated will need intubation and a respirator, and they have a high mortality rate. This patient also was suffering from malnutrition and dehydration and was totally dependent on her parents for her care. By the way, she was a single parent with two young kids. Her exam was fairly straightforward given all this background. Her voice was muted due to weakness of her laryngeal muscles. She had essentially no shoulder or hip muscles and was emaciated. Fortunately, her lungs were clear, and I didn't think she had aspirated or developed inflammation of her lungs, which can be a devastating independent association with this disease. Also her heart seemed strong and had a regular rhythm, which was important because the heart muscle and conductive system can be involved, leading to a higher mortality rate. In any case, it was clear this patient needed an immediate intervention, and she was hospitalized for two weeks, placed on a feeding tube going from her nose to her stomach, and given intravenous fluids and large doses of Solu-Medrol (methylprednisolone, a steroid similar to prednisone). Eventually she underwent a biopsy of one of her quadriceps muscles, confirming the diagnosis. As she gained strength, physical, occupational, and speech therapy played important roles in helping her regain her mobility, independence, and ability to speak and swallow. She was released from the hospital with a feeding tube in place and on 60 mg of prednisone. We soon started her on methotrexate and started to taper her prednisone. Within months, her feeding tube was removed; she was eating normally and back to work. Two years later, she is on methotrexate 30 mg and has a CPK of 133; she works full time and runs several miles daily. She is one of my heroines and one of the reasons why I love rheumatology!

Not every patient with polymyositis has such a severe disease. Most will start with subtle weakness (usually only in their hips and shoulders or proximal muscles), moderate to severe muscle aching or cramping, and mild elevations of their CPKs. Some patients eventually will not be able to rise from chairs without assistance and may have trouble combing their hair. As I described with my patient, they may have trouble swallowing, aspirate, and lose the use of their intercostal muscles, which help expand the chest and enable breathing. Again, it is a systemic disease, so patients don't feel well. There is also a long differential diagnosis of muscle weakness and a slightly shorter list of weakness and elevated CPK. I always make sure I rule out hypothyroidism, which is one of the few metabolic problems that cause weakness with an elevated CPK, and check their medication lists, especially for cholesterol-lowering drugs, which are notorious for causing weakness and elevated CPKs. In fact, when we find elevated CPKs in any patient, we review the medication list. Other causes of weakness and elevated CPKs include muscular dystrophies and muscle injuries. Many of these diagnoses can be sorted out by exam and history, but often they require EMGs, biopsies, and sometimes MRIs of the affected muscles. Having a bright and reliable neurology consultant is invaluable.

Dermatomyositis is similar to polymyositis but differs in specific ways. Several years ago, I had a twenty-seven-year-old man referred to me who could not walk down the hallway of my office rolling his oxygen tank without becoming extremely short of breath. He was extremely weak, especially at his hips and shoulders. He had cracked and rough hands despite being a drug representative with no history of manual labor, had purplish nodules with surrounding hyperpigmentation on his knuckles, and had a reddish rash on his face and chest—all classic findings in dermatomyositis. The roughening of his hands has been called *mechanic's hands*, and the nodules and hyperpigmentation, *Gottron's nodules* and *patches*. The lung changes are similar to those we have described in many diseases— inflammation leading to severe scarring, poor oxygenation, and sometimes death. The course is usually slow and long but can be sudden and explosive. Dermatomyositis and polymyositis are not always associated with lung disease, but those patients who do have it often have specific antibodies (called *antisynthetase*). This patient seemed to be failing fast and had a poor prognosis. I feared the worst and aggressively treated him with prednisone and Cytoxan. Today, he coaches his kids' soccer team, runs, lifts weights, and is on a low dose of methotrexate. He is another reason my job is fun.

Treatment for both polymyositis and dermatomyositis starts with steroids and often simultaneously or eventually with methotrexate. Steroids may be given initially intravenously and then orally in high doses and then slowly tapered. Some people use Imuran, but I am not a fan of this drug. If the patients fail this regimen, intravenous immunoglobulins (IVIG) given for five days every month or Rituxan can be effective. Occasionally we use Cytoxan for lung disease, and cyclosporine and tacrolimus (two drugs that work similarly to suppress the immune system) have also been successful treating the muscle disease.

There are a variety of other forms of muscle disease that we see, including vacuolar or inclusion body myositis, named after its pathological findings on biopsy. It may be caused by several medications or be idiopathic, like most of these diseases—meaning the doctors are idiots because they don't know the cause and it's pathologic. Unlike polymyositis, which usually involves only proximal muscles, it can involve both proximal (hips and shoulders) and distal muscles. Patients may also have some sensory findings, like numbness, not found in polymyositis, which is a pure muscle disease. The treatment is similar, but patients tend to be resistant to most medications.

Probably the most common cause of muscle disease I see lately is cholesterol-lowering drugs. They can cause muscles breakdown and aches, cramps, and weakness. It may take several months to resolve after stopping the drugs, and CPKs may stay elevated for many months. Most patients on these drugs do not develop muscle disease, and monitoring CPKs is helpful but not foolproof. Many of the people who develop problems on these drugs have a metabolic myopathy, meaning that they have a genetic enzyme deficiency that prevents their muscles from fully metabolizing oxygen. This deficiency does not cause a noticeable problem unless the muscle is stressed by another outside factor, such as a drug or illness. Unfortunately, there are very few labs that can test for these enzyme deficiencies.

Occasionally, statin drugs can cause rhabdomyolysis with severe muscle breakdown and muscle fiber death leading to profound weakness and kidney failure. The CPKs are often astronomically high (over one hundred thousand I.U./L) and patients are often hospitalized. Withdrawal of the statin drug, hydration and supportive therapy is usually effective but dialysis is somethimes necessary.

Recently, I saw a patient with profound weakness that potentially could have had three different causes. Rosalie was sitting in a wheelchair when I entered the room and raised her arm to belly-button level as a greeting. She was fifty years old, diabetic, had short black hair, a perky smile and exuded energy despite her obvious disability. She had lost the ability to raise her arms and brush her hair six weeks before the visit and could no longer rise from a stting postion. She had stopped taking her statin (cholesterol lowering) drug two months previously and was being treated for severe hypothyroidism. Two weeks before our visit her CPK was thirteen thousand eight hundred and she was still severely hypothyroid. By the time I saw her her primary care doctor had started her on forty mg. of prednisone and normalized her thyroid. She was minimally better but her CPK has dropped to seventy-eight hundred I.U./L. I thought the most likely diagnosis was stain induced myopathy but there was a remote possibility of hypothyroid myopathy or even polymyositis. I stoopped her steroids and ordered a variety of antibodies including one that Johns Hopkins and RDL laboratory had been investigating for the diagnosis of statin induced myopathy called HMGcoase. To prepare for a muscle biopsy, I ordered an MRI of her quadriceps muscles. It revealed extreme edema and a subsequent biopsy showed muscle fiber death or necrosis without inflammation making polymyositis unlikely. There was a catch, however! She had been on prednisone prior to the biopsy and inflammation may have been treated. Even more worrisome, two weeks later off steroids her CPK was ninety-eight hundred I.U. /L. I always thought that withdrawal of the statin drug was all that was needed to treat statin myopathy so why did she get worse? To my surprise and fascination, the HMGcoase antibody returned at a high level. It turns out that Johns Hopkins have been investigating a group of similar patients and found that statin drugs can cause a severe immune-mediated muscle disease that requires significant immune suppression for recovery. Steroids are helpful but IVIG or rituxan seem most effective. So, while waiting for her insurance's response to my request for IVIG, I started the patient on sixty mg. of prednisone and 30 mg. of methotrexate. To both the patient and my delight, her CPK fell to 1600 I.U./L and the patient is now able to rise unaided from a chair, walk short distances and brush her hair. The insurance is still thinking about our request after initial refusal and several appeals. I am learning something new every day and am hopeful that this lady will have a full recovery. Sometimes, in rheumatology, diagnosis and treatment are based on preliminary studies and successes in a few similar cases.

Pearls

- It is characterized by proximal muscle weakness, cramps, and aches (without sensory changes).
- CPKs are usually high but may be normal.
- Rule out other causes, especially hypothyroidism. There should always be a TSH in the chart.
- Diagnosis is made definitively by biopsy but an EMG, myositis-specific antibodies, and an MRI of muscles may be helpful.
- A patient may present with severe (interstitial) lung disease before diagnosis has been established.
- Skin findings, such as red facial and chest rash, purplish nodules and patches (Gottron's) on fingers, and rough, peeling palms (mechanic's hands) may be initial clues for dermatomyositis.
- Pulmonary-function tests, chest x-ray, and high-resolution CT should be performed at baseline and intermittently.
- Initial treatment is usually high-dose steroids and methotrexate. Patients should be weaned off steroids when stabilized and maintained on methotrexate or alternatively CellCept or Imuran.
- For resistant cases, cyclosporine, tacrolimus, IVIG, or Rituxan may be effective.
- Cytoxan may be used in severe lung disease.
- Inclusion body or vacuolar myositis may involve distal as well as proximal muscles and may have some sensory changes. It is a different species!
- Inclusion body myositis is resistant to most drugs, but they all are worth a try. Cyclosporine may be effective.
- Statin induced myositis may last for months or even longer

References

1. my.clevelandclinic.org/disorders/polymyositis/hic_polymyositis.
aspx

2. www.uptodate.com

3. www.rheumatology.org/Practice
(Patient Education—Diseases and Conditions)

4. Plotz, P. H., M. Dalakas, R. L. Leff, et al. Current Concepts in the Idiopathic Inflammatory Myopathies: Polymyositis, Dermatomyositis, and Related Disorders. *Ann Intern Med* 111:143.

5. Bohan, A., and J. B. Peter. Polymyositis and Dermatomyositis (First of Two Parts). *N Engl J Med* 292:344.

6. Bohan, A., and J. B. Peter. Polymyositis and Dermatomyositis (Second of Two Parts). *N Engl J Med* 292:403.

7. Griggs, R. C., V. Askanas, S. DiMauro, et al. Inclusion Body Myositis and Myopathies. *Ann Neurol* 38:705.

8. Hengstman, G. J., H. J. ter Laak, W. T. Vree Egberts, et al. Anti-signal Recognition Particle Autoantibodies: Marker of a Necrotising Myopathy. *Ann Rheum Dis* 65:1635.

10. Wortmann, R. L. The Dilemma of Treating Patients with Inclusion Body Myositis. *J Rheumatol* 19:1327.

11. Soueidan, S. A., and M. C. Dalakas. Treatment of Inclusion-Body Myositis with High-Dose Intravenous Immunoglobulin. *Neurology* 43:876.

12. Oddis, C. V., A. M. Reed, R. Aggarwal, et al. Rituximab in the Treatment of Refractory Adult and Juvenile Dermatomyositis and Adult Polymyositis: A Randomized, Placebo-Phase Trial. *Arthritis Rheum* 65:314.

13. Rios Fernández, R., J. L. Callejas Rubio, D. Sánchez Cano, et al. Rituximab in the Treatment of Dermatomyositis and Other Inflammatory Myopathies: A Report of 4 Cases and Review of the Literature. *Clin Exp Rheumatol* 27:1009.

14. Qushmaq, K. A., A. Chalmers, and J. M. Esdaile. Cyclosporin A in the Treatment of Refractory Adult Polymyositis/Dermatomyositis: Population Based Experience in 6 Patients and Literature Review. *J Rheumatol* 27:2855.

15. Wilkes, MR., S. M. Sereika, N. Fertig, et al. Treatment of Antisynthetase-Associated Interstitial Lung Disease with Tacrolimus. *Arthritis Rheum* 52:2439.

16. Pisoni, C. N., M. J. Cuadrado, M. A. Khamashta, et al. Mycophenolate Mofetil Treatment in Resistant Myositis. *Rheumatology* (Oxford) 46:516.

17. Yamasaki, Y., H. Yamada, M. Yamasaki, et al. Intravenous Cyclophosphamide Therapy for Progressive Interstitial Pneumonia in Patients with Polymyositis/Dermatomyositis. *Rheumatology* (Oxford) 46:124.

18. Anandacoomarasamy, A., G. Howe, and N. Manolios. Advanced Refractory Polymyositis Responding to Infliximab. *Rheumatology* (Oxford) 44:562.

19. Newman, E. D., and D. W. Scott. The Use of Low-dose Oral Methotrexate in the Treatment of Polymyositis and Dermatomyositis. *J Clin Rheumatol* 1:99.

20. Metzger, A. L., A. Bohan, L. S. Goldberg, et al. Polymyositis and Dermatomyositis: Combined Methotrexate and Corticosteroid Therapy. *Ann Intern Med* 81:182.

Chapter Fifteen

Sjögren's Syndrome

Dry as a Bone

When I first started seeing Jeanie, a forty-five-year-old realtor, she would always sit with a large water bottle in her hand, taking sips of water through a straw, and talk in a raspy voice. Her eyes were often bloodshot, and she often complained of fatigue and achy joints. In her frank and earthy way, she would graphically describe how her dry vagina was ruining her sex life. Recently, she seems a little perkier, is sipping less, and generally has fewer complaints, although she just lost three or four teeth to gum disease. I have been treating her with Evoxac to stimulate her salivary and lacrimal (tear duct) glands, but she still needs special eye drops three or four times a day and over-the-counter Biotene oral products. She rarely speaks of her sexual problems anymore, and Plaquenil has alleviated much of her fatigue and joint pain.

Sjögren's syndrome has been in the news in 2012 because Venus Williams, the famous and talented tennis star, has been diagnosed with it, and it has definitely affected her playing career. Usually, we consider it a companion disease. In other words, it is secondary to another of our diseases, such as rheumatoid arthritis or lupus, but it can be primary or stand alone. Like all these diseases, it is a systemic inflammatory disease that can cause inflammation of any organ, and patients do not feel well. The classic and most common complaints associated with the syndrome are dry eyes and mouth. Patients often carry around water bottles and are constantly drinking during our visit. They may not be aware they have dry eyes but will complain of itchy or gritty eyes and remember that an eye doctor told them they had dry eyes. Paradoxically some may say they have excessive tearing. Other patients will admit that they have an excess of dental caries or severe gum disease and may be losing teeth. Saliva contains antibodies that fight infections, and when it is diminished, people are predisposed to caries and gum disease. Tears have similar effects on the eyes, and a lack of them predisposes patients to eye infection and irritation. In fact, Sjögren's patients have inflammation of many of their glands besides their salivary and lacrimal. They often will complain of inability to sweat and dry vaginas. Their glands, especially their parotids in their neck, can be swollen. The most common complaint outside of glandular problems is intense fatigue, which certainly could affect daily living, never mind a very demanding high-level tennis career. We have at least two medications that can stimulate salivary and lacrimal (tear) glands in some patients—Evoxac (cevimeline) and Salagen (pilocarpine). They are more effective in stimulating saliva and may cause excessive sweating, drooling, dizziness, or nausea. In severe cases they have major impact on quality of life. We also encourage patients to use Biotene oral products and eyedrops and lubricants, especially without preservatives. Ophthalmologists will prescribe anti-inflammatory eyedrops, which contain steroids or cyclosporine (Restasis). They also will occasionally perform surgical procedures, such as punctal occlusion, which consists of plugging the holes that drain the tears, so there is an overflow. In some resistant cases, they can prescribe sclera prostheses. The fatigue sometimes can be treated with medications, such as plaquenil and occasionally low-dose prednisone.

Generally, we think of Sjögren's as a minor nuisance, causing dry eyes and mouth, and fatigue, but it can be associated with an inflammatory arthritis and rarely can affect the lungs, skin, gastrointestinal tract, liver, and nervous system in dramatic fashion. Two or three years ago, I had a new patient referred to me by a smart internist who'd made the diagnosis of Sjögren's syndrome on a patient who had severe orthostatic hypotension. That meant that each time this man sat or stood up his blood pressure dropped so low he would pass out. He had an extensive workup, and the only abnormality anyone could find were two antibodies called *anti-Rho* and *anti-La*, which are associated with about 50–60 percent of Sjögren's patients. The patient's internist then asked him if he had dry eyes and mouth, and sure enough he did! Sjögren's can affect the autonomic nervous system, which supplies the nerve stimulation to our blood vessels. When this system is affected, our arteries and intestines lose their ability to contract, so blood pressures fall, and food is not moved along. This patient had both these problems. He arrived to my office on a stretcher because he couldn't sit up without passing out and gave a history of severe constipation and difficulty swallowing. With his other history and findings, I suspected autonomic neuropathy because of his Sjögren's and treated him with high-dose prednisone and low-dose fludrocortisone, which is a type of steroid that affects sodium and fluid metabolism (a mineralocorticoid). He gradually responded and was able to sit up and walk, but despite trying a variety of immunosuppressive drugs, I could not wean him off moderate doses of prednisone until I tried Rituxan. Now he is riding his motorcycle and is on minimal prednisone. He is another of my rheumatology heroes.

Sjögren's has a high incidence of lymphoma, and any persistently swollen lymph gland should be watched with suspicion. Also, unexplained neurological problems or severe inflammatory lung disease can sometimes be traced to Sjögren's, but all in all, those who describe it as a nuisance companion disease are usually right.

Pearls

- There are many more common causes of dry eyes and dry mouth.
- Anti-SSA and anti-SSB occur in 50–60 percent of patients but occur in other diseases as well. AntiSSA alone is a pretty good diagnostic indicator; anti-SSB is not.
- Diagnosis is based on clinical criteria, including an eye exam performed by an ophthalmologist with ocular surface staining with Lissamine green (for the conjunctiva) and fluorescein (for the cornea).
- The most definitive test is a lip biopsy, looking at salivary glands, but other helpful tests include anti-SSA and anti-SSB, parotid sialogram, and ultrasound of salivary gland.
- Most common symptom other than dryness is extreme fatigue.
- Arthritis and neurological, pulmonary, and skin manifestations are not unusual.
- It is in the differential diagnosis of interstitial lung disease and multiple sclerosis.
- It is often a companion disease but may stand alone.
- Eyedrops and gels applied around the clock are helpful.
- Plugging the tear ducts (punctal plugging) is sometimes helpful.
- Steroid eyedrops may be used transiently to reduce inflammation.
- Restasis drops (topical cyclosporine) may be helpful.
- Dry eyes left untreated may lead to infections and visual problems.
- Evoxac, or cevimeline (a personal favorite), is excellent for mouth dryness and has some effect on the eyes. Salagen, or oral pilocarpine, is helpful for dry mouth.

- Sugar-free candies and gum are helpful for saliva production.
- Biotene products are useful.
- Saliva contains antibodies, and without it, gum disease and caries will lead to a loss of teeth.
- Take dry mouth seriously.
- There is an increased incidence of lymphoma in Sjögren's. Beware of a persistently enlarged gland!
- Vaginal dryness may be managed with topical estrogens and lubricants.
- Plaquenil may be helpful for fatigue and joint pain.
- Steroids are often used for lung and skin disease.
- Rituxan is promising for severe cases with extraglandular problems.

References

1. Fox, Robert I., and Carla Fox. *Sjögren's S Syndrome: Practical Guidelines for Diagnosis and Treatment.*

2. Wallace, Daniel J. *The Sjögren's Book.*

3. www.rheumatology.org/Practice (Patient Education—Diseases and Conditions)

4. Shiboki, S. C., et al. American College of Rheumatology Classification Criteria for Sjögren's Syndrome: A Date Driven Expert Consensus Approach in the Sjogren's International Collaborative Clinical Alliance Cohort. *Arthritis Care RES* (Hoboken) 64 (4 Apr.): 475–87.

5. Ramos-Casals, M., A. G. Tzioufas, and J. Font. 2005. Primary Sjögren's Syndrome: New Clinical and Therapeutic Concepts. *Ann Rheum Dis* 64:347.

6. Vitali, C. Classification Criteria for Sjögren's Syndrome. *Ann Rheum Dis* 62:94.

7. Niemelä, R. K., R. Takalo, E. Pääkkö, et al. Ultrasonography of Salivary Glands in Primary Sjogren's Syndrome: A Comparison with

Magnetic Resonance Imaging and Magnetic Resonance Sialography of Parotid Glands. *Rheumatology* (Oxford) 43:875.

8. Aung, W., I. Yamada, I. Umehara, et al. Sjögren's Syndrome: Comparison of Assessments with Quantitative Salivary Gland Scintigraphy and Contrast Sialography *J Nucl Med* 41:257.

9. Kassan, S. S., and H. M. Moutsopoulos. Clinical Manifestations and Early Diagnosis of Sjögren Syndrome. *Arch Intern Med* 164:1275.

10. Daniels, T. E., and J. P. Whitcher. Association of Patterns of Labial Salivary Gland Inflammation with Keratoconjunctivitis Sicca: Analysis of 618 Patients with Suspected Sjögren's Syndrome. *Arthritis Rheum* 37:869.

11. Malladi, A. S., K. E. Sack, S. C. Shiboski, et al. Primary Sjögren's Syndrome as a Systemic Disease: A Study of Participants Enrolled in an International Sjögren's Syndrome Registry. *Arthritis Care Res* (Hoboken) 64:911.

12. Provost, T. T., and R. Watson. Cutaneous Manifestations of Sjögren's Syndrome. *Rheum Dis Clin North Am* 18:609.

13. Alexander, E. L., F. C. Arnett, T. T. Provost, and M. B. Stevens. Sjögren's Syndrome: Association of Anti-Ro (SS-A) Antibodies with Vasculitis, Hematologic Abnormalities, and Serologic Hyperreactivity. *Ann Intern Med* 98:155.

14. Dalvi, V., E. B. Gonzalez, and L. Lovett. Lymphocytic Interstitial Pneumonitis (LIP) in Sjögren's Syndrome: A Case Report and a Review of the Literature. *Clin Rheumatol* 26:1339.

15. Gyöngyösi, M., G. Pokorny, Z. Jambrik, et al. Cardiac Manifestations in Primary Sjögren's Syndrome. *Ann Rheum Dis* 55:450.

16. Skopouli, F. N., C. Barbatis, and H. M. Moutsopoulos. Liver Involvement in Primary Sjögren's Syndrome. *Br J Rheumatol* 33:745.

17. Delalande, S., J. de Seze, A. L. Fauchais, et al. Neurologic Manifestations in Primary Sjögren Syndrome: A Study of 82 Patients. *Medicine* (Baltimore) 83:280.

18. Dyck, P. J. The Clinical Heterogeneity of Immune Sensory and Autonomic Neuropathies with (or without) Sicca. *Brain* 128:2480.

19. Wu, A. J. Optimizing Dry Mouth Treatment for Individuals with Sjögren's Syndrome. *Rheum Dis Clin North Am* 34:1001.

20. Ramos-Casals, M., P. Brito-Zerón, A. Sisó-Almirall, et al. Topical and Systemic Medications for the Treatment of Primary Sjögren's Syndrome. *Nat Rev Rheumatol* 8:399.

21. Petrone, D., J. J. Condemi, R. Fife, et al. A Double-Blind, Randomized, Placebo-Controlled Study of Cevimeline in Sjögren's Syndrome Patients with Xerostomia and Keratoconjunctivitis Sicca. *Arthritis Rheum* 46:748.

22. Papas, A. S., Y. S. Sherrer YS, M. Charney, et al. Successful Treatment of Dry Mouth and Dry Eye Symptoms in Sjögren's Syndrome Patients with Oral Pilocarpine: A Randomized, Placebo-Controlled, Dose-Adjustment Study. *J Clin Rheumatol* 10:169.

23. Meijer, J. M., P. M. Meiners, A. Vissink, et al. Effectiveness of Rituximab Treatment in Primary Sjögren's Syndrome: A Randomized, Double-Blind, Placebo-Controlled Trial. *Arthritis Rheum* 62:960.

24. St. Clair et al. Rituximab Therapy for Primary Sjögren's: An Open Label Clinical Trial and Mechanistic Analysis. *Arthritis Rheum* 65 (4 Apr.): 1097–106.

Chapter Sixteen

Polymyalgia Rheumatica (PMR)

She's Ninety and Feels Like a Hundred but until Last Week Felt Like Sixty

Thinking of Sadie always makes me chuckle. She was one of my longtime patients and was ninety years old when she arrived for the first time in a wheelchair. She had always been active, bright, and young in spirit, but that day she complained of feeling old. When I reminded her that she was ninety, she responded that until recently she'd felt like she was sixty and had limitless energy. Now she was so stiff she could hardly move, her hips and shoulders ached, and she felt like she was a hundred. She had slight swelling of her hands and limited range of motion of her shoulders. I suspected she had PMR and became even more convinced by a very high ESR and CRP. I prescribed 5 mg of prednisone three times a day, and within seventy-two hours she was back to her vigorous "sixty-year-old" self, and the next time I saw her, she asked me to dance with her.

I consider patients with this disease among my easiest to diagnose and treat. First, they are elderly—usually between sixty and seventy but sometimes as young as fifty. Secondly, the majority have high sedimentation rates (ESRs) and/or high C-reactive proteins (CRPs), which are measures of systemic inflammation, although unfortunately there are a few exceptions. Finally, these patients respond almost miraculously and completely to 10–25 mg of prednisone. I tell them if they are not 80–100 percent better in seventy-two hours, stop the prednisone because we have the wrong diagnosis. Their symptoms are usually shoulder and hip stiffness and pain often accompanied by fatigue and lack of appetite and sometimes weight loss. The disease can be confused with rheumatoid arthritis or fibromyalgia because patients can have a variety of swollen joints or just diffuse aches and pains. As in most rheumatological diseases, it is caused by the immune system overproducing certain factors that stimulate inflammatory cells, making them multiply and circulate and attack the shoulder and hips and sometimes other joints. Unlike rheumatoid arthritis, it does not destroy the joints left untreated but can be quite debilitating. One of my eighty-year-old PMR patients had severely swollen and painful hands. The swelling was diffuse, massive, and nonpitting, preventing him from feeding, dressing, or cleaning himself. The patient was an ex-marine and was humiliated by his condition, which is a subset of PMR. Within seventy-two hours of starting 20 mg of prednisone, his problem was resolved. The response is so dramatic patients are very grateful and impressed, but the tricky part is the long-term treatment. Many primary care doctors correctly make the diagnosis but make two classic mistakes. They start the patients at an unnecessarily high dose of prednisone, which is not terrible, but they taper the patient off the steroids within weeks, and all the symptoms return. Although it's great for my business, it is disheartening for the patient and unnecessary. I usually start patients on 15 mg of prednisone for three months and then taper the prednisone by 1 mg every two weeks until they reach 10 mg and then taper 1 mg every three weeks. Sometimes at around 5 mg,

Polymyalgia Rheumatica (PMR)

it becomes tricky because patients begin to flare, so I raise them up 2–5 mg from the dose at which they started to flare and taper 1 mg or even 0.5 mg a month. I call it the "PMR tango." Most of my patients will eventually be weaned off prednisone, but a small minority remains on a small dose. When I first started treating PMR in the mideighties, most patients would eventually fracture hips and vertebrae because long-term prednisone causes osteoporosis, especially in elderly patients. These days, equipped with that knowledge and effective treatment for osteoporosis, it rarely happens. I order a bone-density exam after the diagnosis has been made and usually treat them with 1,200 mg of calcium, 800 IUs of vitamin D, and a bisphosphonate (an antiosteoporosis drug). One of the unique and more humorous situations I have encountered involves a ninety-five-year-old PMR patient who still competes in five and ten Ks and relay marathons. In one of his international races, there was a question of possible urine testing for steroids, and I had him bring his prescription with him, so he wouldn't be disqualified. I want his genes!

PMR is often a diagnosis of exclusion and 10–20 percent of patients eventually develop RA. Approximately 20 percent of PMR patients will develop giant cell or temporal arteritis (see below), which can be a medical emergency. I warn all my PMR patients that if they develop the headache from hell or sudden visual loss, they are to increase their prednisone to 60 mg and call me immediately. They have forty-eight to seventy-two hours before the blindness becomes permanent.

Sometimes, if a patient does not respond to low-dose prednisone and has typical PMR symptoms and a high ESR or CRP, consider giant cell arteritis, a malignancy, or infection. I recently followed one such patient for six months who became symptomatic any time I lowered his prednisone dose below 15 mg. He suddenly developed right-sided rib pain and was found to have metastatic lung cancer. He was a nonsmoker and had no cough or shortness of breath!

There are a few patients who insist that they are allergic to even small doses of Prednisone making treatment of diseases like Polymyalgia Rheumatica very frustrating. Initially, I thought these claims were bogus—how could anyone be allergic to Prednisone? There are no 'nevers' in medicine and trial and error proved me wrong in these cases so I have had to become creative. Based on a pearl given to me by Frank Quismiorio, one of my mentors, I treat these patients with Medrol or Methylprednisolone, a more potent steroid similar to Prednisone and have had surprising success. I'm not sure I can quote any studies to support this approach but it has worked for me in a handful of difficult cases. Again, rheumatologists often have to think out of the box.

Pearls

- Average age of onset is sixty-five to seventy. For patients below 50, look for another diagnosis.
- Shoulder and hip girdle stiffness and subjective weakness and malaise are the most common symptoms.
- Always check sed rate and CRP. They are usually but not always high. (Approximately 10 percent are negative.)
- If it is the correct diagnosis, patients will respond dramatically to 10–25 mg of prednisone (I choose 15 mg) in twenty-four to seventy-two hours.
- If response is not dramatic or needs higher doses, the diagnosis is incorrect.
- Remember ESRs and CRPs are nonspecific, and if the response or course is questionable, check for malignancy or infection.
- Elevated fibrinogen may be an indication of disease activity.
- Beware of giant cell arthritis!
- Treatment starts with 10–20 mg of prednisone for three months and then slowly taper over a year and a half.

- Sometimes when the taper reaches lower doses and the patient flares, you may have to increase prednisone back up 1–10 mg and taper more slowly (0.5 mg./monthly?).
- If patient is 'allergic to even a low dose of Prednisone—try Medrol.
- Treat for osteoporosis prophylactically with calcium, vitamin D, and a bisphosphonate since therapy will involve more than three months of steroids.
- Obtain a baseline DEXA.

References

1. www.rheumatology.org/Practice
(Patient Education—Diseases and Conditions)
2. Salvarani, C., F. Cantini, and G. G. Hunder. Polymyalgia Rheumatica and Giant-Cell Arteritis. *Lancet* 372:234.
4. Salvarani, C., N. Pipitone, A. Versari, and G. G. Hunder. Clinical Features of Polymyalgia Rheumatica and Giant Cell Arteritis. *Nat Rev Rheumatol* 8:509.
5. Myklebust, G., and J. T. Gran. A Prospective Study of 287 Patients with Polymyalgia Rheumatica and Temporal Arteritis: Clinical and Laboratory Manifestations at Onset of Disease and at the Time of Diagnosis. *Br J Rheumatol* 35:1161.
6. Salvarani, C., S. Gabriel, and G. G. Hunder. 1996. Distal Extremity Swelling with Pitting Edema in Polymyalgia Rheumatica: Report on Nineteen Cases. *Arthritis Rheum* 39:73.
7. Proven, A., S. E. Gabriel, W. M. O'Fallon, and G. G. Hunder. Polymyalgia Rheumatica with Low Erythrocyte Sedimentation Rate at Diagnosis. *J Rheumatol* 26:1333.
8. Dasgupta, B., M. A. Cimmino, H. M. Kremers, et al. 2012 Provisional Classification Criteria for Polymyalgia Rheumatica: A European League Against Rheumatism/American College of Rheumatology Collaborative Initiative. *Arthritis Rheum* 64:943.

9. Kimura, M., Y. Tokuda, H. Oshiawa, et al. Clinical Characteristics of Patients with Remitting Seronegative Symmetrical Synovitis with Pitting Edema Compared to Patients with Pure Polymyalgia Rheumatica. *J Rheumatol* 39:148.

10. Haga, H. J., G. E. Eide, J. Brun, et al. Cancer in Association with Polymyalgia Rheumatica and Temporal Arteritis. *J Rheumatol* 20:1335.

11. Espinosa, G., J. Font, F. J. Muñoz-Rodríguez, et al. Myelodysplastic and Myeloproliferative Syndromes Associated with Giant Cell Arteritis and Polymyalgia Rheumatica: A Coincidental Coexistence or a Causal Relationship? *Clin Rheumatol* 21:309.

12. Salvarani, C., F. Cantini, L. Boiardi, and G. G. Hunder. Polymyalgia Rheumatica and Giant-Cell Arteritis. *N Engl J Med* 347:261.

13. Weyand, C. M., J. W. Fulbright, J. M. Evans, et al. Corticosteroid Requirements in Polymyalgia Rheumatica. *Arch Intern Med* 159:577.

14. Hernández-Rodríguez, J., M. C. Cid, A. López-Soto, et al. Treatment of Polymyalgia Rheumatica: A Systematic Review. *Arch Intern Med* 169:1839.

15. Feinberg, H. L., J. D. Sherman, C. G. Schrepferman, et al. The Use of Methotrexate in Polymyalgia Rheumatica. *J Rheumatol* 23:1550.

16. Ferraccioli, G., F. Salaffi, S. De Vita, et al. Methotrexate in Polymyalgia Rheumatica: Preliminary Results of an Open, Randomized Study. *J Rheumatol* 23:624.

Chapter Seventeen

Systemic Vasculitis

Giant Cell, or Temporal, Arteritis (GCA)

Headaches and Sudden Blindness

Giuseppe was a nice but very frightened Italian seventy-five-year-old who just died two months ago. He had kidney failure before I ever saw him, and I am not sure it was related to his vasculitis or his death. Six months ago, he lost 80 percent of his vision in his right eye and was found to have anterior ischemic optic neuropathy, which means his optic nerve was not getting enough blood. Giant cell arteritis is one of the most common causes of this condition, and his ophthalmologist astutely started this patient on 80 mg of prednisone before referring him to me. The patient's vision improved dramatically, but in two days he became irritable and weak, and his primary care doctor reduced his prednisone to 40 mg. Within three days the patient had permanently lost 80 percent of the vision in his right eye. Yet after I raised his prednisone dose to 60 mg on a Thursday, the patient called me on a Saturday asking for a dose reduction but relented when I reminded him of the consequences of the last reduction. A temporal artery biopsy obtained that Monday after two weeks of steroids was positive. I tried to balance the patient's discomfort against the risks of tapering the prednisone too quickly and compromised as best as I could. Subsequently, Giuseppe was very diligent about his medication but was very anxious and needed constant reassurance. Unfortunately, by the last time I saw him, he was on dialysis and was weak and anemic. I never learned his cause of death but remember him as a sweet, frightened man with a bad but treatable disease.

The biggest concern we have in patients with PMR is the rare complication of giant cell, or temporal, arteritis (GCA). This condition can lead to sudden blindness in one or two eyes, stroke, or severe pain in the arms or legs and is often preceded by the headache from hell, especially in the temple area. It also can cause unexplained fevers and severe jaw pain. If the sudden blindness is treated with high-dose prednisone (60–80 mg) and low-dose aspirin in the first twenty-four to forty-eight hours, it can be reversed. I have had at least one thoughtful patient who had PMR and developed blindness in one eye on a Friday and didn't want to bother anyone over the weekend, so she waited until Monday to call, and by that time her blindness was irreversible. It is considered one of the few rheumatology emergencies. Not everyone who has giant cell arteritis (GCA) has PMR; just as not everyone who has PMR has GCA. Nevertheless, I tell patients with PMR if they have sudden blindness, increase their prednisone to 60 mg daily and call me immediately. Also consider severe headaches emergencies because they are often a warning sign. Just what exactly is happening in GCA? As usual the immune system is overproducing inflammatory cells. They in turn cause inflammation in the aorta (the big artery coming out of the heart) and many of its branches, one of which eventually feeds the one providing blood to the eye.

Systemic Vasculitis

GCA is a member of a group of diseases called *vasculitides* or a condition called *vasculitis*. They all can be devastating, even fatal. Not everyone with GCA starts off with blindness, headaches, PMR, or jaw pain. Since it can affect any of the branches of the arch of the aorta, it may present with a variety of bizarre symptoms, and although it often causes extremely high CRPs and ESRs, occasionally they may be normal as well. Patients may complain of severe limb pain or vertigo or develop sudden hypertension or abdominal pain because of diminished blood supply. One of my favorite patients was an elderly lady who I saw in the hospital late one night. She had a few-week history of extreme vertigo and had had intermittent muscle aches with a vague history of at least one elevated ESR, but recently all her labs had been normal. Her astute primary care doctor (PMD) had placed her on prednisone at some point for the presumptive diagnosis of PMR, so he was concerned that the vertigo was an unusual manifestation of giant cell arteritis, and the prednisone was keeping the ESR and CRP artificially low. I examined the patient thoroughly and felt her temporal artery pulses, which were bounding and nontender, and concluded that it was unlikely she had GCA. The patient had the same silly sense of humor as I did, and we laughed and giggled into the wee hours of the night. By the time I was ready to leave, I had doubts about my original conclusion and decided to err on the cautious side and obtain a biopsy of one of her temporal arteries, and lo and behold, it was positive! Temporal artery biopsies are very specific in that if they are positive, you can be certain of the diagnosis, but they are not very sensitive since a large number can be negative in active disease. Some people recommend biopsying both sides to maximize the yield; I rarely find it is worthwhile, but that is a personal opinion.

Treatment always starts with high-dose steroids and then a slow taper over one and a half years. Unfortunately, no other medication has been found to be effective, although there are some case reports and early studies that may support the use of Actemra (tocilizumab). I usually start with 60 mg of prednisone and a baby aspirin daily. Some physicians advocate 80 mg to start, but I find that most patients have trouble tolerating 60 mg, never mind 80 mg. Occasionally, if convenient on the first visit, many physicians load the patients with 250–1,000 mg intravenously of Solu-Medrol, which is a slightly more potent steroid than prednisone and tends to improve prognosis. There are different regimens of tapering. I find it depends on the patient's tolerance of prednisone, their underlying diseases (such as diabetes or glaucoma, which prednisone will make worse), and the disease response. Many physicians after the first two weeks will taper by 10 mg every two weeks until they reach 40 mg and then 5 mg every two weeks until they reach 30 mg and then 2.5 mg every two weeks until they reach 20 mg and then 1 mg every two weeks. I prefer waiting three months before initiating the first taper. I start by reducing the patient to 50 mg and then by 5 mg a week until the patient reaches 30 mg. Then I taper by 2 mg a week until they reach 20 mg and then taper 1 mg every week. At 15 mg the reduction is 1 mg every two weeks, and by 10 mg, it's every three to four weeks. A rise in the ESR or CRP, a relapse, or complications from coexisting diseases, such as diabetes or glaucoma, are guides to adjusting doses up or down. I find the most common complaints with high-dose steroids are irritability, insomnia, and weakness. I've had spouses call me and insist I take the patient off steroids because he or she has become unbearable. As mentioned previously we worry about osteoporosis in any patient that is going to be on steroids for any prolonged period. Easy bruising and poor wound healing become a major problem with the passage of time. All these side effects become daunting until you weigh them against the risk of blindness, stroke, or loss of a limb. I have had several patients who have required several stents and arterial bypasses in their arms or legs to preserve a limb. Despite all these grave possibilities, patients tend to do well if treated promptly and adequately. Patience is a virtue with this disease because if the prednisone taper is too quick, the disease may return with a vengeance.

Recently, I have treated two patients who were either steroid resistant or intolerant with Actemra. One was a bad diabetic and Prednisone was wreaking havoc with her blood sugars. My two patients have done surprisingly well. Until recently, it was steroids or bust and some patients did!

Pearls

- The average age of onset is seventy. Below fifty, it's very unlikely.
- Patients feel sick and usually but not always have a very high sed rate and/or CRP.
- Although headaches, visual loss, and jaw pain (claudication) are the most recognized symptoms, vertigo, extremity pain (claudication), stroke, and fever are other complaints.
- The headache is extremely severe and persistent and often but not always temporal.
- Temporal pulses may be diminished, and the temple area may be tender.
- It is in the differential diagnosis of fever of unknown origin.
- It may affect any artery coming off the aorta but does not affect the cerebral arteries.
- If blindness is not treated by high-dose steroids in twenty-four to seventy-two hours, vision loss may be permanent.
- Although only 20 percent of polymyalgia rheumatica (PMR) patients will develop GCA, always warn them about the possibility, and instruct them to increase their prednisone to 60 mg and then call their doctor if they develop sudden blindness.

- GCA may develop years after polymyalgia has been in remission.
- Biopsy the tender temporal artery or the one with diminished pulse.
- There may be skip lesions, so a negative biopsy does not rule GCA out.
- Biopsy may be useful up until two weeks after initiation of steroids.
- If other arteries may be involved, consider aortic angiogram, MRA, or CT angiogram of the aorta.
- Treat initially with pulse doses of IV Solu-Medrol (125–500 mg) for three days and follow by 1 mg/kg of prednisone for three months and then slow taper over one and a half years.
- Add a daily baby aspirin.
- Remember prophylaxis for osteoporosis.
- Occasionally, patients who are intolerant of Prednisone tolerate Medrol at doses between 4-20 mg.

References

1. Myklebust, G., and J. T. Gran. A Prospective Study of 287 Patients with Polymyalgia Rheumatica and Temporal Arteritis: Clinical and Laboratory Manifestations at Onset of Disease and at the Time of Diagnosis. *Br J Rheumatol* 35:1161.

2. Achkar, A. A., J. T. Lie, G. G. Hunder, et al. How Does Previous Corticosteroid Treatment Affect the Biopsy Findings in Giant Cell (Temporal) Arteritis" *Ann Intern Med* 120:987.

3. Gabriel, S. E., W. M. O'Fallon, A. A. Achkar, et al. The Use of Clinical Characteristics to Predict the Results of Temporal Artery Biopsy among Patients with Suspected Giant Cell Arteritis. *J Rheumatol* 22:93.

4. Hunder, G. G., D. A. Bloch, B. A. Michel, et al. The American College of Rheumatology 1990 Criteria for the Classification of Giant Cell Arteritis. *Arthritis Rheum* 33:1122.

5. Calamia, K. T., and G. G. Hunder. Giant Cell Arteritis (Temporal Arteritis) Presenting as Fever of Undetermined Origin. *Arthritis Rheum* 24:1414.

6. Nuenninghoff, D. M., G. G. Hunder, T. J. Christianson, et al. 2003. Incidence and Predictors of Large-Artery Complication (Aortic Aneurysm, Aortic Dissection, and/or Large-Artery Stenosis) in Patients with Giant Cell Arteritis: A Population-Based Study over 50 Years. *Arthritis Rheum* 48:3522.

7. Salvarani, C., and G. G. Hunder. Giant Cell Arteritis with Low Erythrocyte Sedimentation Rate: Frequency of Occurrence in a Population-Based Study. *Arthritis Rheum* 45:140.

8. Weyand, C. M., J. W. Fulbright, G. G. Hunder et al. Treatment of Giant Cell Arteritis: Interleukin-6 as a Biologic Marker of Disease Activity. *Arthritis Rheum* 43:1041.

9. Hunder, G. G. Giant Cell Arteritis and Polymyalgia Rheumatica. In *Textbook of Rheumatology*, 5th edition, edited by W. N. Kelly, E. D. Harris, S. Ruddy, and C. B. Sledge, xx–xx. Philadelphia: WB Saunders.

10. Delecoeuillerie, G., P. Joly, A. Cohen de Lara, and J. B. Paolaggi. Polymyalgia Rheumatica and Temporal Arteritis: A Retrospective Analysis of Prognostic Features and Different Corticosteroid Regimens (11 Year Survey of 210 Patients). *Ann Rheum Dis* 47:733.

11. Kyle, V., and B. L. Hazleman. Treatment of Polymyalgia Rheumatica and Giant Cell Arteritis. II. Relation between Steroid Dose and Steroid Associated Side Effects. *Ann Rheum Dis* 48:662.

12. Hunder, G. G., S. G. Sheps, G. L. Allen, and J. W. Joyce. Daily and Alternate-Day Corticosteroid Regimens in Treatment of Giant Cell Arteritis: Comparison in a Prospective Study. *Ann Intern Med* 82:613.

13. Mazlumzadeh, M., G. G. Hunder, K. A. Easley, et al. Treatment of Giant Cell Arteritis Using Induction Therapy with High-Dose

Glucocorticoids: A Double-Blind, Placebo-Controlled, Randomized Prospective Clinical Trial. *Arthritis Rheum* 54:3310.

14. Mahr, A. D., J. A. Jover, R. F. Spiera, et al. Adjunctive Methotrexate for Treatment of Giant Cell Arteritis: An Individual Patient Data Meta-analysis. *Arthritis Rheum* 56:2789.

15. Unizony, S., L. Arias-Urdaneta, E. Miloslavsky, et al. Tocilizumab for the Treatment of Large-Vessel Vasculitis (Giant Cell Arteritis, Takayasu Arteritis) and Polymyalgia Rheumatica. *Arthritis Care Res* (Hoboken) 64:1720.

16. Salvarani, C., L. Magnani, M. Catanoso, et al. Tocilizumab: A Novel Therapy for Patients with Large-Vessel Vasculitis. *Rheumatology* (Oxford) 51:151.

Takayasu's Arteritis

The Young and the Pulseless

This disease is extremely rare—I think I have seen only two or three cases, but one stands out from the rest. Ryan was a spunky woman in her twenties who had two to three kids and had severe fatigue and severe joint, extremity, chest, and abdominal pain. The pains were debilitating and were associated with intermittent bowel blockages and shortness of breath. I tried high-dose prednisone for months with little effect, and she developed the chipmunk face and muscle atrophy associated with long-term high-dose steroid use. With her personality and great attitude, she looked like a cherub. We tried methotrexate, Imuran, and (I believe) cyclosporine (and maybe CellCept) with little success. We sent her to the Cleveland Clinic—the mecca for vasculitis—because her abdominal pain and GI symptoms were becoming unbearable, and she was becoming malnourished because she couldn't eat. There, she underwent a by-pass of her mesenteric arteries and seemed to be doing significantly better. I lost contact with her when I moved my practice to Oregon but remember her fondly because of her humor, great attitude, and bravery in a bad situation. She was another of my rheumatology heroes! If you're still out there, Ryan, I hope you're doing well.

Since we have been talking about giant cell arteritis, which is a vasculitis, I think it is only appropriate that we discuss the vasculitis that pathologically and clinically most resembles it—Takayasu's arteritis. Once again, the aorta and the big vessels coming off of it become inflamed and either narrowed or blocked. In contrast to GCA, the age of onset is between ten and forty years of age. Most of the symptoms can be logically deduced by what organ or part of the body those arteries supply. Mesenteric arteries supply the gastrointestinal tract, so patients will complain of abdominal pain after or independent of meals. It's like developing angina after exertion when your coronary arteries are blocked. If the arteries to your arms are narrowed, any activities using your arms will cause pain. If the arteries to your kidneys are blocked, you might develop severe hypertension. You get the idea. Since Takayasu's is a systemic disease where inflammatory factors are circulating in the blood, patients feel ill. They often have severe fatigue, fevers, and weight loss, and may have joint pain and even frank arthritis. In fact, this observation may be generalized to all systemic vasculitides. If the patients don't feel ill, it is not a systemic vasculitis! Also, vasculitis is serious business and can be fatal. The course can be horrendous, and until recently, many vasculitis patients have had short lifespans, and I'm not sure that has changed much in Takayasu's. Interestingly, unlike giant cell arteritis, this disease usually starts when patients are in their twenties. Also, it more often involves more blood vessels and has been called *pulseless disease* because patients have absent pulses in their extremities. The aorta and all the major blood vessels branching off of it may become occluded or dissect because of inflammation. The systemic complaints may precede the occlusive disease by several decades. In fact, the Japanese described some patients with abnormalities in their retinas that were similar to those found in diabetics. These findings can be a clue to early diagnosis.

Diagnosis is based on clinical findings but definitively on classic findings on angiography of the aortic arch or a magnetic resonance angiogram. Sedimentation rate and CRP are elevated and are one way to monitor disease activity.

The standard treatment is of course high-dose steroids, but patients often require bypass grafts of various arteries. If steroids fail, we try all the usual suspects, including methotrexate, Imuran, CellCept, and Arava. There have been some small successes with TNF antagonists.

Pearls

- Average age of onset is ten to twenty years old.
- Patients are fatigued and usually have joint pain.
- Symptoms relate to the occluded artery coming off the aorta.
- They are often truly pulseless, but also check for bruits.
- They have a high ESR and CRP.
- Diagnosis confirmed by angiogram, CT angiogram, or MRA visualizing the aorta and its branches.
- Steroids are the mainstay of treatment, but methotrexate, CellCept, and most recently Remicade are possible alternatives.
- Patients may require bypass surgery of a variety of arteries.

References

1. Arend, W. P., B. A. Michel, D. A. Bloch, et al. The American College of Rheumatology 1990 Criteria for the Classification of Takayasu Arteritis. *Arthritis Rheum* 33:1129.
2. Kerr, G. S. Takayasu's Arteritis. *Rheum Dis Clin North Am* 21:1041

3. Yamada, I., F. Numano, and S. Suzuki. Takayasu Arteritis: Evaluation with MR Imaging. *Radiology* 188:89.

4. Yamada, I., T. Nakagawa, Y. Himeno, et al. Takayasu Arteritis: Evaluation of the Thoracic Aorta with CT Angiography. *Radiology* 209:103.

5. Kissin, E. Y., and P. A. Merkel. Diagnostic Imaging in Takayasu Arteritis. *Curr Opin Rheumatol* 16:31.

6. Hoffman, G. S., R. Y. Leavitt, G. S. Kerr, et al. 1994. Treatment of Glucocorticoid-Resistant or Relapsing Takayasu Arteritis with Methotrexate. *Arthritis Rheum* 37:578.

7. Salvarani, C., Magnani L, Catanoso M, et al. Tocilizumab: A Novel Therapy for Patients with Large-Vessel Vasculitis. *Rheumatology* (Oxford) 2012; 51:151.

8. Salvarani, C., L. Magnani, M. G. Catanoso, et al. Rescue Treatment with Tocilizumab for Takayasu Arteritis Resistant to TNF-α Blockers *Clin Exp Rheumatol* 30:S90.

9. Valsakumar, A. K., U. C. Valappil, V. Jorapur, et al. 2003. "Role of Immunosuppressive Therapy on Clinical, Immunological, and Angiographic Outcome in Active Takayasu's Arteritis. *J Rheumatol* 30:1793.

10. Hoffman, G. S., P. A. Merkel, R. D. Brasington, et al. Anti-tumor Necrosis Factor Therapy in Patients with Difficult to Treat Takayasu Arteritis. *Arthritis Rheum* 50:2296.

Polyarteritis Nodosa (PAN)

A Limp Wrist, Some Red Dots, and a Lot of Laughs

Esther was one of my first patients in Oregon. She's hard to forget because of her wittiness and natural warmth. Fourteen years ago, at age sixty-four, she developed a wrist drop (could not raise it), fevers, weight loss, and new-onset hypertension and was extremely ill. She also had red dots, called *petechiae*, on her legs. I suspected PAN but wasn't sure until an angiogram of the arteries to her kidneys established the diagnosis. I initially treated with high doses of prednisone but eventually added Cytoxan. Over the next two years, she recovered almost completely except for tingling in her hands and feet because of a residual peripheral neuropathy. Today, she is almost eighty and retains her warm sense of humor. She is here for her biannual visit to monitor her blood work and health. I feel like I'm visiting an old friend or favorite aunt. She inquires about my cat, Bob, and wife, Leanne, and I tease her about her annual shopping trip to Medford with her friend Joan.

PAN is the classic vasculitis. When I was in training, it seemed to be in the differential diagnosis of every ICU patient with a catastrophic illness that involved multiple body organs. The very possibility of this diagnosis struck fear in most students and physicians because it was often hard to diagnosis and fatal. Certainly, the prognosis has changed with more knowledge over the years but not as much as it has in many other diseases. It is systemic, so again patients have fevers, fatigue, poor appetite, and muscle and joint aches. Remember—if it is systemic, patients don't feel well. Like the other vasculitides, patients' symptoms depend on what blood vessel is affected. It affects medium- and large-sized blood vessels and multiple organs. Patients may have purpura or bruise-like marks on their skin or in extreme cases gangrene of extremities. They may have a variety of other nonspecific skin lesions, like ulcers, blisters, and red spots. Neurological problems, such as wrist drop, foot drop, or numbness or tingling, especially on one side of the body, are common. Sudden onset of severe hypertension may reflect renal artery involvement. Mesenteric artery involvement in the GI tract can cause severe abdominal pain. Muscle pain and weakness with or without muscle enzyme abnormalities are common. Rarely it affects blood vessels in the lungs, liver, heart, ovaries, or testicles and may or may not lead to symptoms. Most important, it is a systemic illness and can be fatal.

Laboratory tests reflect inflammation with high ESRs and CRPs and often anemia. Definitive diagnosis is made by biopsying an affected organ or by angiogram. I have always felt squeamish about two of the biopsy sites recommended rarely in this disease—the sural nerve and the testicle. The former because it is painful, has a low yield, and may leave residual pain. The latter because it's the testicle!

Treatment as usual starts with high-dose steroids and often leads to Cytoxan, with Imuran as an alternative. Biologics, such as TNF antagonists, are being investigated.

Pearls

- It is a multiorgan disease with fatigue, fevers, rash, hypertension, and muscle and joint pain.
- Wrist drop and other isolated neuropathies can be found.
- ESR and CRP are elevated. RF and ANA and possibly ANCA may be present.
- It may be associated with hepatitis B.
- A biopsy or angiogram (CT or MRA) may be diagnostic.
- A biopsy of an affected organ, especially the liver or muscle if possible, is most productive.
- Sometimes a blind biopsy of the sural nerve or testis is helpful, but I generally avoid them.

- High doses of steroids followed by Cytoxan or Imuran are the standard of care.
- There may be some role for TNF antagonists.

References

1. Sato, O., and D. L. Cohn. "Polyarteritis and Microscopic Polyangiitis." In *Rheumatology*, edited by J. H. Klippel and P. A. Dieppe, xx–xx. St. Louis: Mosby.

2. Pagnoux, C., R. Seror, C. Henegar, et al. Clinical Features and Outcomes in 348 Patients with Polyarteritis Nodosa: A Systematic Retrospective Study of Patients Diagnosed between 1963 and 2005 and Entered into the French Vasculitis Study Group Database. *Arthritis Rheum* 62:616.

3. Guillevin, L., A. Mahr, P. Callard, et al. Hepatitis B Virus-Associated Polyarteritis Nodosa: Clinical Characteristics, Outcome, and Impact of Treatment in 115 Patients. *Medicine* (Baltimore) 84:313.

4. Tervaert, J. W., and C. Kallenberg. Neurologic Manifestations of Systemic Vasculitides. *Rheum Dis Clin North Am* 19:913.

5. Levine, S. M., D. B. Hellmann, and J. H. Stone. Gastrointestinal Involvement in Polyarteritis Nodosa (1986–2000): Presentation and Outcomes in 24 Patients. *Am J Med* 112:386.

6. Jennette, J. C., R. J. Falk 2012 Revised International Chapel Hill Consensus Conference Nomenclature of Vasculitides. *Arthritis Rheum* 65:1.

7. Guillevin L., F. Lhote, P. Cohen, et al. Corticosteroids plus Pulse Cyclophosphamide and Plasma Exchanges versus Corticosteroids plus Pulse Cyclophosphamide Alone in the Treatment of Polyarteritis Nodosa and Churg-Strauss Syndrome Patients with Factors Predicting Poor Prognosis: A Prospective, Randomized Trial in Sixty-Two Patients. *Arthritis Rheum* 38:1638.

8.Fauci, A. S., P. Katz, B. F. Haynes, and S. M. Wolff. Cyclophosphamide Therapy of Severe Systemic Necrotizing Vasculitis. *N Engl J Med* 301:235.

9.Ribi, C., P. Cohen, C. Pagnoux, et al. Treatment of Polyarteritis Nodosa and Microscopic Polyangiitis without Poor-Prognosis Factors: A Prospective Randomized Study of One Hundred Twenty-Four Patients. *Arthritis Rheum* 62:1186.

10.Al-Bishri, J., N. le Riche, and J. E. Pope. Refractory Polyarteritis Nodosa Successfully Treated with Infliximab. *J Rheumatol* 32:1371.

11.Guillevin, L., Cohen, A. Mahr, et al. Treatment of Polyarteritis Nodosa and Microscopic Polyangiitis with Poor Prognosis Factors: A Prospective Trial Comparing Glucocorticoids and Six or Twelve Cyclophosphamide Pulses in Sixty-Five Patients. *Arthritis Rheum* 49:93.

12.Guillevin, L., A. Mahr, P. Callard, et al. Hepatitis B Virus-Associated Polyarteritis Nodosa: Clinical Characteristics, Outcome, and Impact of Treatment in 115 Patients. *Medicine* (Baltimore) 84:313.

Granulomatosis with Polyangiitis (Wegener's Disease), Microscopic Polyangiitis, and Eosinophilic Granulomatosis with Polyangiitis (Churg-Strauss Syndrome)

Sinuses, Lungs, and Kidneys, Asthma, and Amusing Characters

Gerald is my longest-standing granulomatosis with polyangiitis (GPA) patient. Unfortunately, he is now wheelchair-bound because of multiple strokes and dementia, probably unrelated to his disease.

He was a very entertaining, outgoing, big guy with limited GPA before his strokes. He first came to me carrying the diagnosis of rheumatoid arthritis based on inflammation of his joints, a positive rheumatoid factor, and high ESRs. Since the diagnosis was credible, I placed him on methotrexate, and he did fairly well until he developed severe sinus and ear problems. A positive ANCA and sinus biopsy established the diagnosis of GPA. Rheumatoid factors and inflammatory arthritis may be found in a percentage of GPA patients and lead to incorrect diagnoses. Interestingly, methotrexate is effective in both rheumatoid arthritis and limited GPA, so I was inadvertently using the correct medication, but he eventually required prednisone and higher doses of methotrexate. When the diagnosis was first made at a university center, they treated him with Cytoxan for a few months. He developed bladder cancer probably as a result of Cytoxan a few years ago. He is mute and completely dependent on his poor wife for everything. I miss him and pity his wife. My other longstanding limited GPA patient has been relatively stable on methotrexate but has lost his sense of smell and taste and intermittently has drainage from his ears or nose when his disease is active.

GPA is a member of a group of vasculitides called *ANCA-associated diseases* because many patients test positive for these unique antibodies (antineutrophic cytoplasmic antibodies), which come in different forms or patterns depending on the disease. These patients typically have sinus, upper respiratory, lung, and/or kidney involvement. Neurological, eye, joint, ear, and skin involvement are relatively common depending on the disease and patient. Of course these patients are sick with systemic complaints. Granulomatosis with polyangiitis (GPA) and eosinophilic granulomatosis with polyangiitis (EGPA) patients usually will complain of sinus and nasal drainage, ear difficulties, and poor sense of taste and smell. They may develop inflammation of their nasal cartilage leading to its collapse and a "saddle nose" deformity. Inflammation of the eye can lead to pain, redness, visual changes, or weakness of the eye muscles. In the limited form of GPA, these may be the only symptoms, but in the generalized form, patients may have devastating involvement of their lungs and kidneys with severe shortness of breath, cough, and eventually—if untreated—respiratory and kidney failure. In the past, these diseases were often fatal, but prognosis has improved dramatically with prompt and proper treatment. EGPA patients usually have a history of asthma and have a surplus of eosinophils. Skin lesions, heart problems, neuropathies, and GI problems are more common in EPGA than in GPA or microscopic polyangiitis (MP). Kidney and lung manifestations are similar in GPA and MP, but the histopathology seen on biopsy is different. Again, all the clinical manifestations are caused by inflammation of small- and medium-sized blood vessels, and one can predict the symptoms by the organ involved.

Diagnosing these diseases may be based on clinical criteria, laboratory findings (especially ANCAs), and radiological findings in the lungs and sinuses, such as cavities, but the definitive diagnosis is often made by a lung, kidney, or sinus biopsy. I particularly think of these diagnoses when encountering a sick patient with severe lung, upper respiratory, kidney, and/or sinus disease.

Like most vasculitides, treatment starts with high-dose steroids. However, because many years ago it became obvious that these patients did not survive long on steroids alone, over the last several decades, Cytoxan by mouth or intravenously has been started early in the disease with good success. Still, although the disease was better controlled, patients were dying from complications of Cytoxan, such as lymphoma or bladder cancer. Therefore, patients were switched early in their course to methotrexate, Imuran, or recently CellCept with fair to good results. Still, a fair number of patients suffered complications from early treatment with Cytoxan. Therefore, some patients with mild or limited disease were treated initially with methotrexate or CellCept instead of Cytoxan also with good results. However, this regimen was thought inadequate in patients with severe disease, especially with kidney involvement. Cytoxan seemed to be the only option. The rheumatology community was in a bind until recently when the FDA approved Rituxan for treatment of ANCA-associated vasculitides. We finally have a drug that seems to work equally as well as Cytoxan without its long-term, devastating complications. Cytoxan is still probably the drug of choice to induce remission for extremely severe cases.

As in most rheumatology diseases, it is much easier to put out little fires than big ones, so I tell these patients I need to see them regularly (every six to twelve weeks) to monitor their disease activity and check for drug toxicity.

These diseases are fairly rare, so it surprises me that I have followed even six to seven patients during the last fourteen years and saw several tragic cases the previous decade. Each one seems to teach me something new about the disease, the patient, and the referring doctors. I remember consulting on an ICU patient who was in kidney and respiratory failure, comatose, with a history of sinus problems. His white cell count, ESR, and CRP were high, and I suspected GPA and ordered an ANCA, which was negative. I then ordered a kidney biopsy, which was consistent with but not diagnostic of GPA. The patient was failing high-dose steroids, so I ordered Cytoxan, but the ICU staff insisted that because of the ANCA negativity, the diagnosis was in question, and Cytoxan was too risky. The patient died shortly thereafter. The autopsy revealed mainly liquefied lungs and kidneys but a definitive diagnosis of GPA. ANCA is specific for GPA but is seen in about 82–94 percent, not 100 percent, of patients. We treat patients, not labs, and biopsies trump labs!

Systemic Vasculitis

One of my EPGA patients is a fiftyish-year-old woman with a long history of asthma, intermittent pneumonia, and sinus problems associated with joint pain and fatigue. She was treated with both prednisone and methotrexate but continued to have relapses, which required higher doses of steroids. Finally, about a year ago, I started her on Rituxan, and she hasn't had a relapse yet!

Pearls

- ANCA-related vasculitis may be very serious, even fatal.
- Wegener's granulomatosis is now granulomatosis with polyangiitis (GPA).
- It usually involves the upper respiratory tract, and sinus, nasal, and ear drainage are common.
- Eye involvement is also common.
- Look for the saddle nose.
- The limited form just involves the upper respiratory tract.
- Other forms may be fatal and aggressive and involve the kidneys and lungs.
- Check ANCA, ESR, and CRP.
- ANCA (CANCA or anti-PR3) is most commonly associated with GPA.
- ANCA is helpful with diagnosis but does not correlate with disease activity. Use CRP and ESR.
- Patients may have other antibodies, such as RF, and may have inflammatory arthritis and be mistaken for RA.
- Check chest and sinus x-rays.
- Wherever possible, if diagnosis is in doubt, obtain biopsy of involved lung or sinus. Kidney biopsy may be helpful but too nonspecific.
- Granulomas are diagnostic.

- Treat aggressively.
- Start with steroids and add methotrexate or CellCept for mild disease.
- Treat with Cytoxan or preferably Rituxan for severe disease with lung and renal involvement.
- Steroids alone are not adequate unless treating a minor flare.
- Eosinophilic granulomatosis with polyangiitis (Churg-Strauss disease) is associated with asthma and eosinophil elevation in the blood and tissues.
- Usually patients have lung infiltrates, upper respiratory disease, joint pain, and often cardiac involvement but may have neurological or GI findings.
- Fevers are common.
- In 55 percent of patients P-ANCA or MPO-ANCA antibodies are found.
- ANCA does not correlate with activity; ESR and CRP do.
- It has the same treatment regimen as in GPA.
- Microscopic polyangiitis (MPA) has kidney and lung involvement like GPA but different histology on biopsy.
- ANCA (P-ANCA or MPO) is present in 70 percent of patients.
- Biopsy when possible.
- Treatment is similar to other ANCA-related vasculitis.

References

1. Falk, R. J., W. L. Gross, L. Guillevin, et al. Granuloatosis with Polyangiitis (Wegener's): An Alternative Name for Wegener's Granulomatosis." *Arthritis Rheum* 63:863.
2. Watts, R., S. Lane, T. Hanslik, et al. Development and Validation of a Consensus Methodology for the Classification of the ANCA-Associated Vasculitides and Polyarteritis Nodosa for Epidemiological Studies. *Ann Rheum Dis* 66:222.

3. Harper, S. L., E. Letko, C. M. Samson, et al. Wegener's Granulomatosis: The Relationship between Ocular and Systemic Disease. *J Rheumatol* 28:1025.

4. Pagnoux, C., A. Mahr A, P. Cohen, and L. Guillevin. 2005. Presentation and Outcome of Gastrointestinal Involvement in Systemic Necrotizing Vasculitides: Analysis of 62 Patients with Polyarteritis Nodosa, Microscopic Polyangiitis, Wegener Granulomatosis, Churg-Strauss Syndrome, or Rheumatoid Arthritis-Associated Vasculitis. *Medicine* (Baltimore) 84:115.

5. Weidner, S., S. Hafezi-Rachti, and H. D. Rupprecht. Thromboembolic Events as a Complication of Antineutrophil Cytoplasmic Antibody-Associated Vasculitis. *Arthritis Rheum* 55:146.

6. Stone, J. H. Wegener's Granulomatosis Etanercept Trial Research Group: Limited versus Severe Wegener's Granulomatosis: Baseline Data on Patients in the Wegener's Granulomatosis Etanercept Trial. *Arthritis Rheum* 48:2299.

7. Guillevin, L., B. Durand-Gasselin, R. Cevallos, et al. Microscopic Polyangiitis: Clinical and Laboratory Findings in Eighty-Five Patients. *Arthritis Rheum* 42:421.

8. Hagen, E. C., M. R. Daha, J. Hermans, et al. Diagnostic Value of Standardized Assays For Anti-neutrophil Cytoplasmic Antibodies in Idiopathic Systemic Vasculitis. EC/BCR Project for ANCA Assay Standardization. *Kidney Int* 53:743.

9. Finkielman, J. D., A. S. Lee, A. M. Hummel, et al. ANCA are Detectable in Nearly All Patients with Active Severe Wegener's Granulomatosis. *Am J Med* 120:643.e9.

10. Pagnoux, C., P. Guilpain, and L. Guillevin. Churg-Strauss Syndrome. *Curr Opin Rheumatol* 192 5.

11. Guillevin, L., P. Cohen, M. Gayraud, et al. Churg-Strauss Syndrome. Clinical Study and Long-Term Follow-up of 96 Patients. *Medicine* (Baltimore) 78:26.

12. Masi, A. T., G. G. Hunder, J. T. Lie, et al. The American College of Rheumatology 1990 Criteria for the Classification of Churg-Strauss Syndrome (Allergic Granulomatosis and Angiitis). *Arthritis Rheum* 33:1094.

13. Abril, A., K. T. Calamia, and M. D. Cohen. The Churg Strauss Syndrome (Allergic Granulomatous Angiitis): Review and Update. *Semin Arthritis Rheum* 33:106.

14. Keogh, K. A., and U. Specks. Churg-Strauss Syndrome: Clinical Presentation, Antineutrophil Cytoplasmic Antibodies, and Leukotriene Receptor Antagonists. *Am J Med* 115:284.

15. Peikert, T., J. D. Finkielman, A. M. Hummel, et al. Functional Characterization of Antineutrophil Cytoplasmic Antibodies in Patients with Cocaine-Induced Midline Destructive Lesions. *Arthritis Rheum* 58:1546.

16. Bosch, X., A. Guilabert, G. Espinosa, and E. Mirapeix. Treatment of Antineutrophil Cytoplasmic Antibody Associated Vasculitis: A Systematic Review." *JAMA* 298:655.

17. Gayraud, M., L. Guillevin, P. le Toumelin, et al. Long-Term Follow-up of Polyarteritis Nodosa, Microscopic Polyangiitis, and Churg-Strauss Syndrome: Analysis of Four Prospective Trials Including 278 Patients. *Arthritis Rheum* 44:666.

18. De Groot, K., N. Rasmussen, P. A. Bacon, et al. Randomized Trial of Cyclophosphamide versus Methotrexate for Induction of Remission in Early Systemic Antineutrophil Cytoplasmic Antibody-Associated Vasculitis. *Arthritis Rheum* 52:2461.

19. Pagnoux, C., A. Mahr, M. A. Hamidou, et al. Azathioprine or Methotrexate Maintenance for ANCA-Associated Vasculitis. *N Engl J Med* 359:2790.

20. J ones, R. B., J. W. Tervaert, T. Hauser, et al. Rituximab versus Cyclophosphamide in ANCA-Associated Renal Vasculitis. *N Engl J Med* 363:211.

21. Stone, J. H., P. A. Merkel, R. Spiera, et al. Rituximab versus Cyclophosphamide for ANCA-Associated Vasculitis. *N Engl J Med* 363:221.

22. De Groot, K., L. Harper, D. R. Jayne, et al. Pulse versus Daily Oral Cyclophosphamide for Induction of Remission in Antineutrophil Cytoplasmic Antibody-Associated Vasculitis: A Randomized Trial. *Ann Intern Med* 150:670.

23. Harper, L., M. D. Morga, M. Walsh, et al. Pulse versus Daily Oral Cyclophosphamide for Induction of Remission in ANCA-Associated Vasculitis: Long-Term Follow-up. *Ann Rheum Dis* 71:955.

24. Langford, C. A., C. Talar-Williams, and M. C. Sneller. Use of Methotrexate and Glucocorticoids in the Treatment of Wegener's Granulomatosis. Long-Term Renal Outcome in Patients with Glomerulonephritis. *Arthritis Rheum* 43:1836.

25. Falk, R. J., and J. C. Jennette. Rituximab in ANCA-Associated Disease. *N Engl J Med* 363:285.

26. Specks, U. Methotrexate for Wegener's Granulomatosis: What Is the Evidence? *Arthritis Rheum* 52:2237.

27. De Groot, K., N. Rasmussen, P. A. Bacon, et al. Randomized Trial of Cyclophosphamide versus Methotrexate for Induction of Remission in Early Systemic Antineutrophil Cytoplasmic Antibody-Associated Vasculitis. *Arthritis Rheum* 52:2461.

Behcet's Disease

No, This Is Not Herpes

Risa first came to me in a panic about a year ago. She was a very pretty twenty-three-year-old who was just two weeks away from her wedding and honeymoon and had huge painful ulcers on the roof of her mouth and in her vagina. Her father was a doctor and suspected Behcet's, even though it was rare and she belonged to the wrong ethnic group. She had very few other symptoms, and I was skeptical. Years ago, I had been taught that Behcet's was a devastating vasculitis seen mainly in Middle Eastern people. Over the years, I have learned otherwise, so when I saw the angry-looking ulcers in her mouth and vagina and ruled out infections such as herpes, I was less skeptical. Besides, Risa was begging me to do something so that she could have a happy wedding and honeymoon. Predictably, the more stressed she became, the worse and more painful the ulcers became. I performed this weird procedure called a *pathergy test*, where I inserted a twenty-gauge needle into her forearm and the next day found a little papule, or bump, at the site of insertion. Strangely, this finding clinched the diagnosis, and I treated her with a tapering dose of prednisone and colchicine as well as topical steroids successfully. Her wedding and honeymoon were a smashing success. She occasionally needs colchicine for a few weeks but otherwise has been asymptomatic over the last year. I dread pregnancy or other stresses.

This vasculitis was one of the rare diseases our professors in medical school told us about and then said you'll never see it. Theoretically, it sounded horrifying. Patients of Middle Eastern origin, especially Turks, would develop painful ulcers in their mouth and genitals. They often also had rashes, iritis, meningitis, or a variety of devastating neurological problems, venous and arterial blood clots, and severe kidney disease. Treatment was with all the usual suspects, including prednisone, Cytoxan, Imuran, and Colchicine, CellCept, and cyclosporine were added and most recently Rituxan, methotrexate, and TNF antagonists. Most Behcet's patients we see these days have what one of my colleagues calls "designer Behcet's," where patients of a variety of nationalities develop just oral and genital ulcers and rashes and perhaps some joint pain. They do not seem to have the more life-threatening organ involvement, although they may have fevers, malaise, and elevated ESRs and CRPs. I do not mean to diminish the impact of their symptoms because the ulcers can be huge and extremely painful. I have several such patients, but one has to be aware of the differential diagnosis and be sure not to miss the obvious.

I recently saw a twenty-four-year-old Middle Eastern man who had a three-month history of oral and genital ulcers and was sent to me as a Behcet's. A careful history revealed that his girlfriend had the same problem, and his antibodies for recent herpes 2 were positive. During my training, I saw one of the severe, classic Behcet's patients and really never want to see one again. The designer versions are just fine.

Pearls

- Oral and genital ulcers, rash, and pathergy test make the diagnosis.
- Classically Middle Eastern, but "designer Behcet's," not so much.
- It's a vasculitis, so expect high ESR and CRP.
- Rule out herpes, lichen planus, and other causes of ulcers.
- "Designer Behcet's" is a kinder, gentler version of a historically terrible disease.
- Severe vasculitis may have kidney disease, meningitis, arterial thrombosis (clots), and arthritis.

- Oral and genital ulcers may respond to colchicine, but oral, IV, or topical steroids may be necessary.
- More severe manifestations may require Imuran, Cytoxan, methotrexate, CellCept, cyclosporine, TNF antagonists, or Rituxan.

References

1. Sakane, T., M. Takeno, N. Suzuki, and G. Inaba. Behçet's Disease. *N Engl J Med* 341:1284.

2. 1990 Criteria for diagnosis of Behçet's disease. International Study Group for Behçet's Disease. *Lancet* 335:1078.

3. Davatchi, F., M. Schirmer, C. Zouboulis, et al., on Behalf of the International Team for the Revision of the International Study Group Criteria for Behcet's Disease. Evaluation and Revision of the International Study Group Criteria for Behcet's Disease. Proceedings of the American College of Rheumatology Meeting, November 2007, Boston, MA. Abstract 1233.

4. Barnes, C. G., and H. Yazici. Behçet's Syndrome. *Rheumatology* (Oxford) 38:1171.

5. Saadoun, D., B. Wechsler, K. Desseaux, et al. Mortality in Behçet's Disease. *Arthritis Rheum* 62:2806.

6. Yurdakul, S., C. Mat, Y. Tüzün, et al. A Double-Blind Trial of Colchicine in Behçet's Syndrome. *Arthritis Rheum* 44:2686.

7. Hatemi, G., A. Silman, D. Bang, et al. Management of Behçet Disease: A Systematic Literature Review for the European League against Rheumatism Evidence-Based Recommendations for the Management of Behçet's Disease. *Ann Rheum Dis* 68:1528.

8. Hatemi, G., A. Silman, D. Bang, et al. EULAR Recommendations for the Management of Behçet Disease. *Ann Rheum Dis* 67:1656.

1. Barnes, C. G. Treatment of Behcet's Syndrome. *Rheumatology* (Oxford) 45:245.

2. Rozenbaum, M., I. Rosner, and E. Portnoy. Remission of Behçet's Syndrome with TNF-alpha Blocking Treatment. *Ann Rheum Dis* 61:283.

3. Sarwar, H., H. McGrath, Jr., and L. R. Espinoza. Successful Treatment of Long-Standing Neuro-Behçet's Disease with Infliximab. *J Rheumatol* 32:181.

Kawasaki Disease, or Mucocutaneous Lymph Node Syndrome

Babies on Motorcycles

There is a whole group of vasculitides that I will just mention or omit completely because they are rare and beyond the scope of this book. Kawasaki is usually seen in small children and is associated with high fever, red eyes, swollen glands, strawberry tongue (swollen and red), rash, swollen and red palms and soles, cardiac abnormalities, and a variety of systemic complaints. I have never seen a case but have heard a few described. Treatment is usually with intravenous immunoglobulins and moderate doses of aspirin. Occasionally, steroids are used. Pictures of children with this disease are pretty remarkable.

Pearls

- It is a vasculitis of babies.
- Classic findings are fevers, strawberry tongue, red palms and soles, and cardiac abnormalities.
- Treat with IVIG and ASA.

References

1. Burns, J. C., and M. P. Glodé. Kawasaki Syndrome. *Lancet* 364:533.

2. Melish, M. E. Kawasaki Syndrome: A 1986 Perspective. *Rheum Dis Clin North Am* 13:7.

3. Newburger, J. W., M. Takahashi, J. C. Burns, et al. The Treatment of Kawasaki Syndrome with Intravenous Gamma Globulin. *N Engl J Med* 315:341.

Leukocytoclastic, or Hypersensitivity, Vasculitis (LCV)

Detective Novels, Wit, and a Rash

Helen just died last year, and I miss her. She was ninety-two and once told me that if she was thirty to forty years younger, my wife would have major competition. She loved mystery novels, especially those by P. D. James. Her razor-sharp wit and twinkling eyes made visits very entertaining and kept me on my toes. Unfortunately, she had some strange bone marrow disease and was on a variety of medications. Prior to seeing me, she developed a red, raised, bruise-like rash on her legs that was painful to the touch. A few of the "bruises" ulcerated. A skin biopsy established the diagnosis of LCV. When I saw her for the first time, I was convinced that one of her medications was the cause, but there was a remote possibility that it was due to her bone marrow disease. With the cooperation of her hematologist, her medications were changed, and she was placed on a tapering dose of prednisone. The rash resolved, but we could never taper her below 10 mg of prednisone. She was a character and always lit up my day.

LCV may be the most common form of vasculitis. It may be purely cutaneous without systemic involvement. Palpable purpura or bruises will appear exclusively on the legs. Usually drugs or infections are the cause. Biopsy to confirm the diagnosis is often definitive but rarely required. Withdrawal of the offending drug is effective. Sometimes steroids are used. A variant of hypersensitivity vasculitis called *Henoch-Schonlein purpura* often occurs in children. Patients develop purpura, joint pain, kidney disease (usually just protein in the urine but in severe cases kidney failure), severe abdominal pain with GI bleed or blockage, and a variety of other systemic complaints. Biopsies from skin or other organs may be definitive because of the presence of IGA in small blood vessels (arterioles and venules) but is rarely necessary. In this case, patience is a virtue because most cases will resolve spontaneously and are treated symptomatically with NSAIDs, acetaminophen, and hydration, although in severe kidney disease or with GI complications, hospitalization and steroids may be necessary. Adults may develop this condition, but it is rare. My last case was a thirteen-year-old who had skin disease and protein in his urine after having an upper respiratory tract infection. He didn't look particularly sick and didn't test positive for any other diseases in the differential diagnosis. We treated him symptomatically and did not biopsy his rash, and over two weeks his symptoms resolved. Eight years later he is a successful computer nerd in college and never has had a recurrence, although his aunt has adult-onset Still's disease—whatever that means. (You are soon to find out.)

Pearls

- Classic finding is purpura or a bruise-like rash on legs, which can ulcerate.
- In adults, the most common cause is drug reaction.
- It may require steroids as well as discontinuing the offensive drug.
- In children, hypersensitivity vasculitis (Henoch-Schonlein purpura) usually involves purpura, protein in urine, arthritis, and abdominal pain (and rarely GI bleed).
- This variant only requires supportive treatment unless kidney or GI involvement is severe; then treat with steroids.
- Biopsy of skin, kidneys, or colon may show presence of IGA in an arteriole or venule.

References

1. Calabrese, L. H., and G. F. Duna. Drug-Induced Vasculitis. *Curr Opin Rheumatol* 8:34.

2. Calabrese, L. H., B. A. Michel, D. A. Bloch, et al. The American College of Rheumatology 1990 Criteria for the Classification of Hypersensitivity Vasculitis. *Arthritis Rheum* 33:1108.

3. Michel, B. A., G. G. Hunder, D. A. Bloch, and L. H. Calabrese. Hypersensitivity Vasculitis and Henoch-Schönlein Purpura: A Comparison between the 2 Disorders. *J Rheumatol* 19:721.

Vasculitis Potpourri

I will now give you some one-liners about a variety of vasculitides. Most of them however are no joke!

Vasculitis associated with various collagen vascular diseases—including RA, lupus, dermatomyositis, and scleroderma—usually involves the skin but may involve the nervous system, GI tract, or almost any other system.

Cryoglobulinemia—cryoglobulins are proteins in the blood that precipitate out in the cold and dissolve when rewarmed. They are often associated with infections, such as hepatitis C, and can resemble hypersensitivity vasculitis or lupus. Patients can be any age and can be quite sick. Raynaud's, skin ulcers, arthritis, and kidney disease are common manifestations. Steroids, plasmapheresis, Rituxan, or some of the other usual suspects and treatment of any underlying disease can be effective. I can only remember one elderly gentleman with this condition, who was extremely tall and slow-moving, whom I treated when I was in training. He had an underlying hematological malignancy, chronic skin ulcerations, and arthritis and seemed to do well on low-dose prednisone and Imuran.

Pearls

- Check for cryoglobulins in hepatitis C especially in patients with arthritis, raynaud's phenomenon and vasculitis.
- Specimen must be stored and tested at body temperatures.
- These proteins precipitate out in cold.
- Consider them in severe Raynaud's and vasculopathy.
- Treat with steroids, Imuran, Rituxan, and/or plasmapheresis.
- Treat underlying disease.

References

1. Trendelenburg, M., and J. A. Schifferli. Cryoglobulins Are Not Essential. *Ann Rheum Dis* 57:3.
2. Dammacco, F., and D. Sansonno. Therapy for Hepatitis C Virus-Related Cryoglobulinemic Vasculitis. *N Engl J Med* 369:10
3. Ferri, C., M. Sebastiani, D. Giuggioli, et al. Mixed Cryoglobulinemia: Demographic, Clinical, and Serologic Features and Survival in 231 Patients. *Semin Arthritis Rheum* 133:355.

Primary central nervous system vasculitis affects only the brain, but patients are sick with headaches and neurological symptoms and have high ESR and CRP and abnormal spinal taps. Diagnosis is made by brain angiogram or MRA and sometimes definitively by brain biopsy. Many benign conditions mimic this vasculitis with abnormal angiograms caused by arterial spasm. I had a case of a woman with a "thunderclap" headache only after orgasms. She had an abnormal angiogram with spasm. After careful questioning, I discovered that she was using daily nasal sprays that constrict blood vessels because she had chronic sinus problems. With discontinuation of the medication, her headaches disappeared, and her angiogram normalized.

Pearls

- Almost always have high ESR and CRP and abnormal spinal tap.
- Diagnosis made by angiogram, MRA, and definitively by biopsy of nondominant temporal lobe (brain).
- Differentiate from cerebral vasospasm and infection.
- Patients with vasospasm almost always have normal ESR, CRP, spinal tap.

References

1. Calabrese, L. H., G. F. Duna, and J. T. Lie. Vasculitis in the Central Nervous System. *Arthritis Rheum* 40:1189.
2. Calabrese, L. H., A. J. Furlan, L. A. Gragg, and T. J. Ropos. Primary Angiitis of the Central Nervous System: Diagnostic Criteria and Clinical Approach. *Cleve Clin J Med* 59:293.
3. Calabrese, L. H., D. W. Dodick, T. J. Schwedt, and A. B. Singhal. Narrative Review: Reversible Cerebral Vasoconstriction Syndromes. *Ann Intern Med* 146:34.

Relapsing polychondritis (RPC) is a systemic autoimmune inflammatory disease that characteristically causes inflammation of the cartilage of the ears, nose, respiratory tract, and joints. One third of the cases are associated with a systemic vasculitis. Most patients complain of painful, swollen ears, but they can develop nasal cartilage inflammation, leading to a saddle nose deformity. Rarely the trachea or windpipe can collapse, leading to acute respiratory failure. Since many patients have an associated vasculitis, they can have kidney, neurological, heart, or really any organ involvement. My two most memorable patients both had big, painful, swollen ears but otherwise were completely different. The first was a pretty young lady of thirty who had chronic ear swelling and pain and eventually developed flattening of her nose because of cartilage inflammation. She had some difficulty breathing because of upper respiratory inflammation and became anorectic with severe weight loss. I am still not sure whether her anorexia and weight loss were psychological or because of vasculitis of the GI tract. In any case, I tried steroids, methotrexate, Imuran, and Cytoxan without much success. She eventually developed heart disease, significant arthritis, and neuropathy but seemed to stabilize on a combination of Remicade and CellCept. She is still extremely brittle and recently had a bleed inside her brain after a motor vehicle accident. I am holding my breath.

The second patient was a sixty-year-old retired wrestling coach who would always put me in some kind of wrestling hold when I entered the room and then massage my neck and ask me if I drank my sixty-four ounces of daily water requirement. He was short and stocky and had a shy smile and wry sense of humor. However, as the months passed, he became very fearful and obviously demented and would cower in the corner when I entered. After some research, I realized that RPC could cause dementia and treated him with high doses of prednisone and with Imuran. After a year, he began to smile again and place me in the wrestling holds. I am not sure he is back to baseline, but after five years, he is off medications and doing well.

Pearls

- It's not just about the ear!
- The nose and the trachea can be involved, leading to respiratory failure.
- It may have associated vasculitis with neurological, cardiac, or kidney involvement.
- ESR and CRP can be elevated.
- Rarely, it can cause dementia.
- It can be a companion disease or stand alone.
- Treatment starts with prednisone, but Dapsone, methotrexate, Imuran, CellCept, or TNF antagonists may be helpful. I use Dapsone after prednisone.

References

1. www.rheumatology.org/Practice (Patient Education—Diseases and Conditions)

2. Kent, P. D., C. J. Michet, Jr., and H. S. Luthra. Relapsing Polychondritis." *Curr Opin Rheumatol* 16:56.

3. Michet, C. J. Vasculitis and Relapsing Polychondritis. *Rheum Dis Clin North Am* 16:441.

4. Stewart, K. A., and D. J. Mazanec. Pulse Intravenous Cyclophosphamide for Kidney Disease in Relapsing Polychondritis. *J Rheumatol* 19:498.

5. Lipnick, R. N., and C. W. Fink. Acute Airway Obstruction in Relapsing Polychondritis: Treatment with Pulse Methylprednisolone. *J Rheumatol* 18:98.

6. Park, J., K. M. Gowin, and H. R. Schumacher, Jr. Steroid Sparing Effect of Methotrexate in Relapsing Polychondritis. *J Rheumatol* 23:937.

8. Trentham, D. E., and C. H. Le. Relapsing Polychondritis. *Ann Intern Med* 129:114.

9. Richez, C., C. Dumoulin, X. Coutouly, and T. Schaeverbeke. Successful Treatment of Relapsing Polychondritis with Infliximab. *Clin Exp Rheumatol* 22:629.

10. Carter, J. D. Treatment of Relapsing Polychondritis with a TNF Antagonist. *J Rheumatol* 32:1413.

11. Wallace, Z. S., and J. H. Stone. Refractory Relapsing Polychondritis Treated with Serial Success with Interleukin 6 Receptor Blockade. *J Rheumatol* 40:100.

12. Peng, S. L., and D. Rodriguez. Abatacept in Relapsing Polychondritis. *Ann Rheum Dis* 72:1427.

13. Leroux, G., N. Costedoat-Chalumeau, B. Brihaye, et al. Treatment of Relapsing Polychondritis with Rituximab: A Retrospective Study of Nine Patients. *Arthritis Rheum* 61:577.

Susac's Syndrome

This Is Not Marching Band Music

Linda is a 44year old attractive brunette with an impish smile whom I have been treating for a questionable diagnosis of Lupus for years. She is a very upbeat accomplished writer, musician and was training to be a police officer when her plans got derailed. About a year ago she developed visual problems and personality changes. Knowing that no one would want a blind, psychotic police officer she dropped out of her program. A retinal specialist found optic neuritis and retinal ischemia or poor blood flow to her retina. A MRI revealed areas of poor blood flow to her brain (white matter lesions). I thought these findings might be due to her Lupus and treated her with Prednisone and Cellcept with success but the symptoms and findings kept recurring and worsening. She began having episodes of disorientation, anger and was losing her sight rapidly. To make matters worse, she was losing her hearing. I rationalized that she was a bass guitarist in a rock band but I was worried. Her Lupus antibodies were negative and she had two sisters with multiple sclerosis so I referred her to neurology. After a thorough workup that ruled out MS, the neurologist with her retinologist's blessing sent her to a neuro-ophthalmologist who diagnosed Susac's syndrome. Visits to the Mayo clinic and correspondence with Robert Rennebohm the director of the Susac's Syndrome consult service at the Cleveland clinic, led the patient to believe she truly had this syndrome despite some dissenting opinions and some inconsistencies in her findings.

Under Dr. Rennebohms supervision, I started her on a protocal that includes Prednisone, IV Solumedrol, Cellcept and IVIG (intravenous immunoglobulins). Her treatment regimen is state of the art but as usual so far not everything is going as planned. She had severe nausea and hemolytic anemia (antibodies cannibalizing her red blood cells) secondary to the IVIG. I could not give her the intravenous Solumedrol because at doses higher than 30 mg. of Prednisone her blood pressure went through the roof and she became psychotic. I am hoping a new regimen of Cellcept, Prednisone low doses of Solumedrol and a different brand IVIG do the trick. More sleepless nights....

Susac's syndrome is an extremely rare autoimmune microvascular endotheliopathy meaning the lining of capillaries or very small blood vessels are inflamed and swollen leading to ischemia or poor blood flow. The organs usually involved are the eyes (retina), brain (especially the cental corpus callosum) and the ears. Patients may have headaches, cognitive dysunction, personality changes, psychosis, deafness, tinnitus (ringing), weakness, loss of balance, visual field cuts or blindness.

Diagnosis is based on the clinical triad of ear, eye and brain findings with radiological and hearing test confirmation. Retinal fluorescein angiography shows branch retinal artery occlusion and leakages. MRIs of the brain reveal white matter and deep grey matter lesions, central corpus callosum abnormalities and leptomeinges enhancement. Hearing tests demonstrate low frequency losses. Linda had some but not all, these findings.

The only time I have encountered Susacs in the past is on lists of differential diagnoses for retinal ischemia and deafness. Dr. Rennebohm kindly and quickly educated me so that I could be comfortable treating Linda. Her treatment regimen is state of the art but as usual so far not everything is going as planned. She has severe nausea and hemolytic anemia secondary to the IVIG and I could not give her the intravenous Solumedrol because at doses higher than 30 mg. of Prednisone her blood pressure goes through the roof and she becomes psychotic. I am hoping the abbreviated regimen of Cellcept, Prednisone and IVIG does the trick.

Pearls

- Susac's syndrome involves ears, brain and eyes
- It is a microvasacular endotheliopathy
- Branch retinal artery occlusion
- Visual field cuts, even blindness
- Low frequency hearing loss
- MRI findings of white and gray matter lesions, cental corpus callosum lesions and leptomeninges inflammation
- Personality changes, cognitive dysfunction and even psychosis and dementia
- Weakness and loss of balance
- Treatment includes Prednisone, Cellcept, IV Solumedrol and IVIG

References

1. Susac, Jo editorial: Susac's syndrome Am. J. Neuroradiology, 2004 25:35 351-352
2. Rennebohm R, Susac Jo Egan RA Daroff RB
3. Susac's Syndrome—update J. Neurol Sci 2010 Dec. 15; 299 (1-2): 86-91
4. Rennebohm Rm, Lubowm, rusin J, Martin L., Grzybowski, DM Susac, Jo, Aggressive immunosuppressive treatment of Susac's Syndrome in adolescent: using treatment of dermatomyositis as model. Pediatric Rheumatology online J. 2008, Jan. 29; 6:3

Chapter Eighteen

Sarcoidosis

No, It's Not TB or Lymphoma but Can Be a Whole Lot of Trouble

Jorge is a forty-year-old psychologist who I have followed for about two years. He is a pretty mellow guy who rarely complains, so when he does, I take it very seriously. Initially, he had some non-specific joint and abdominal complaints, and he was found to have enlarged glands on a screening chest x-ray. A CT of his abdomen revealed lesions on his liver and pancreas. His doctors correctly worried about infection or lymphoma, a blood cancer. However, a biopsy of one of the glands between his lungs established the diagnosis of sarcoidosis, and he was referred to me. He really was not very symptomatic initially, and I hesitated to prescribe any medications. I mostly worried about his lungs and respiratory status, which could deteriorate pretty quickly. However, his breathing tests were all normal, and the CT of his lungs was pretty benign. So I just followed him for several months until he started to complain of increasing joint and abdominal pain. I tried Plaquenil, methotrexate, Arava, and Imuran. He either could not tolerate the medication, or they were ineffective.

More recently, he developed painful red eyes (iritis), typical for sarcoidosis. Despite months of topical and occasional oral steroids, it
kept recurring. Therefore, after a prolonged wrestling match with his
insurance, I started him on Humira with good results. However, several months later his kidney function deteriorated rapidly. I searched
the literature and found that sarcoidosis rarely affected the kidneys.
In fact, recently I attended a lecture on rare manifestations of sarcoidosis by a leading expert and it wasn't even mentioned! So, I
stopped the Humira and obtained an ultrasound which showed a
mass on one of his kidneys. Two biopsies revealed kidney cancer
and sarcoid kidney. The kidney cancer probably wouldn't have been
found as early if his sarcoidosis hadn't affected his kidney function.

His cancer was resected successfully but he continued to have
kidney dysfunction. High doses of Prednisone normalized his kidneys but caused him to have high blood sugars and gain about 40
pounds. His head and face almost looked deformed by the excess
weight. Unfortunately, every time we reduced his Prednisone dose,
his kidney disease flared. We tried Imuran, Cellcept and Tacrolimus
but he could not tolerate any of them. So without any studies to
back me, I prescribed intravenous IGG and voila, his kidney function
stabilized at 80% off steroids.... so far. Sometimes you just have to
think out of the box. Jorge is 44 and a great guy and I just couldn't
give up on him.

More recently, my aunt, who is an extremely young and vibrant
seventy-eight-year-old, lost about forty pounds over a year uninten-
tionally and became weak and feeble. Not only could she not play
her daily tennis match, she required help walking any distance and
became almost housebound. Her blood work revealed abnormal
liver function, and a CAT scan demonstrated masses on her liver.
My cousins freaked! Their father, her husband, had just died of liver

cancer. Fortunately, a biopsy helped her doctors diagnose sarcoidosis, and after a few months of tapering doses of prednisone, she has gained back all her weight and energy and will start playing tennis this week. (By the way, she just started dating a fifty-three-year-old!)

Two days ago, I saw Laura, a tall twenty-four-year-old brunette with an infectious laugh. She had a six-week history of purplish painful nodules on her legs, predominantly her shins, and had developed migratory arthritis involving her hands, knees, and ankles. Interestingly, she had a nodule on the second knuckle (MCP) of her right hand that was biopsied a year ago and diagnosed as a rheumatoid nodule. Her primary care doctor had done an extensive workup, and Laura had tested negative for rheumatoid arthritis and lupus. The doctor prescribed doxycycline for two weeks, and Laura's nodules and arthritis improved somewhat. Doxycycline has some anti-inflammatory qualities. Laura's mother studied the Internet and suggested very astutely that her daughter's purplish nodules were erythema nodosum. It is a form of panniculitis, or inflammation of subcutaneous fat, that can be associated with a variety of diseases, infections, and medications. One of the associated diseases is sarcoidosis, so although Laura was asymptomatic, I ordered a chest x-ray. One of the cardinal findings in this disease is hilar adenopathy, or enlargement of the lymph nodes between the lungs and lo and behold, Laura's chest x-ray showed these classic findings. Unfortunately, TB, lymphoma, and other diseases can produce similar findings; therefore, I recommended a pulmonary specialist perform a lymph node biopsy. Laura's adventure had just begun. The biopsy revealed granulomas, or a group of cells most consistent with sarcoidosis. So after a tapering dose of prednisone, she is off medications and asymptomatic.

Sarcoidosis is a rare disease that affects multiple organs, which are infiltrated by groups of cells called *granulomas*. Patients characteristically have enlarged glands throughout their bodies but especially in their lungs. They often have strange rashes, fevers, iritis, muscle inflammation and weakness, inflammation and scarring of their lungs, and arthritis. However, any system can be involved, including the heart, the nervous system, muscles, the GI tract (especially the liver and spleen), and kidneys. Patients may be very sick when we first see them, with severe shortness of breath, fatigue, and weakness, or be asymptomatic. If a routine chest x-ray reveals enlarged lymph nodes or masses, a biopsy is needed to establish the diagnosis of sarcoidosis after ruling out tuberculosis, lymphoma, and fungal disease. The skin, muscles, or the liver are among other good sources for biopsy. Lymphoma may be mistaken for sarcoidosis because of the multiple swollen glands and multisystem involvement.

One of the saddest cases I treated was a middle-aged gentleman who was referred to me by one of the top researchers in sarcoidosis. He had a terrible, ulcerating total body rash, inflammation of his lungs with hilar lymphadenopathy (swollen glands in the area between the lungs), fevers, and horrible inflammatory arthritis involving most joints. The expert had performed a lung biopsy, which suggested but was not diagnostic of sarcoidosis, and started him on high-dose steroids, with some improvement. The patient also had an enlarged spleen and liver, which can also be seen in sarcoidosis and generally felt awful. Sarcoidosis is a systemic disease! After a few months, the patient relocated to Oregon, and I began treating him. Despite more steroids, Imuran, methotrexate, Plaquenil, and a few doses of Remicade, the patient's skin and joints became so bad he could hardly walk, and his whole body was an open sore. I began to suspect the diagnosis was incorrect. There is an old rule in medicine that if a disease is not responding or acting like you would expect it to after a time, reconsider both your treatment and diagnosis. Therefore, I sent the patient to the dermatology department in a major medical center for possible biopsy. The patient had a particularly malignant lymphoma and died shortly thereafter. This case reinforced two lessons I thought I had already learned: never accept anybody's diagnosis until you establish it yourself, and always rule out lymphoma, tuberculosis, and fungal infection in suspected sarcoidosis cases.

Most of my sarcoidosis cases are pretty benign and easy. They often just have swollen glands, mild arthritis, and iritis and can be treated symptomatically with eyedrops, but if the iritis is recurrent or the arthritis is severe, they may require systemic steroids (methotrexate, Imuran, CellCept, Plaquenil, Humira, or Remicade). Another big group of these patients may mainly have lung disease, which can be quite severe and life threatening and requires aggressive treatment, often involving high-dose steroids. Usually these patients are followed mainly by pulmonary doctors. I monitor sarcoidosis patients with annual or semiannual chest x-rays and pulmonary-function tests but have a low threshold for obtaining CT scans of their lungs. I have one patient who has enlarged salivary glands, fevers, a probable granuloma on her chest x-ray, joint pain, bilateral carpal tunnel syndrome (common in sarcoidosis), and a positive angiotensin converting enzyme (ACE) test. This test is seen in many sarcoid patients, but there are many false positives. No one wants to biopsy this patient's glands or lungs, and she has not tested positive for tuberculosis or a variety of fungi. I am pretty sure she has sarcoidosis but not definitively, so I gave her an intramuscular shot of steroid and started her on Plaquenil, and she seems to be responding. Nevertheless, I have some nervous reservations and always have lymphoma in the back of my mind.

Like all the diseases I follow, different patients follow different courses and have different organs involved. Some patients have predominantly lung or muscle involvement and require high doses of prednisone, and others have asymptomatic liver, muscle, or lymph gland involvement and are just treated symptomatically. Arthritis may be treated with NSAIDs alone or with Plaquenil, methotrexate, Humira, or Remicade. As I mentioned above, iritis is often just treated with steroid eyedrops alone but may require systemic treatment. Sarcoidosis's course and prognosis are variable, as is the treatment.

Pearls

- If sarcoid is suspected, always order a chest x-ray, looking for hilar adenopathy (swollen glands between the lungs).
- Swollen glands and lung involvement are common, but muscle, skin, liver, and neurological problems do occur.
- It is a multisystem systemic disease.
- It is in the differential diagnosis of iritis, so always order a chest x-ray and often a chest CT.
- ACE levels are unreliable but may be a clue.
- Biopsy may give the definitive diagnosis.
- Beware of lymphoma masquerading as sarcoid.
- Rule out TB and fungus definitively.
- Monitor pulmonary-function tests and CT and chest x-rays regularly.
- Involve a good pulmonary consultant.
- Check muscle strength and CPK.
- If the disease does not respond to the usual treatment, reevaluate and consider lymphoma.
- TNF antagonists may be helpful, but Enbrel does not work.
- Patients do not always have to be on medications, especially steroids, although they may be necessary at times.
- Plaquenil, methotrexate, Imuran, and CellCept are reasonable alternatives to steroids.
- Treat lung disease aggressively, usually with high-dose steroids.

References

1. www.uptodate.com

2. Winston, Charles. *The Sarcoidosis Handbook.*

3. Mitchell, Donald, David Moller, Stephen G. Spiro, and Athol Wells. *Sarcoidosis.*

4. Iannuzzi, M. C., B. A. Rybicki, and A. S. Teirstein. "Sarcoidosis." *N Engl J Med* 357:2153.

5. Thomas, K. W., and G. W. Hunninghake. Sarcoidosis. *JAMA* 289:3300.

6. Newman, L. S., C. S. Rose, and L. A. Maier. Sarcoidosis. *N Engl J Med* 336:1224.

7. Suda, T., A. Sato, M. Toyoshima, et al. Weekly Low-Dose Methotrexate Therapy for Sarcoidosis. *Intern Med* 33:437.

8. Lower, E. E., and R. P. Baughman. Prolonged Use of Methotrexate for Sarcoidosis. *Arch Intern Med* 155:846.

9. Emery, P., F. C. Breedveld, E. M. Lemmel, et al. A Comparison of the Efficacy and Safety of Leflunomide and Methotrexate for the Treatment of Rheumatoid Arthritis. *Rheumatology* (Oxford) 39:655.

10. Pritchard, C., and K. Nadarajah. Tumour Necrosis Factor Alpha Inhibitor Treatment for Sarcoidosis Refractory to Conventional Treatments: A Report of Five Patients. *Ann Rheum Dis* 63:318.

Chapter Nineteen

Amyloidosis

A Renegade Protein Run Amok

Giuseppe was a seventy-six-year-old Italian jokester. He always seemed to gaze downward as he joked with an impish smile. He had a leathery, worn, angular, long face that I would have expected to see on an Italian peddler in a movie. He slurred his words with an accent probably because he had a huge tongue, characteristic of his disease. He had a long history of osteomyelitis (a bone infection) of his leg and one year previous to our first visit had developed swollen hands. His physician made the diagnosis of carpal tunnel syndrome, and during surgery a biopsy of the tendon sheath revealed amyloid. He was referred to me because of his swollen hands. An x -ray showed a very destructive infiltrative process in the bones of the hands consistent with amyloidosis. Interestingly, his urine had an excess of protein, and I wondered if the amyloid had infiltrated his kidneys or whether he had a type of blood cancer called *multiple myeloma*, which can be associated with amyloidosis. Blood and urine tests confirmed the cancer, and three years later, he is still alive and reportedly doing well on a new, promising regimen for multiple myeloma. I hope he has maintained his sense of humor.

Amyloidosis is another strange and rare disease that can affect multiple systems. It can be devastating. Any organ may be infiltrated by an alien protein until it is totally destroyed. It's like one of those scary science-fiction movies. There are several kinds of amyloid proteins; each seems to have a predilection for specific organs. Protein in the urine, a thickened heart, neuropathy, bleeding, an enlarged spleen or liver, muscle or joint infiltration, and enlarged tongues are all possible manifestations.

They are caused by deposits of an abnormal protein, which can be diagnosed definitively by biopsies of the affected organ, bone marrow, or the abdominal fat pad. The latter is fairly easy and accessible by using a large needle and aspirating the fat just under the skin in the abdomen. I used to perform this particular biopsy in the office years ago and had a few successes. The tissue has to be processed in a specific way when it is obtained. It has certain distinctive characteristics when examined under the microscope, one of which is its ability to bind to a special stain called *Congo red*. If I suspect amyloidosis, I always specifically ask for that stain. There are also some imaging techniques, such as echocardiograms, which can be very suggestive of the diagnosis, and something called *serum amyloid p component scintigraphy*, which can measure the extent of amyloid involvement. Systemic amyloidosis can be associated with a blood cancer or with untreated, chronic inflammatory diseases, such as rheumatoid arthritis or Crohn's disease. Amyloid deposits are found in the brains of Alzheimer's patients. Although there are some promising new therapies (RNAi therapy), treating the underlying disease seems to be the only effective one and only temporarily. Early in my career, we would see rheumatoid arthritis patients who would develop sudden protein in their urine, and amyloidosis was always in the differential diagnosis. But with better treatment of RA these days, I haven't seen one in years. Still, it's important to look for an underlying cause of amyloidosis once the diagnosis has been established since treating the underlying disease is the best and almost only option.

Finally, my most recent amyloidosis patient had amyloid found on his vocal cords after several months of hoarseness. He has had an extensive workup to rule out systemic rather than just localized amyloidosis. Fortunately, it seems that it is confined to his cords, and he is being treated with focal radiation. Patients with localized amyloidosis generally have it in the upper respiratory tract and have a good prognosis since it rarely spreads. Nevertheless as with most educated or curious patients these days, my patient and his wife did extensive reading on amyloidosis and were terrified about his prognosis until it was confirmed that he had localized disease. However, there is nothing that is 100 percent certain in medicine.

Pearls

- It is a protein that infiltrates multiple organs but is occasionally localized.
- It may be associated with any chronic inflammatory disease, such as rheumatoid arthritis or inflammatory bowel disease.
- It may be associated with multiple myeloma.
- It should be considered in any patient with unexplained malabsorption, protein in the urine, or neuropathies.
- Prognosis is poor unless patient has localized disease or an underlying treatable disease, such as multiple myeloma.
- Treat underlying disease.
- There are promising new treatments on the horizon (RNAi therapy).

References

1. www.uptodate.com

2. Bellotti, V., M. Nuvolone, S. Giorgetti, et al. The Workings of the Amyloid Diseases. *Ann Med* 39:200.

3. van Gameren, I. I., B. P. Hazenberg, J. Bijzet, and M. H. van Rijswijk. Diagnostic Accuracy of Subcutaneous Abdominal Fat Tissue Aspiration for Detecting Systemic Amyloidosis and Its Utility in Clinical Practice. *Arthritis Rheum* 54:2015.

4. Kyle, R. A., and E. D. Bayrd. Amyloidosis: Review of 236 Cases. *Medicine* (Baltimore) 54:271.

5. Hazenberg, B. P., P. C. Limburg, J. Bijzet, and M. H. van Rijswijk. A Quantitative Method for Detecting Deposits of Amyloid A Protein in Aspirated Fat Tissue of Patients with Arthritis. *Ann Rheum Dis* 58:96.

6. Saraiva, M. J. Sporadic Cases of Hereditary Systemic Amyloidosis. *N Engl J Med* 346:1818.

7. Hazenberg, B. P., and M. H. van Rijswijk. Where Has Secondary Amyloid Gone? *Ann Rheum Dis* 59:577.

9. Obici, L., S. Raimondi, F. Lavatelli, et al. Susceptibility to AA Amyloidosis in Rheumatic Diseases: A Critical Overview. *Arthritis Rheum* 61:1435.

10. Lachmann, H. J., H. J. Goodman, J. A. Gilbertson, et al. "Natural History and Outcome in Systemic AA Amyloidosis. *N Engl J Med* 356:2361.

11. Livneh, A., D. Zemer, P. Langevitz, et al. Colchicine in the Treatment of AA and AL Amyloidosis. *Semin Arthritis Rheum* 23:206.

12. Keersmaekers, T., K. Claes, D. R. Kuypers, et al. Long-Term Efficacy of Infliximab Treatment for AA-Amyloidosis Secondary to Chronic Inflammatory Arthritis. *Ann Rheum Dis* 68:759.

13. Okuda, Y., and K. Takasugi. Successful Use of a Humanized Anti-interleukin-6 Receptor Antibody, Tocilizumab, to Treat Amyloid A Amyloidosis Complicating Juvenile Idiopathic Arthritis. *Arthritis Rheum* 54:2997.

Chapter Twenty

Osteoporosis

Fragile—Handle with Care

Sylvia started seeing me about ten years ago when she was sixty-five. She was noted to have severe osteoporosis on a bone density exam, had a strong family history, and already had one collapsed vertebra. She had lost one inch of height and was a little bent (kyphosis). I started her on Fosamax (alendronate) 70 mg weekly, 1,200 mg of calcium, and 800 IUs of vitamin D. Her bone density improved imperceptibly over the next four years, and she developed another vertebral fracture. We switched her to Forteo (teriparatide) for two years, and she made substantial gains in her bone density, and after one year's holiday from all antiosteoporotic drugs, we switched her to yearly Reclast (zoledronic acid). Unfortunately, her bone density deteriorated dramatically again, and she fractured several more vertebrae and her left wrist. She was in tremendous pain and was found to have lumbar stenosis as well as the fractures. Because the patient refused retreatment with Forteo, citing a drug company and FDA restriction, we prescribed Prolia. She eventually had surgery for her lumbar stenosis with some relief. However, since that time, she has lost five inches and is permanently bent to seventy-five degrees. She has to strain her neck to look up at me when she is standing at her walker. I have prescribed months of physical therapy without success. She is miserable but accepting and always greets me with a wry smile.

Osteoporosis is a disease of low bone mass, skeletal fragility, and increased risk of fracture. In the simplest terms, bones are always in different phases of construction and deconstruction. Two cells dominate bone physiology and are in equilibrium—the osteoblasts, which are like bricklayers laying down new bone, and the osteoclasts, which are like termites or "Pac-Men" eating away old bone. In osteoporosis the osteoclasts outwork the osteoblasts, so there is a net loss. Most medications we use in osteoporosis inhibit osteoclasts. Early in my career in rheumatology, we didn't pay much attention to osteoporosis—it was mainly addressed by endocrinologists, and there was not much effective treatment. Once bone densitometry machines, or DXAs, were developed to measure bone densities and a group of medications called *bisphosphonates* were discovered and found to be effective, everything changed.

I remember inheriting in the mideighties a group of patients who had been on moderate to large doses of steroids for years. Many developed spinal deformities, fractured vertebrae and hips, and often became at least temporarily disabled. Little old ladies became bedbound or confined to walkers and dependent on narcotics because of collapsed vertebrae or fractured hips. As I mentioned previously, it seemed that everyone with polymyalgia rheumatica eventually developed fractures. Today, we are better educated and better equipped to treat and prevent osteoporosis. We also know that it is not confined to postmenopausal women. More and more men are developing osteoporosis for a variety of reasons.

Osteoporosis for me is divided into prevention and treatment. Premenopausal women or men with risk factors such as long-term steroid use or antiseizure or acid reflux medications, or who have a variety of diseases such as rheumatoid arthritis, hyperparathyroidism, or hyperthyroidism, should be screened with a DXA. Some researchers advocate ordering expensive lab tests, which reflect increased bone breakdown or buildup. I don't. If a premenopausal woman or a man does not have risk factors, I do not screen. If they have risk factors but no osteoporosis, then calcium 1,200 mg and vitamin D 800 IUs is probably adequate therapy. Dietary sources of calcium and vitamin D are preferable but might not be in sufficient quantities. Of course, weight-bearing exercise, smoking cessation, and avoidance of excessive alcohol consumption are important starting points for any osteoporosis prevention or treatment. Along with calcium (citrate is the best absorbed) and vitamin D, these measures may be all that is needed to treat premenopausal woman with osteoporosis, but patients with ongoing risk factors and recurrent fractures probably need more. Unfortunately, there are few good studies of the effectiveness and safety of the available pharmacological therapies for osteoporosis in premenopausal females. Estrogen or oral contraceptives may be effective and bisphosphonates, like risedronate, alendronate, ibandronate, or zoledronic acid, are particularly useful in patients on steroids, although only risedronate and alendronate have been approved by the FDA for use in steroid-induced osteoporosis. Studies have also found that teriparatide, or parathyroid hormone (PTH), is also effective in the same scenario. Calcitonin in a nasal spray form called *Miacalcin* and another group of drugs called *SERMs* (selective estrogen receptor modulators) may be somewhat effective. Miacalcin is particularly effective in reducing the pain from collapsed vertebrae, although it is not a particularly potent antiosteoporosis drug. Recently it has been associated with cancer and may be withdrawn from the market. I have a forty-year female patient with lupus and failing kidneys who has been taking prednisone for years and has severe osteoporosis with at least one fracture. She is a high risk for more fractures, but her low kidney function is a contraindication for bisphosphonates, so I am treating her with denosumab (Prolia), which inhibits osteoclast activity and is safe in kidney failure but has not been studied in premenopausal women.

Risk assessments for osteoporosis should be performed on all postmenopausal women. The World Health Organization has developed a Fracture Risk Assessment Tool, called *FRAX*. It lists weighted risks and assigns them a number and then adds the sum of these numbers to a number assigned to the DXA (hip) T-score and comes up with that patient's relative risk for fracture. I admit I do not use the tool on every patient, but I do screen for all the risk factors (advanced age, previous fracture, steroid use, family history of fracture, low body weight, smoking, excessive alcohol, rheumatoid arthritis, and other disorders associated with osteoporosis). I also obtain a baseline DXA and repeat it every two years if the patient has osteoporosis or osteopenia, which is the precursor to osteoporosis. DXAs are tools to measure bone densities in femoral necks (hips), lumbar spines, and sometimes wrists. They produce something called a *T-score*. The lower the T-score, the worse the bone density; and a score of minus 2.5 diagnoses osteoporosis, which indicates theoretically an increased risk of future fractures. However, the DXA is not completely accurate alone, and thus instruments like the FRAX, which takes into consideration other factors (such as age), are necessary. Quantitative ultrasounds have also been used to assess osteoporosis but have not been particularly accurate. Quantitative CT may be more accurate than DXA in assessing the spine, but it is more expensive, less reproducible, and exposes the patients to more radiation.

I recommend that all postmenopausal women have a daily intake of 1,200 mg of calcium and 800 IUs of vitamin D (preferably through diet) and have a daily routine of weight-bearing exercises. Intensity doesn't matter, and antigravity exercises, like water aerobics or walking in space, do not count. I counsel patients about the risks of smoking and excessive alcohol, especially in the face of established osteoporosis and fractures, and try to avoid sounding too preachy. Once we have established that a postmenopausal patient has osteoporosis or has osteopenia and a high FRAX score, we reiterate all the above dietary and lifestyle changes and suggest that the patient take alendronate (Fosamax) or risedronate (Actonel), which are both bisphosphonates, a class of drugs that inhibits osteoclasts, the termite-like cells in bones described previously. Both are oral drugs that have been found to increase bone density in both the hip and spine. A third drug, ibandronate, which is available in intravenous and oral forms, has been found to be effective only in increasing bone density in the spine, not the hip, so I don't prescribe it. These medications are very effective and have changed the course of osteoporosis treatment dramatically over the last two decades. However, these medications are not without their drawbacks or controversy. A few years ago, there was a big furor about these drugs causing aseptic necrosis of the jaw, which, as you remember, means that the jaw bone would die because of poor circulation. This complication occurred mainly in patients with gum disease and poor dentition and mostly in the cancer population, who were receiving these medications in high doses in an intravenous form. Its incidence was one in ten thousand patients. Nevertheless, patients were being told by their dentists about the risks and often stopped the medication despite the fact they had little gum or dental disease. I had several patients who immediately began to complain of jaw pain and swelling and demanded x-rays and MRIs. Fortunately, none were positive. I believe I have seen one case over the last twenty years picked up by a dentist. It was one of those times that I wished I had a handout depicting the risks of osteoporosis. Ted Pincus, one of the giants in rheumatology, has said that he gives patients handouts outlining the risks of the disease before giving them a handout outlining the risks of a medication. Patients seem to be more concerned about potential risks of medication than the terrible risks of a disease. Before starting patients on a bisphosphonate, I screen for gum or dental disease and will try another class of drug if it's a problem. The most common side effect of oral bisphosphonates is acid reflux (GERD), and patients are told to avoid lying down while taking these meds and to take them thirty minutes before breakfast, so they are absorbed well. If the patient already has a problem with GERD or develops it while on therapy, I switch to zoledronic acid (Reclast), which is an intravenous bisphosphonate, or try other injectables, such as Prolia or Forteo. Other rare side effects include flu-like symptoms with muscle and bone pain, iritis (painful red eyes), low calcium, and atrial fibrillation. I do not use these drugs in patients with moderate to severe kidney malfunction.

Reclast may be more effective than the oral alternatives, and because it is a fifteen-minute infusion every twelve months, it leads to better compliance. There is some evidence that patients are not very compliant in taking the oral bisphosphonates. I prescribe Reclast when patients have failed oral bisphosphonates, have GERD, or have compliance problems. The most recent controversy regarding this class of drug is atypical hip fractures—another rare event but the media was all over it. Understandably, patients wanted to stop their bisphosphonate immediately since they thought that they were taking these drugs to prevent fractures, not create them. The studies indicate that these atypical fractures occur in patients who have been taking these medications for more than five years, and the risks of osteoporotic fractures off these medications much outweigh the risks of these atypical fractures. Because of these findings, most physicians are advocating at least one year of drug holiday after three to five years of therapy. I choose three years.

I monitor the patients' DXA every two years, and if the patients continue to have fractures or their bone density deteriorates despite bisphosphonate therapy, I prescribe Forteo or Prolia. Sometimes my choice is determined by insurance companies, the patients' finances, and phobias. Many patients have needle phobias and won't consider daily subcutaneous injections—that is, Forteo. It is the only available medication that stimulates osteoblasts, or the bone "bricklayers," and is especially good for patients with multiple fractures. In fact, I recommend it for patients who have osteoporosis and already have had a fracture. Prolia is a biologic and is an antibody against RANKL, a protein that stimulates osteoclast receptors. It can be used as mentioned previously in kidney failure patients, may be effective in patients who fail bisphosphonates, and just recently became FDA approved for men. It is injected subcutaneously (under the skin) every six months and may lead to better compliance. Rash and joint or bone pain are occasional adverse effects However, once again there is a less than 2 percent chance of aseptic necrosis of the jaw. One of the more interesting quandaries I have encountered in the last few years is a lupus patient with avascular necrosis of the hips who had severe GERD and osteoporosis and refused all therapy for her osteoporosis because she thought she was at higher risk for jaw osteonecrosis with bisphosphonates and Prolia because of her previous history of osteonecrosis.

The perfect solution would have been Forteo, but she felt she couldn't inject herself daily. I consulted several osteoporosis specialists, and they felt she would be no more at risk than someone who had not had osteonecrosis of the hips. She chose Prolia over Reclast and so far has done well, with no new bone problems.

I no longer prescribe the other medications used in osteoporosis, such as SERMs (raloxifene), estrogen, and calcitonin, except in certain situations because they are not as effective.

Pearls

- Osteoporosis increases the risk of fractures but is not the only factor.
- DXA is important but is not the only measurement that should be used to measure the risk and need for treatment.
- A FRAX score, which incorporates age and other risk factors, may be state of the art.
- Fracture risk rather than a T-score should be the determining factor for treatment.
- Smoking cessation, avoidance of heavy alcohol use, exercise (thirty minutes three times a week), and fall-prevention counselling are important measures to prevent osteoporosis in post-menopausal women.
- Postmenopausal women require 1,200 mg of calcium and 800 IUs of vitamin D either in their diets or with daily supplements or a combination of both.
- It may be safest to prescribe the above mentioned supplements in all patients with osteoporosis regardless of their dietary intake.
- Men may develop osteoporosis, especially with certain risk factors such as smoking, steroids, heavy alcohol use, long-term use of antiseizure drugs or proton pump inhibitors, hormone deficiencies, certain diseases, malignancy or extended bed rest.
- The same risk factors increase the incidence of osteoporosis in all ages of women.
- Reducing fractures rather than increasing bone density should be the determining factor for determining the effectiveness of a therapy.

Osteoporosis

- Consider evaluation for osteoporosis in any patient with an atypical fracture.
- Bisphosphonates are usually first-line treatment for osteoporosis, except in patients with kidney failure, gum or dental disease, or severe GERD.
- Fosamax or Actonel are preferred over Boniva because there are no good studies proving that Boniva prevents hip fractures.
- Reclast is preferred in patients with GERD or a tendency toward noncompliance.
- Prolia and Forteo are safe in kidney failure and are good choices for those who fail or can't tolerate bisphosphonates.
- Forteo is the only drug that stimulates osteoblasts and bone formation and is good for patients with fractures and severe osteoporosis.
- There are some studies that show that Forteo may be just as effective when given daily for three months on and three months off for two years rather than continuously.
- Evista or SERMs may be the drug of choice in women with osteoporosis and a high risk for breast cancer. There is no evidence it reduces the risk of hip fractures.
- Hip fractures have high risk for mortality in elderly patients.
- Patients who are going to be on long-term (more than three months) steroids should have a baseline DXA.
- Any patient over the age of fifty who is going to be treated with prednisone 7.5 mg or more for more than three months should treated pharmacologically (with bisphosphonates?) for osteoporosis.
- Any man over the age of fifty or postmenopausal woman with a T-score of -1.5 or worse and treated with any dose of steroids for long term should be treated pharmacologically.

- Any premenopausal woman who is not on estrogen therapy or man under the age of fifty with a fragility fracture while on prednisone of more than 7.5 mg. for more than 3 months should be treated pharmacologically.

References

1. Lane, Nancy E. *The Osteoporosis Book: A Guide for Patients and Their Families.*

2. www.uptodate.com

3. www.rheumatology.org/Practice
(Patient Education—Diseases and Conditions)

4. Cosman, F., et al. Retreatment with Teriparatide One Year after the First Teriparatide Course in Patients on Long Term Alendronate. *J Bone Miner Res.*24 (6): 1110.

5. Rosen, C. J. Clinical Practice: Postmenopausal Osteoporosis. *N Engl J Med* 353:595.

6. Reginster, J. Y., D. Felsenberg, S. Boonen, et al. Effects of Long-Term Strontium Ranelate Treatment on the Risk of Nonvertebral and Vertebral Fractures in Postmenopausal Osteoporosis: Results of a Five-Year, Randomized, Placebo-Controlled Trial. *Arthritis Rheum* 58:1687.

7. Yamamoto, T., and P. G. Bullough. The Role of Subchondral Insufficiency Fracture in Rapid Destruction of the Hip Joint: A Preliminary Report. *Arthritis Rheum* 43:2423.

8. Poole, K. E., and J. E. Compston. Osteoporosis and Its Management. *BMJ* 333:1251.

9. Kanis, J. A. Diagnosis of Osteoporosis and Assessment of Fracture Risk. *Lancet* 359:1929.

10. WHO Fracture Risk Assessment Tool (FRAX). http://www.shef.ac.uk/FRAX (accessed June 5, 2012).

11. Grossman, J. M., R. Gordon, V. K. Ranganath, et al. American College of Rheumatology 2010 Recommendations for the Prevention and Treatment of Glucocorticoid-Induced Osteoporosis. *Arthritis Care Res* (Hoboken) 62:1515.

12. Sambrook, P., J. Birmingham, P. Kelly, et al. Prevention of Corticosteroid Osteoporosis: A Comparison of Calcium, Calcitriol, and Calcitonin. *N Engl J Med* 328:1747.

13. Cohen, S., R. M. Levy, M. Keller, et al. Risedronate Therapy Prevents Corticosteroid-Induced Bone Loss: A Twelve-Month, Multicenter, Randomized, Double-Blind, Placebo-Controlled, Parallel-Group Study. *Arthritis Rheum* 42:2309.

14. Saag, K. G., R. Emkey, T. J. Schnitzer, et al. Alendronate for the Prevention and Treatment of Glucocorticoid-Induced Osteoporosis. Glucocorticoid-Induced Osteoporosis Intervention Study Group. *N Engl J Med* 339:292.

15. American College of Rheumatology Ad Hoc Committee on Glucocorticoid-Induced Osteoporosis. Recommendations for the Prevention and Treatment of Glucocorticoid-Induced Osteoporosis: 2001 Update. *Arthritis Rheum* 44:1496.

16. Saag, K. G., E. Shane, S. Boonen, et al. Teriparatide or Alendronate in Glucocorticoid-Induced Osteoporosis. *N Engl J Med* 357:2028.

17. Orwoll, E., M. Ettinger, S. Weiss, et al. Alendronate for the Treatment of Osteoporosis in Men. *N Engl J Med* 343:604.

18. McClung, M. R., E. M. Lewiecki, S. B. Cohen, et al. Denosumab in Postmenopausal Women with Low Bone Mineral Density. *N Engl J Med* 354:821.

Chapter Twenty-one

Pediatric Rheumatology / Adult-Onset Still's Disease

Kids Are Not Little Adults, Even Though They Can Get Adult Diseases

I always take a deep breath and prepare my little speech about being an adult rheumatologist before walking into the room to see a pediatric case. I did have some training in pediatric rheumatology, but it was minimal. At the annual American College of Rheumatology meetings, I attend a seminar on pediatric rheumatology every other year. Still, I feel inadequate and like a stopgap, especially if it is something serious. With Jimmy it was no different. He was an eight-year-old boy who had a six-month history of limping intermittently after running into the side of a jungle gym. His parents initially thought it was just a bruise, but after the limping persisted, they took him to his pediatrician. After a negative x-ray, the doctor ordered an MRI and found fluid in Jimmy's left hip. Both ESR and CRP were elevated, indicating systemic inflammation. Juvenile idiopathic arthritis (JIA) was suspected, and Jimmy was referred to me. I found him to be a bright and active little boy who could still run and jump, but his parents said that he would intermittently limp, complain of pain at night, and uncharacteristically avoid sports. I found that there was some subtle loss of range of motion of his hip, and his white blood count was slightly elevated. He also tested negative for rheumatoid arthritis. The diagnosis of pauciarticular (less than five joints) JIA was probable but not certain. I felt that if he still had significant fluid in his hip joint that it should be aspirated under ultrasound or CT guidance and analyzed, and, if appropriate, steroid should be injected. I was not equipped to perform this procedure and referred him to a pediatric rheumatologist in Portland. In the meantime, it was important for Jimmy to see an ophthalmologist to screen for iritis, which can occur asymptomatically in these patients and lead to blindness. I also prescribed Naprosyn in pediatric doses and told his parents that if indeed it was pauciarticular JIA, there was about a 50 percent chance it would go into permanent remission. I obtained some further blood work, including an ANA, and told the parents that I would happy to see Jimmy again if the diagnosis was established and he was on a stable medication regimen. However, in the back of my mind, I was slightly worried by the high white blood cell count and nightly bone pain, which is characteristic of leukemia. I needed pediatric input and an aspiration if possible. His last WBC was normal, and I have not seen Jimmy back for a second visit yet.

I rarely see kids, but since there is no pediatric rheumatologist for about four hundred miles, I will occasionally see mild cases. As in life, kids aren't little adults, and although they can have lupus, RA, ankylosing spondylitis, fibromyalgia, dermatomyositis, scleroderma, vasculitis, and most other diseases, they may have different features and require slightly different treatment. I am not going to spend much time on pediatric disease because it is not my expertise, and I have little experience. If I am at all uncomfortable treating these patients, I send them to a pediatric rheumatologist. In children, inflammatory arthritis is called *juvenile idiopathic arthritis* and is divided into five categories—systemic arthritis, or Still's disease; polyarthritis, involving many joints; pauciarthritis, involving few joints; enthesitis-related arthritis, involving inflammation of the area where ligaments and tendons anchor into bone; and psoriatic arthritis, which is similar to the adult form. Each of these subsets has different features and courses and sometimes different treatments. The one subset I will discuss is systemic JIA, or Still's disease, because there is an adult form that I encounter and treat intermittently. These patients will have fevers of about 102 degrees Fahrenheit, often only in the afternoons. Inflammatory arthritis, a mild, short-lived, salmon-colored rash, and swollen glands are common. Enlarged liver and spleen, and pleural or pericardial effusions (fluid between the linings of the lungs or heart) are also often seen. Many adults with this disease are referred after an extensive workup by infectious disease and hematology because of their fevers and high white blood cell counts. Infection and leukemia are suspected. These patients often have high ESRs, CRPs, platelets, and serum ferritin (an iron measurement). All these measurements reflect inflammation. I recently had a patient who had an elevated ferritin reflecting active disease. He called my office asking why I hadn't treated his elevated iron. Unsatisfied with my answer, he had his internist call me and inquire about phlebotomies or blood-letting to reduce the iron levels, thinking that the patient had an iron storage disease called *hemochromatosis*. I explained that elevated serum ferritin just reflects active disease and not iron overload. In fact the patient's iron saturation was only 34 percent which is in the medium range. She seemed to understand, and I was also able to reassure the patient and eventually convince him that he needed more aggressive treatment for his Still's disease.

Most patients will just complain of fever, fatigue, and muscle or joint pain and may even have elevated muscle enzymes reflecting muscle inflammation. NSAIDs may be adequate to treat fevers and joint pain but usually not. Steroids may be the initial treatment for high fevers and lung or heart inflammation. Sometimes methotrexate is effective. I have used Plaquenil with success, but it is not usually recommended. Anakinra, or Kineret, is probably the most successful biologic, but the TNF inhibitors can also be useful, and Actemra has had some success. Recently Ilaris (canakinumab), another IL-1 inhibitor, was approved for treatment of JIA, and since it is a monthly subcutaneous injection, it may be preferable to Kineret. I have yet to have experience with it and have not seen enough literature to pass judgment.

Pearls

- There are five subtypes of JIA.
- Pauciarticular is most likely to go into remission.
- All subtypes are at risk for uveitis and should be seen regularly by an ophthalmologist, especially for those patients with a positive ANA.
- They are usually different than adult RA, especially radiologically.
- NSAIDs may be appropriate for three months; then if patients do not achieve remission, they should be treated aggressively with methotrexate and/or a biologic.
- Intra-articular steroids are helpful in monoarticular or pauciarticular cases.
- Enthesitis may be hard to diagnose, but check ESR and CRP and look for psoriasis or ankylosing spondylitis.
- Systemic subtype, or Still's disease, is in the differential diagnosis of fever of unknown origin or periodic fevers and may occur in adults.

- In Still's disease, low-grade fevers with two spikes usually occur in the morning and late afternoon.
- In Still's disease, transient, salmon-colored rash, elevated white blood cell count, lymphadenopathy (swollen glands), sore throat, arthritis (may be destructive), enlarged spleen, and in-flamed pleura, myocardium, or pericardium are all possible manifestations.
- Serum ferritin, ESR, CRP, and CPK can all be elevated in Still's.
- In JIA patients with joint disease who fail methotrexate, TNF an-tagonists would be the drugs of choice, but Orencia or Actemra would be alternatives.
- In patients with other systemic features who fail NSAIDs, ste-roids, and methotrexate, IL-1 or IL-6 antagonists would be the drugs of choice.
- Beware of macrophage activating syndrome (MAS)!

References

1. www.uptodate.com
2. www.rheumatology.org/Practice
(Patient Education—Diseases and Conditions)
3. Beukelman, T., N. M. Patkar, K. G. Saag, et al. 2011 American College of Rheumatology Recommendations for the Treatment of Juvenile Idiopathic Arthritis: Initiation and Safety Monitoring of Therapeutic Agents for the Treatment of Arthritis and Systemic Features. *Arthritis Care Res* (Hoboken) 63:465.
4. Irigoyen, P. I., J. Olson, C. Horn, et al. Treatment of Systemic Onset Juvenile Rheumatoid Arthritis with Anakinra. *Arthritis Rheum* 50:S437.
5. Ruperto, N., H. I. Brunner, P. Quartier, et al. Two Randomized Trials of Canakinumab in Systemic Juvenile Idiopathic Arthritis. *N Engl J Med* 367:2396.

6. Yokota, S., T. Imagawa, M. Mori, et al. Efficacy and Safety of Tocilizumab in Patients with Systemic-Onset Juvenile Idiopathic Arthritis: A Randomised, Double-Blind, Placebo-Controlled, Withdrawal Phase III Trial. *Lancet* 371:998.

7. Kimura, Y., P. Pinho, G. Walco, et al. Etanercept Treatment in Patients with Refractory Systemic Onset Juvenile Rheumatoid Arthritis. *J Rheumatol* 32:935.

8. Russo, R. A., and M. M. Katsicas. Clinical Remission in Patients with Systemic Juvenile Idiopathic Arthritis Treated with Anti-tumor Necrosis Factor Agents. *J Rheumatol* 36:1078.

9. Prahalad, S., K. E. Bove, D. Dickens, et al. Etanercept in the Treatment of Macrophage Activation Syndrome. *J Rheumatol* 28:2120.

10. Minden, K., M. Niewerth, J. Listing, et al. Long-Term Outcome in Patients with Juvenile Idiopathic Arthritis. *Arthritis Rheum* 46:2392.

11. Singh-Grewal, D., R. Schneider, N. Bayer, and B. M. Feldman. Predictors of Disease Course and Remission in Systemic Juvenile Idiopathic Arthritis: Significance of Early Clinical and Laboratory Features. *Arthritis Rheum* 54:1595.

12. Cassidy, J. T., and R. E. Petty. Juvenile Rheumatoid Arthritis. In *Textbook of Pediatric Rheumatology*, 4th edition, edited by J. T. Cassidy and R. E. Petty, Philadelphia: WB Saunders Company.

13. Davì, S., A. Consolaro, D. Guseinova, et al. An International Consensus Survey of Diagnostic Criteria for Macrophage Activation Syndrome in Systemic Juvenile Idiopathic Arthritis. *J Rheumatol* 38:764.

14. Flatø, B., G. Lien, A. Smerdel-Ramoya, and O. Vinje. Juvenile Psoriatic Arthritis: Long-Term Outcome and Differentiation from Other Subtypes of Juvenile Idiopathic Arthritis. *J Rheumatol* 36:642.

Chapter Twenty-two

Osteoarthritis and Soft Tissue Injuries

I know osteoarthritis and soft tissue injuries from the inside and outside. Having run twenty-seven marathons and cycled, swam, and run many miles for nearly forty years of my life, I can't remember many painless days. I have suffered a variety of injuries, some of which are now chronic, yet I am able to continue what my friend and fellow marathoner Con Dooley calls "a head-banging lifestyle." Therefore, I have taken special interest in sports medicine, soft tissue injuries, and rehabilitation. In this section, I will review briefly my treatment for some of the common wear-and-tear soft tissue injuries and the most common forms of osteoarthritis (DJD). When I was in training, I spent time at Rancho Las Amigos Hospital—a rehabilitation facility—and would spend hours hanging out in the physical and occupational therapy departments, reading manuals and talking to the therapists. In addition, over the years as I've developed a variety of injuries from my "head-banging" ways, I've read many books and spent hours rehabilitating in physical therapy, where I tried to pick the therapists' brains and observe other patients. Once I discover what works for me, I apply it to others, adjusting to their special needs. Finally, after years of treating patients, I've discovered that medicine is truly a practice—I discard the methods that fail and keep the successes. Common sense is the best guide, and patient feedback is the best validation. Here are some of my pearls.

Warranty Has Expired

Marianne is a fairly accomplished artist in her sixties who I have been following for several years. She has severe osteoarthritis of her hands, especially her thumb, and has mild osteoarthritis of both knees. She is an avid rower and has difficulty gripping the oars because of pain in her right thumb and wrist. NSAIDs, topical or oral, have been only mildly successful, and she has requested too many injections into her first carpometacarpal (CMC) for my comfort. I ordered a functional CMC splint from occupational therapy (OT). It will secure the joint and can be worn during most activities and alleviate pain. I have hundreds of patients wearing such a splint, but it is made of too hard and inflexible a material for rowing. I had OT make a more flexible one for rowing and another one for her art. She is happy with the results but has some pain and swelling in her right knee. She has regained the twenty pounds she lost when she was first diagnosed with arthritis of her knee. I noted the change and gently suggested that it may be part of the problem. In the meantime, I aspirated 15 cc of clear yellow fluid out of her knee and injected it with steroids. I also discussed injecting her knee in the future with Synvisc (see glossary and medication chapter), which was successful a year ago. She promised to lose the weight, buy some new, better support shoes, and consider Synvisc by our next visit. I reiterated that I would rather not inject steroids into her knee again. As far as I know, she is back in her rowing classes and continues her career as an artist.

DJD of the First Carpometacarpal Joint (CMC)

One of the major things that distinguish humans from apes is our ability to oppose our thumb to our forefinger and grasp objects. Over a lifetime we repeat this action many times a day, putting strain on a joint at the base of the thumb just above the wrist called the *first CMC joint*. In some cases the cartilage or padding will wear down, and the adjacent bones will compensate by hypertrophying, often creating a squaring appearance. Patients will complain of a painful and weak grip and begin to lose the ability to grasp things. As a cyclist I have found it painful to grasp the handlebars on long rides and have to put my thumb over rather than around the handlebars. I find NSAIDs only slightly helpful but mostly in the topical form. Injections with steroids can be effective but over time become less and less so and can actually damage the joint if done too often. Surgery is a last resort and is not always effective. I find the easiest and most effective treatment for most patients is a splint made by occupational therapy that is from fiberglass material and wraps just around that joint (not the wrist) and is worn during most activities but not during sleep. Thus, it is called a *functional first CMC splint*. Store-bought or softer versions do not seem very effective, although for some activities the softer versions may be necessary. Unfortunately these splints are not waterproof and are discarded during dishwashing. After months of wearing these splints, some patients are able to function painlessly without them. They protect and put the joint to rest. Clearly, they don't work for everybody—musicians and artists especially—but they are a benign, easy fix for most patients. I have a favorite occupational therapist that fabricates all the splints and adjusts them when needed. Patients avoid ulcers, upset stomachs, kidney problems, unnecessary surgeries, and painful shots, and everybody is happy!

Pearls

- A functional first CMC splint made by an OT is the best therapy for first CMC DJD.
- The first CMC is the most common hand joint involved in DJD.
- Patients often complain of wrist pain.

DJD of the Rest of the Hand

I have a few artists and musicians in my practice who have significant osteoarthritis of their hands. They include a local blues guitarist and an older gentleman who has decided he wants to become a classical pianist. I also intermittently see an older lady who has pretty deformed hands and yet is an outstanding artist. Their symptoms are usually stiffness and to a minor degree pain. They have bony swelling at their two distal knuckles, called *proximal*, and the distal interphalangeal joints (PIPs and DIPs) and sometimes have small, little, bony hooks at the DIPs called Heberden's nodes and Bouchard's at the PIPs. In severe cases, such as the artist, patients can have markedly dislocated knuckles. They should be differentiated from psoriatic arthritis, gout, pseudogout, and rheumatoid arthritis patients. Remarkably almost all patients can remain very functional. I find hot or warm water or paraffin will relieve the stiffness, and kneading clay, dough, or putty during leisure moments maintains flexibility. NSAIDs are helpful for pain and swelling, and I tend to use topicals for tolerability. In elderly more than younger patients, I watch kidney and liver functions carefully, and of course, I am concerned about the possibility of GI bleeds and ulcers in all patients taking NSAIDs. I send rare patients to occupational therapy (OT) for ring splints that wrap above and below the DIPs and PIPs. I have never sent a patient for surgery for DJD of the hand, and I do not prescribe narcotics. As mentioned previously, pain is usually not a major complaint with DJD, but if it is, look for fibromyalgia and treat it, or look for other causes, such as carpal tunnel syndrome, an inflammatory arthritis, or repetitive trauma (such as karate).

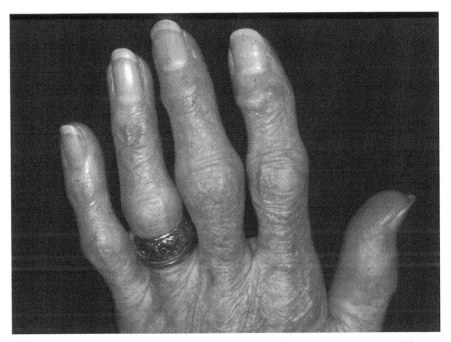

Osteoarthritis or degenerative arthritis with Bouchard's and Heberden's nodes—courtesy of ACR image bank

Pearls

- Most patients complain of mild pain and stiffness.
- If pain is more severe, look for another underlying problem, such as fibromyalgia or an inflammatory process, such as gout, pseudogout, psoriasis, or RA.
- Thermal modalities and topical NSAIDs are usually all that necessary.

References

1. Rheumatic Disease by Jeanne Melvin

2. www.rheumatology.org/Practice
(Patient Education—Diseases and Conditions)

3. www.niams.nih.gov>Health_info (Handbook on www.rheumatology.org/Practice
(Handout on Health: Osteoarthritis)

4. Hochberg, M. C., R. D. Altman, K. T. April, et al. American College of Rheumatology 2012 Recommendations for the Use of Nonpharmacologic and Pharmacologic Therapies in Osteoarthritis of the Hand, Hip, and Knee. *Arthritis Care Res* (Hoboken) 64:465.

5. Zhang, W., G. Nuki, R. W. Moskowitz, et al. OARSI Recommendations for the Management of Hip and Knee Osteoarthritis: Part III: Changes in Evidence Following Systematic Cumulative Update of Research Published through January 2009. *Osteoarthritis Cartilage* 18:476.

6. 2008. "Diclofenac Gel for Osteoarthritis." *Med Lett Drugs Ther* 50:31.

DJD of the Knees

The bane of the knee is obesity. Once I verify that a patient has DJD of the knees, I share with them three basic universal truths. Excess weight will accelerate the deterioration of cartilage in the knee, so weight control is very important. Good support shoes (with ties) and possibly orthotics help the knees track better and may alleviate pain. I advise most patients regardless of age to buy a good pair of motion-control running shoes at a good running shoe store where an expert can analyze their gait and recommend appropriate footwear. Many older patients have flat feet and pronate their ankles, or turn them inward; therefore, they need shoes that have a wedge on the inside, or medial side, of the shoe. Motion-control shoes and good orthotics do so. I have studied or used many brands and types of running shoes, and the barefoot concept does not work for bad feet or knees. My flippers, or flat feet, will not allow me to walk or run without knee pain unless I have good support shoes or orthotics. These days, I can buy good orthotics in a running store for $35 (I prefer Superfeet), whereas years ago my custom-made orthotics cost $400. It's been worthwhile browsing in various running shoe stores and catalogues to see what's available.

Finally, quadriceps strengthening will also help knees track better and give better support. I either instruct patients on how to strengthen these muscles or send them to a PT. Many years ago, we advised patients to avoid weight bearing if they had arthritis of their knees, but the pendulum has swung the other way, and the consensus is "move it or lose it," unless the knee is swollen or inflamed. If the patients have trouble walking, sometimes custom-made knee braces or supports are helpful, but they are inconvenient and unwieldy. I also find that once they need braces, they are only a year away from surgery. Some time ago when running with a buddy, I encountered a former runner with bad knees who was fast walking in the hills at a torrid pace using hiking poles. He told us that the poles were the best investment he had made in years. Since then I have advised patients with bad knees, hips, or peripheral neuropathy to purchase a pair. They unload the joints and help with proprioception. They are more symmetrical than canes, more streamlined and less awkward than crutches, and a lot cooler!

Knee swelling and warmth may mean that the patient has a superimposed inflammatory process, such as pseudogout or gout (or even infection), or more likely some torn or loose cartilage. If NSAIDs do not resolve the problem, the knee needs to be drained and the fluid examined (preferably under a polarizing microscope, which I have in my office). Usually I will also inject the knee with a steroid through the same needle, so there is only one stick. I advise the patient to avoid weight bearing as much as possible for forty-eight hours for the best results. Most patients will have miraculous results that will last for three to six months, but the more severe the arthritis, the less likely it will work and the shorter the duration of relief.

I prescribe topical and occasionally oral NSAIDs for those who need it, avoiding narcotics. Tylenol is rarely effective but may be worth a try. For those who continue to have pain despite trying everything, I sometimes inject their knees with a Hyalgan derivative, usually Synvisc-One. It is a gel made from rooster comb cartilage and works as a good anti-inflammatory or lubricant. I find it works in 60 percent of patients for up to six months and may be given no more frequently than every six months.

Glucosamine and chondroitin, alone or in combination, have its advocates, and as one of my colleagues reminds me, they are effective in dogs and horses, so they must work. Unfortunately, studies not funded by the drug industries have not supported those claims. Still, placebo works in 30 percent of patients, so I tell patients if they want to try it, make sure they try a cheap formulation. I have the same approach with MSM and anti-inflammatory diets and supplements. Remember, testimonials are not scientific, although for some patients they are powerful, and I try to remain open as long as the therapy is not harmful. Placebo is powerful.

Finally when the patient's quality of life is impacted and the patient has virtually no cartilage left, I recommend a knee replacement. Most orthopedic surgeons do not want to perform surgery on patients too young. The replacements last up to twenty years but much less in someone who is hard on them, such as a young person who may have to have to have multiple revisions. My ninety-one-year-old mother needed knee replacements when she was around eighty years old, and now she is virtually immobile but refuses surgery because of her age. Her quality of life has suffered dramatically as a consequence, so I recommend not waiting past eighty to have this procedure done. As a runner I am acutely aware that once you have your knee replaced, you shouldn't run, or you may loosen the prosthesis or prematurely wear it down. Still, some people do and claim that their orthopedic surgeon approved. Nevertheless, as a runner I would wait until I can't possibly shuffle with my buddies before having it done. There is also a whole spectrum of pain tolerance among patients. There is the fibromyalgia patient whose pain level is twelve out of ten with minimal osteoarthritis, and then there is my friend Carol who is still running fifty-mile races on knees that are bone on bone. She no longer finishes first.

Pearls

- Move it or lose it—keep mobile! Cycling and swimming and elliptical are helpful but use different muscles than walking.
- Weight loss, good support shoes, and quadriceps strengthening are important starting points for therapy.

- Topical NSAIDs may be helpful.
- Oral NSAIDs are also helpful, but monitor kidney and liver function and watch for GI bleeds. I prefer topicals, especially in elderly patients, and avoid them all in the face of kidney disease.
- Intra-articular steroids are effective in acute flares, but always aspirate the joint and check the fluid for crystals and cell count.
- Do not inject steroids more than three or four times a year and at no less than three month intervals.
- Hyaluronate intra-articular injections are effective in some patients and may last up to six months.
- Braces help some patients for a limited period of time.
- Hiking poles are cool and symmetrical and may give better balance than canes.
- If patients have an end-stage knee and are over sixty, refer them to orthopedics before they are too old or debilitated, or their quality of life will suffer when they are elderly.

References

1. Sharma, L., J. Song, D. T. Felson, et al. The Role of Knee Alignment in Disease Progression and Functional Decline in Knee Osteoarthritis. *JAMA* 286:188.

2. Losina, E., R. P. Walensky, W. M. Reichmann, et al. Impact of Obesity and Knee Osteoarthritis on Morbidity and Mortality in Older Americans. *Ann Intern Med* 154:217.

3. Steultjens, M. P., J. Dekker, and J. W. Bijlsma. Avoidance of Activity and Disability in Patients with Osteoarthritis of the Knee: The Mediating Role of Muscle Strength. *Arthritis Rheum* 46:1784.

4. van Dijk, G. M., J. Dekker, C. Veenhof, et al. Course of Functional Status and Pain in Osteoarthritis of the Hip or Knee: A Systematic Review of the Literature. *Arthritis Rheum* 55:779.

5. Brouwer, G. M., A. W. van Tol, A. P. Bergink, et al. Association between Valgus and Varus Alignment and the Development and Progression of Radiographic Osteoarthritis of the Knee. *Arthritis Rheum* 56:1204.

6. Hochberg, M. C., R. D. Altman, K. T. April, et al. American College of Rheumatology 2012 Recommendations for the Use of Nonpharmacologic and Pharmacologic Therapies in Osteoarthritis of the Hand, Hip, and Knee. *Arthritis Care Res* (Hoboken) 64:4657. Diclofenac Gel for Osteoarthritis. *Med Lett Drugs Ther* 50:31

7. Tugwell, P. S., G. A. Wells, and J. Z. Shainhouse. Equivalence Study of a Topical Diclofenac Solution (Pennsaid) Compared with Oral Diclofenac in Symptomatic Treatment of Osteoarthritis of the Knee: A Randomized Controlled Trial." *J Rheumatol* 31:2002.

8. Lambert, R. G., E. J. Hutchings, M. G. Grace, et al. Steroid Injection for Osteoarthritis of the Hip: A Randomized, Double-Blind, Placebo-Controlled Trial." *Arthritis Rheum* 56:2278.

9. Clegg, D. O., D. J. Reda, C. L. Harris, et al. Glucosamine, Chondroitin Sulfate, and the Two in Combination for Painful Knee Osteoarthritis. *N Engl J Med* 354:795.

10. Reginster, J. Y. The Efficacy of Glucosamine Sulfate in Osteoarthritis: Financial and Nonfinancial Conflict of Interest. *Arthritis Rheum* 56:2105.

11. Altman, R. D., and R. Moskowitz. Intraarticular Sodium Hyaluronate (Hyalgan) in the Treatment of Patients with Osteoarthritis of the Knee: A Randomized Clinical Trial. Hyalgan Study Group. *J Rheumatol* 25:2203.

12. Jüni, P., S. Reichenbach, S. Trelle, et al. Efficacy and Safety of Intraarticular Hylan or Hyaluronic Acids for Osteoarthritis of the Knee: A Randomized Controlled Trial. *Arthritis Rheum* 56:3610.

DJD of the Hips

The Age of Bionics

Recently, I saw a ninety-one-year-old patient who was referred to me with severe knee and back pain. She was a former CEO of a big company and was still a very active and intellectually sharp woman. She played tennis and golf regularly until recently. X-rays and MRIs of her back and knee revealed moderate degenerative arthritis, but injections in these areas were ineffective. When I examined her, I found that her hip had lost significant range of motion, and a subsequent x-ray showed severe osteoarthritis with complete obliteration of the joint space. She is now scheduled for hip replacement. Hip arthritis can refer pain to the knee and buttock, and unless the joint is examined, the diagnosis will be missed.

On the other hand, many of the patients who complain of hip pain don't have hip problems. The vast majority will be complaining of buttock pain, which is referred from the back. A good history and exam should be able to distinguish the two, but I have patients who insist the pain is coming from their hips despite my reassurance and a negative x- ray. In these cases, only an MRI of their hips and a second opinion will satisfy. It's frustrating but rare and certainly not cost effective. On the flip side, as mentioned above, some patients complaining of knee pain actually have referred pain from their hip, and since they have no pain there, they have a hard time believing that it is a hip problem. There are many causes of hip pain that aren't arthritis, such as polymyalgia rheumatica in an elderly patient, trochanteric bursitis, tendonitis, and inguinal hernias. A good exam and history and sometimes but not always x-rays should easily distinguish osteoarthritis from the others. Once DJD is established, I have patients work on flexibility and strengthening, sometimes prescribing physical therapy. Mobility is essential, and if walking is difficult,

I recommend my latest favorite innovation—hiking poles, for all the reasons I mentioned previously. A good pair of walking or running shoes is always helpful. Patients should avoid slippers or flip-flops; both put the patients at risk for falling and give no support.

NSAIDs or Tylenol around the clock can be helpful, but in elderly patients especially I am concerned about kidney or liver disease or gastrointestinal bleeding with long-term use. Again, I avoid narcotics except for short-term use. Just as in the knees, the studies supporting the use of glucosamine, chondroitin, MSM, and so forth are shaky, but if they are cheap, they may be worth a try if the patient is motivated. Sometimes a relative's, friend's, or celebrity's advice has more powerful effect than a doctor's.

Very rarely I will inject the hip with steroids and lidocaine. Although I use anatomy landmarks to guide my injections and have had some good success, ultrasound or CT-guided injections are probably more accurate.

When the patient has an end-stage hip and all medical options have been exhausted, I refer them to an orthopedic surgeon for a hip replacement. Recently, patients seem to prefer minimally invasive versions, but I am not well versed in the different options for surgery so won't comment. Again, the degree of pain is not always a good indicator for surgery because the pain may be multifactorial. Some of the pain may be coming from the spine and may be amplified by fibromyalgia or depression, so surgery may not be the best solution. I try to refer to thoughtful, conservative surgeons who will analyze all these factors before recommending surgery.

Pearls

- Move it or lose it—keep walking and active. Cycling and swimming and elliptical are helpful but use different muscles than walking.

- Hiking poles may be superior walking aids.
- Weight control, stretches, and strengthening are helpful.
- NSAIDs are helpful, but watch kidney and liver function and beware of GI bleeds.
- Glucosamine and chondroitin have conflicting support in studies. Try six months of an inexpensive version, and if ineffective, discontinue it.
- When the hip is end stage and quality of life is threatened, an orthopedic referral is the best choice.

References

1. www.uptodate.com
2. www.rheumatology.org/Practice
(Patient Education—Diseases and Conditions)
3. www.niams.nih.gov>health_info (Handout on Health: Osteoarthritis)
4. Hochberg, M. C., R. D. Altman, K. T. April, et al. American College of Rheumatology 2012 Recommendations for the Use of Nonpharmacologic and Pharmacologic Therapies in Osteoarthritis of the Hand, Hip, and Knee. *Arthritis Care Res* (Hoboken) 64:465.
5. Zhang, W., M. Doherty, N. Arden, et al. EULAR Evidence Based Recommendations for the Management of Hip Osteoarthritis: Report of a Task Force of the EULAR Standing Committee for International Clinical Studies Including Therapeutics (ESCISIT). *Ann Rheum Dis* 64:669.

Lumbar Spondylosis, or DJD of the Lumbar Spine

Mortality Sucks (so Does Back Pain)

I have had a bad back for over twenty years. For the first few years, I could not escape the pain. If I stood or sat for too long, I felt like I was performing seppuku—the Japanese suicide ritual where one runs a sword through one's gut. The pain would radiate from my back through my midsection and eventually into my buttocks and down my legs. It literally made me sick and took the wind out of my sails. It was always in the background and sucked any joy or happiness from my life. I was diagnosed with lumbar spondylosis with multiple bulging discs, one of which was torn and leaking. I also had sacroiliac dysfunction, which or may or may not have been related. The sacroiliac (SI) joints are in the back of the pelvis and move symmetrically with walking. Occasionally one gets stuck, and the muscles around it spasm, and the ligaments stretch, causing pain. Not only was my running career off the tracks, but I found it difficult to manage chronic-pain patients and maintain my composure and a clear head. I began to see fewer patients and spend my evenings lying on the floor. My social life was severely limited, and my disposition soured. I rode my bicycle and swam for exercise, but even these activities became difficult. I tried NSAIDs, but they were minimally effective, and I wasn't sure whether the nausea and diarrhea they caused were better than the pain relief. I tried muscle relaxants, but after a lost afternoon where my office manager could not rouse me from a deep sleep in my office chair until all the patients had rescheduled, I decided they were not the solution. Narcotics gave me "brain farts," where I had major lapses in memory—very dangerous for a doctor treating patients. So I was stuck with nonpharmacological options. I tried hanging upside down like a bat at a chiropractor's

267

office four days a week for six months, without success, although I met some interesting people who swore it helped them. I tried acupuncture with and without electrical stimulation and Chinese herbs, with no relief. I had chiropractors crack my back and adjust my SI joints, without effect, even though they were very optimistic. Two psychotherapists helped me grapple with my neurosis and deconstruct my childhood. I studied research and literature on back pain and visited orthopedic surgeons. The first surgeon gave me the best advice in retrospect, even though I despised and resented it initially. After examining me and looking at my x-rays, he told me, "Have a good attitude, and it will get better." I wanted a quick, easy fix. How callous and unsympathetic could he be? So I spent the next few years raging against the pain and making some huge missteps, including rollerblading down a hill without kneepads, fracturing my kneecap, and tearing my posterior cruciate ligaments in one knee. I was a mess and at wits end. I let a neurosurgeon talk me into a minimally invasive needle procedure on one of my discs, with poor results. My world was closing in on me—I felt I lived in a shrinking box where I could do less and less. It brought me to the brink—I was staring at the abyss. Finally, I decided I needed to change course, attitude, or perspective. I started a new physical therapy program focusing on my core strength and maintaining flexibility. I bought a new custom-made road bicycle and road big miles over the weekends. I swam and took spin cycling classes during the week. I worked hard at managing my stress better, changed all the furniture in my house to accommodate my back, started running slowly and minimally when my knee recovered, and finally, swallowed my ego and let friends carry my heavy bags when grocery shopping. I also walked miles during the evenings, avoided sitting for long periods, and poured out my heart and soul into a semifictional first novel. I started to improve but was still in pain after a year or two. Finally, I moved from LA to Ashland and no longer spent half my life in a car. I began to run more and continued my flexibility and core work and eventually began riding my bicycle to work. Within two years my constant pain had disappeared, and within three I ran another marathon.

Dealing with chronic back pain is a marathon, and if you surrender to it early and become passive, you will not be successful. I have treated many patients with acute and chronic back pain. Most acute pain resolves within weeks. There can be many causes, such as muscle strain and spasm of a variety of muscles (including the piriformis), herniated or torn discs, "pinched nerves" or radiculopathy, SI joint dysfunction, a fractured or collapsed vertebra, kidney infection, and a variety of inflammatory conditions. It's important that physicians take a good history and examine the patients, or they may prescribe the wrong treatment. When I was teaching years ago, I found that many physicians could describe the patient's MRI but not the back exam because they hadn't even performed one. Patients often focus on the bulging discs on their MRIs as a sign that they are untreatable without surgery. Most of us over fifty have bulging discs—it is part of the degenerative process. In the early 1990s, there was a study where they performed a large number of MRIs on patients who were divided into two groups: one with back pain and one without. The radiologists were blinded; in other words, they weren't told who did or didn't have back pain. Interestingly, just as many people who had back pain had normal MRIs as people who didn't, and the reverse was also true. So back pain is multifactorial, and bulges do not tell the whole story. Depression, poor stress management, and core muscle strength, bad ergonomics at work and play, and physical strain and abnormal anatomy, among other factors, all play a part and must be addressed.

About once a month, someone limps into my office shaped like an S, with a strained smile and a dull look in his or her eyes.

Inevitably, the patient has an acute back problem. A good history and exam usually narrows the differential diagnosis and helps focus treatment. If it is an older patient on steroids, I would rule out a collapsed vertebra. If it is a younger, active patient, chances are that he or she has an acute muscle strain, SI joint dysfunction, or disc problem. Many years ago these patients would be put on strict bed rest for two weeks, but the duration has been found to be counterproductive because it promotes muscle atrophy. I usually put patients on two days' strict bed rest—tell them to enlist a "slave," like a husband or a wife, and avoid any sitting position for more than twenty minutes. During those two days, I prescribe 10–15 mg of Valium a day as a muscle relaxant and give them a tapering dose of steroids, MedrolPak), as a potent anti-inflammatory. The Valium also keeps them sedated and sleeping and counteracts the stimulatory effects of high-dose steroids. Usually I follow those two days with physical therapy, which includes back school (the do's and don't's of backcare), core strengthening, McKenzie (extension) exercises, occasional modalities, and, where appropriate, ergonomic and postural evaluation and therapy and work hardening. I emphasize to the patient that the work has just begun, and they must continue this program at home, especially if the back pain has been recurrent or has been present for more than three months. If the patient can't afford physical therapy, I recommend Pilates and/or yoga and a walking program. Occasionally, I will prescribe NSAIDs but almost never narcotics, except for a very short duration; otherwise many potential problems, including narcotic dependence and hyperalgesia, may arise. Some practitioners disagree.

If the back pain has been chronic, I make sure the patient has had a thorough workup ruling out inflammatory back disease such as that seen in ankylosing spondylitis. I ask a lot of questions: Was the onset in the teens or twenties? Is it worse in the morning? Does it wake the patient from sleep? Does exercise make it better? Does morning stiffness last more than thirty minutes? Do NSAIDs help? Does it radiate into the buttocks? Are there any other joints or symptoms associated with it? These serve to confirm or rule out a diagnosis. A good exam will rule out many other causes, such as SI dysfunction, a short leg, and fibromyalgia. I do not initially order x-rays and will only order an MRI if I suspect neurological compromise. If the patient does not respond to my initial treatment, I may reconsider. Many of the older patients may have lumbar stenosis, meaning either the disc bulge or herniation or a bony outgrowth is narrowing the spinal canal and squeezing the spinal cord, creating pain and often neurological symptoms. These patients have often lost their ability to bend backward, walk in a flexed posture, and have leg pain or cramps with any prolonged walking. Their activity levels become increasingly limited. Half of these patients will respond to therapy and spinal injections; the others will require surgery. Most patients with plain lumbar spondylosis will respond to a combination of physical therapy, home programs, alterations in lifestyle and ergonomics, attitude adjustment, and occasional spinal injections. I find a pain specialist helpful when they concentrate on focal injections in the spine and spinal stimulators and avoid prescribing more and more narcotics. I have one such specialist whom I trust. NSAIDs and muscle relaxants are helpful in some patients, but long-term use is questionable. I find Lidoderm patches and TENS units helpful in some difficult patients. Lumbar braces and supports are helpful in some situations, such as long trips and postsurgical situations, but may cause muscle atrophy in the long run. Certainly, I have seen patients where all bets are off—they have the worst stenosis or spondylosis possible and are not surgical candidates, so you try everything or anything. When every measure has failed, the patient has some neurological compromise, or has a definite fixable anatomic abnormality on their MRI, I refer

them to a back surgeon. I have some favorites who do not think surgery first. I find that once a patient has had one surgery, he or she is
more likely to have more, especially if a fusion has been done. Since
surgery is not my expertise, I will keep my comments to a minimum,
but there are some patients for whom it is necessary and the outcome is swift and almost miraculous. Since surgery is irreversible
and can have rare horrendous outcomes, these patients should be
selected carefully.

Finally, attitude does count in back pain, and fibromyalgia and
depressed patients are less likely to have good outcomes unless
these problems are addressed. The orthopedic surgeon who told
me to have a good attitude was wise and compassionate after all.

Pearls

- Examine the back!
- Make sure SI joints are moving symmetrically.
- Proper ergonomics at home and work are important.
- Back friendly furniture is also key.
- For acute back pain, rest for two days (no longer), preferably in a
  supine position.
- Analgesics, anti-inflammatories, and muscle relaxants are help-
  ful for the short term, but long-term use may be harmful.
- Narcotics make central pain syndrome worse.
- Radiological findings don't correlate well with symptoms.
- Flexibility and core strengthening are equally important.
- Good attitude and patience go a long way.
- Good physical therapists are great allies.
- Epidurals are sometimes helpful for radiculopathies (nerve com-
  pression) or stenosis.
- Surgery is a last resort.

References

1. McKenzie, Robin A. *Treat Your Own Back.*

2. McKenzie, Robin A. *The Lumbar Spine Mechanical Diagnosis and Therapy.*

3. Katz, J. N., and M. B. Harris. Clinical Practice: Lumbar Spinal Stenosis. *N Engl J Med* 358:818.

4. Weinstein, J. N., T. D. Tosteson, J. D. Lurie, et al. Surgical versus Nonsurgical Therapy for Lumbar Spinal Stenosis. *N Engl J Med* 358:794.

5. Pinto, R. Z., C. G. Maher, M. L. Ferreira, et al. Epidural Corticosteroid Injections in the Management of Sciatica: A Systematic Review and Meta-analysis. *Ann Intern Med* 157:865.

6. Chou, R., A. Qaseem, V. Snow, et al. Diagnosis and Treatment of Low Back Pain: A Joint Clinical Practice Guideline from the American College of Physicians and the American Pain Society. *Ann Intern Med* 147:478.

7. Russel, A. S., W. Maksymowych, and S. LeClercq. Clinical Examination of the Sacroiliac Joints: A Prospective Study. *Arthritis Rheum* 24:1575.

8. Riddle, D. L., and J. K. Freburger. Evaluation of the Presence of Sacroiliac Joint Region Dysfunction Using a Combination of Tests: A Multicenter Intertester Reliability Study. *Phys Ther* 82:772.

9. Deyo, R. A., and J. N. Weinstein. Low Back Pain. *N Engl J Med* 344:363.

10. Jensen, M. C., M. N. Brant-Zawadzki, N. Obuchowski, et al. Magnetic Resonance Imaging of the Lumbar Spine in People without Back Pain. *N Engl J Med* 331:69.

Cervical Spondylosis, or Osteoarthritis of the Cervical Spine

Your Mother Was Right about Posture

Joan challenged me the first day I saw her. She was a seventy-two-year-old writer who had a ten-year history of neck pain. She had tried all kinds of medications, acupuncture, heat, cold, and even a neck brace without success. She was skeptical that I could help but was giving it one last shot. As a doctor, it's hard to say, "I can't help you." In most cases, there is always something. Joan was a tall, elegant-looking lady with rounded shoulders, thin upper body, slightly flexed neck, and generally poor posture from hours of sitting in front of a computer. Her MRI showed moderate osteoarthritis of her cervical spine but nothing dramatic. I checked her ESR and CRP to make sure she didn't have PMR, and they were normal. I suggested to her that if we could work on her posture, ergonomics, and strengthen her upper back and neck muscles, she might improve. It would take months of hard work at physical therapy, but it could be done. At first she was resistant and skeptical but reluctantly agreed to a two-month trial. In the meantime, I gave her some Lidoderm (like novocaine) patches to place on her neck. To my mild surprise, she returned to my office three months later with almost perfect posture and a smile. It never hurts to know a skilled physical therapist!

Like low back pain, the cause of neck pain is multifactorial. Patients can have horrendous x-rays or MRIs and have minimal pain or be in agony with normal x-rays. I know I'm in trouble when patients are talking about their "bulging discs" and implying that they are untreatable. Most neck patients get better with time and the appropriate treatment, including some adjustments in lifestyle and posture. My approach to patients who have an acutely painful neck is to take a good history and examine the patient. I look for a history of trauma or an inflammatory disease, such as RA or psoriatic arthritis. I perform a careful neurological exam, looking for any abnormality indicating a compromised or damaged nerve or spinal cord. If the patient has predominantly muscle spasm, I will advise heat and rest and give either Valium or another muscle relaxant for two days and a seven-day course of tapering steroids or a longer course of NSAIDs. I also perform a thorough rheumatology exam, looking for fibromyalgia or inflammatory arthritis. In chronic cases, I check their posture. Many patients have rounded shoulders and forward flexion of their neck, especially if they have been sitting at a desk looking at a computer all day. Strengthening their core and upper back muscles and better awareness of their position in space, especially at the end of the workday, may help. Ergonomic evaluation of the work place is productive. One of my trick questions is to ask how many pillows the patient uses at night and whether they read in bed. The answer should be one and no because prolonged flexion of the neck can lead to strain and exacerbate underlying arthritis. Physical therapy, including traction, stretches, exercises, and modalities such as ultrasound and phonophoresis, can be helpful. They can go over daily ergonomics with the patient and help the patient make adjustments. Chiropractors and osteopaths may make adjustments and work on the patient's musculature, but again, I advise against "cracking." Topical NSAIDs and Lidoderm patches may provide good relief. TENS (Transcutaneous nerve stimulator) units for home use can be effective. Relieving or addressing stress or depression may often be keys to relieving the pain. Cymbalta and other antidepressants may be the key. It is also important to discover what activities or positions trigger or exacerbate the pain and make changes. In RA, psoriasis, or ankylosing spondylitis, sudden onset of neck pain may mean subluxation or dislocation of the top two vertebrae because of stretching or tearing of their anchoring ligaments. It can lead to cord compression and quadriplegia. I consulted on a patient with ankylosing spondylitis who was involved in a motor accident and had sudden onset of neck pain. By the time I saw him a few days later, he was clearly weak and had very active reflexes. His x-rays in the ER were read as normal, but when we obtained x-rays and subsequent MRI with his neck in flexion and extension, it was obvious that he had fractured through a fused upper cervical spine and was on his way to becoming a quadriplegic. Most neck patients do not have such tragic outcomes. In fact, I find with the proper exercise and postural training almost every patient improves. Your mother was probably wiser than you think when she was constantly correcting your posture.

Pearls

- Posture and ergonomics are key.
- Core strengthening, especially the upper back, is extremely important.
- Good physical therapy, occasionally with traction, can make all the difference.
- Massage is also a consideration.
- Medications rarely help in the long term, but try topical NSAIDs.
- Focal facet and other injections may help.
- Address psychological stresses.

References

1. McKenzie, Robin A. *Treat Your Own Neck.*
2. McKenzie, Robin A. *The Cervical and Thoracic Spine Mechanical Diagnosis and Therapy.*
3. Carette, S., and M. G. Fehlings. "Clinical practice: Cervical Radiculopathy." *N Engl J Med* 353:392.

4. Binder, A. L. "Cervical Pain Syndromes." In *Oxford Textbook of Rheumatology*, edited by P. J. Maddison, 1060. Oxford: Oxford Medical Publications.

5. Bronfort, G., R. Evans, A. V. Anderson, et al. Spinal Manipulation, Medication, or Home Exercise with Advice for Acute and Subacute Neck Pain: A Randomized Trial. *Ann Intern Med* 156:1.

6. Hoving, J. L., B. W. Koes, H. C. de Vet, et al. Manual Therapy, Physical Therapy, or Continued Care by a General Practitioner for Patients with Neck Pain: A Randomized, Controlled Trial. *Ann Intern Med* 136:713.

7. Walker, M. J., R. E. Boyles, B. A. Young, et al. The Effectiveness of Manual Physical Therapy and Exercise for Mechanical Neck Pain: A Randomized Clinical Trial. *Spine* (Philadelphia) 33:2371.

8. Thiel, H. W., J. E. Bolton, S. Docherty, and J. C. Portlock. Safety of Chiropractic Manipulation of the Cervical Spine: A Prospective National Survey. *Spine* (Philadelphia) 32:2375.

9. White, A. R., and E. Ernst. A Systematic Review of Randomized Controlled Trials of Acupuncture for Neck Pain. *Rheumatology* (Oxford) 38:143.

DJD of the Shoulders, Ankles, and Feet

The Catcher Who Could No Longer Throw

Rick is a barrel-chested, jovial ex-semiprofessional catcher. In the past, he always greeted me with a smile and a half-hearted handshake, raising his hand to belly button level. I knew almost immediately when I first saw him that he either had a rotator cuff tear or DJD of the shoulder or both. He had both. I tried treating him with physical therapy and joint injections, with mild, transient relief. His MRI showed a complete loss of cartilage in his shoulder as well as complete tears in two of his rotator cuff tendons. He was already taking a hefty dose of narcotics, and I had nothing else to offer, so I referred him to a shoulder surgeon. He can now raise his arm to chest level and has little pain.

Osteoarthritis of the shoulder is rare unless the patient has a history of trauma or an inflammatory process, such as RA or pseudogout. Most shoulder problems are related to rotator cuff tendonitis or tears, subacromial bursitis, or referred pain from the neck. Patients may have acromioclavicular joint osteoarthritis (where the collarbone ends and meets the shoulder) or dislocation. Arthritis of this joint may cause impingement of the rotator cuff tendons. If indeed the patient has DJD of the shoulder, strengthening exercises, NSAIDs, Lidoderm or NSAID patches, and occasional steroid injections are helpful. Occasionally in severe DJD, I have performed a suprascapular nerve block (this nerve provides sensation to the shoulder) with mixed success, but when patients have lost most of their cartilage and mobility, a total shoulder arthroplasty is probably best. Interestingly, I have a group of older patients who either are not surgical candidates or who refuse surgery and have recurrent huge effusions in their shoulders. I have aspirated as much as 540 cc of fluid from one of my patient's shoulder. I find that these patients usually have rotator cuff tears as well as a history of some sort of inflammatory arthritis, such as RA. They often look like they are wearing a one-sided football pad. Fortunately, their accumulation of fluid does not happen often, and it is usually responsive to an injection of steroids not given more than three to four times a year. Their response is usually miraculous, and patients are extremely grateful. I never inject steroid in a joint more often than once every three months, and if patients seem to need it more often, I refer them for possible surgery.

Pearls
- Strengthen rotator cuff, deltoids and all surrounding muscles.
- Occasional intra-articular injections are sometimes helpful.
- AC joint DJD may cause impingement.
- Total shoulder arthroplasty may be the only option for severe DJD of shoulder.

References

1. Anderson, B. C. *Office Orthopedics for Primary Care: Diagnosis*, third edition. Philadelphia: Elsevier Saunders Company.
2. Arkkila, P. E., I. M. Kantola, J. S. Viikari, and T. Rönnemaa. Shoulder Capsulitis in Type I and II Diabetic Patients: Association with Diabetic Complications and Related Diseases. *Ann Rheum Dis* 55:907.
3. Johnson, T. R. The Shoulder. In *Essentials of Musculoskeletal Care*, edited by R. K. Snider, xx–xx. Rosemont, IL: American Academy of Orthopaedic Surgeons.

Fractured Ankles and a Suicide

Even though Gregg came from a completely different background than me and had polar-opposite political and religious beliefs, we really connected. I had taught his daughter for a short time when she was a medical student and found her to be bright and delightful. He was a big man with a great family and a successful business. He had fractured his ankles jumping out of an airplane in Vietnam. I encouraged him to lose weight, put him in ankle braces, and injected his ankles intermittently over the years. He seemed to manage and remain active, but a few years ago he committed suicide for unknown reasons. He was a great guy. It is sad.

Ankle DJD is also extremely rare and occurs in the same settings as outlined above. Trauma with an associated fracture (caused by jumping out of buildings or helicopters) was the cause in two of my patients, and RA in another. I usually advise patients to keep their weight at a minimum, wear good support shoes, and wear a good ankle brace (often laced). Occasional steroid injections may be helpful, and when all else fails, I refer them to a surgeon for a fusion. In 2013, I am not sure about the reliability of an ankle replacement, although some of my patients have had short-term success.

My late father was disabled by an ankle problem that turned into severe DJD and eventual dislocation of his ankle. He had severe flat feet and tore the tendon that helps maintains ankle stability and prevents it from dislocating. The posterior tibial tendon is on the inside part of the ankle, and when it is torn, there is substantial pain and deformity. If the tear is missed, as it was in my dad, patients will eventually develop disability and severe arthritis. If there is a sudden increase in ankle pain and the patient develops a severe valgus (turns inward) deformity of the ankle, I always order an MRI. I never forget my dad.

Pearls

- Weight loss is important.
- Good support shoes are helpful.
- Ankle braces, which can fit into shoes, may alleviate pain and increase mobility.
- Hiking poles are helpful.
- Don't miss posterior tibial tendon ruptures.
- Posterior tibial tendonitis is a common overuse injury in patients with flat feet.
- Ankle fusion is still more successful than replacement, but the latter is getting better and may be the better option in the future.

References

1. Supple, K. M., J. R. Hanft, B. J. Murphy, et al. Posterior Tibial Tendon Dysfunction. *Semin Arthritis Rheum* 22:106.

2. Rees, J. D., A. M. Wilson, and R.L. Wolman. Current Concepts in the Management of Tendon Disorders. *Rheumatology* (Oxford) 45:508.

3. Gluck, G. S., D. S. Heckman, and S. G. Parekh. Tendon Disorders of the Foot and Ankle, Part 3: The Posterior Tibial Tendon. *Am J Sports Med* 38:2133.

DJD of the Feet

Pointy Shoes and Crooked Toes

Rose is one of hundreds of women I have seen over the years with the same profile and same problem. She is always immaculately dressed even at eighty and complains bitterly of her sore feet. Her big toe is at almost a V-shaped angle to her foot, and her toes look like claws. She hides her narrow-pointed high heels under her seat because she knows I won't approve. She is considering a bunionectomy on both feet but is hesitant about surgery at her age. When she asks me about alternatives, I smile and point at her shoes. It has become a ritual that won't change.

Finally, DJD of the feet is quite common, especially in women who wear shoes with narrow toe boxes. Hallux valgus is a form of osteoarthritis where the big toe loses cartilage and becomes increasingly crooked, almost forming a bony V where it attaches to the foot. Most people refer to it as a *bunion*. It can be painless or painful, and it can widen the foot so that it is harder to fit into shoes and be a source of cosmetic embarrassment. Good shoes with a wide toe box are often the answer, but a good podiatrist is helpful.

Arthritis of other toes can be a nuisance, unseemly, or very painful. Good cushioned shoes are again often the answer, and I find a good pair of running shoes is least expensive and most effective. However, many women are unhappy with this suggestion, and men sometimes need to wear work boots. Orthotics can be helpful and need not be custom made or expensive. Again, podiatrists are good people and helpful. It's important to take a good history and perform a good exam before assuming that foot pain is caused by arthritis. Plantar fasciitis, fractures, neuropathy, nerve entrapment, and Morton's neuroma are just a few of the common findings that should be ruled out. X-rays just tell part of the story and do not necessarily correlate with pain.

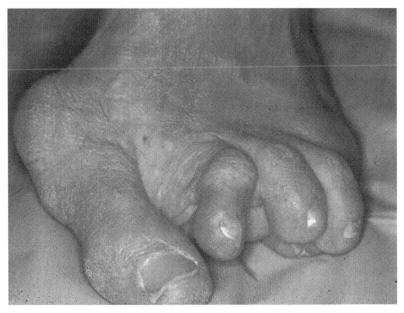

DJD or osteoarthritis with hallux valgus deformity (bunion)
and cock-up toes — courtesy of ACR image bank

Pearls

- Wear shoes with a wide toe box and good cushioning.
- A small doughnut pad at the metatarsal or first MTP may be helpful.
- Podiatrists are good people and often quite skilled.
- Surgery may be one answer, but it is not always the only one.

References

1. www.uptodate.com
2. www.niams.nih.gov>Health_info
(Handout on Health: Osteoarthritis)
3. Mann R., and M. Coughlin. Adult Hallux Valgus. In *Surgery of the Foot and Ankle*, edited by M. Coughlin and R. Mann, 150. St. Louis: Mosby.

Miscellaneous Soft Tissue Problems

Zumba Can Be Dangerous

Maria is my forty-five-year-old lupus patient who had a stroke a few years ago and completely recovered. She has been on steroids intermittently over the years, and all of her tissues are very thin. After several flailing arm movements while dancing the Zumba a week ago, she developed a sudden aching in her shoulder and has had trouble putting on her brassiere ever since. When I examined her, she could only raise her right arm above her chest with assistance and had pain when I lifted her arm above her shoulder from the side. She had partial relief from a steroid injection and two months of physical therapy. An MRI revealed a complete tear of one of her rotator cuff tendons. I referred her to a shoulder surgeon but he is reluctant to repair the tendons because the steroids have made them so friable. She has had two more months of physical therapy and can now put on her bra and has significantly less pain.

Rotator cuff tendonitis is probably the most common shoulder problem I see. Patients will complain of an ache radiating into their upper arm, especially when lifting their arm. They often have pain when I lift their arm up from the side and when it comes down. They also have weakness or pain when I push their arm outward with their elbow bent. The rotator cuff is a group of four muscles that surround the head of the humerus (the ball in the socket of the shoulder) and also attach to the scapula, or "wing." They stabilize the shoulder and act as a pulley system for its movement. If any of these muscles become inflamed or torn, movement becomes painful or difficult. A patient with a full tear usually cannot lift his arm from the side without help. Most patients will improve with a steroid injection in the subacromial space at the side of shoulder supplemented by a good physical therapy program. However, some patients cannot afford or refuse physical therapy, and I then recommend either buying a book on rotator cuff exercises or Googling them. Physical therapy alone and NSAIDs may suffice, but the injection and therapy seems to have the best outcome. If the patient does not respond after a few months, then I will obtain an x-ray and eventually an MRI. Several times a year, I have a patient call almost daily after the injection and a few weeks of physical therapy complaining of intense pain. The patient may have a tear, but usually it is fibromyalgia amplifying the pain. Inevitably, I will order an MRI, and if it is a tear or other major pathology, I will refer him or her to orthopedics. I will also treat any underlying fibromyalgia or depression. Other shoulder problems include subacromial bursitis, which involves a bursa in the shoulder and can mimic rotator cuff tendonitis. A bursa is a fluid-filled sac-like structure between bones and soft tissue, especially muscles. If it becomes inflamed the surrounding structures may develop pain. Many physicians seem to use bursitis as a throwaway term to placate their patients when they really don't know what's going on. There are a few bursas surrounding the shoulder, and ice, NSAIDs, or occasionally an injection will take care of any inflammation. Repetitive or unaccustomed movements or strain of the shoulder often are the cause of these problems. Pitchers and third basemen are very susceptible. However, aging and degeneration of tissue also can lead to inflammation and tears.

Frozen shoulder is another common problem and is often seen in diabetics. Neither the patient nor physician can lift the patient's arm very far. Often x-rays are normal, and there are no signs of inflammation. Patients often have developed adhesions in their shoulder capsule but occasionally have chronic inflammation or structural damage. In most cases steroid injections and PT are effective. Occasionally, manipulation of the shoulder under anesthesia is necessary.

Pearls

- Rotator cuff tendonitis can be fairly accurately diagnosed by a good clinician—painful arc when raising the arm from the side or externally rotating the arm when the elbow is flexed and the palm is against the abdomen are good signs.
- If the patient can't raise the arm but the clinician can raise it for him or her, think rotator cuff tear.
- A steroid injection into the subacromial space, together with physical therapy, is the best treatment.

References

1. Robinson, Jerry, and Joseph Horrigan. *Seven Minute Rotator Cuff Solution.*

2. Cook, Chad E. *Orthopedic Manual Therapy.*

3. Van der Windt, D. A., B. W. Koes, B. A. de Jong, and L. M. Bouter. Shoulder Disorders in General Practice: Incidence, Patient Characteristics, and Management. *Ann Rheum Dis* 54:959.

4. Rees, J. D., A. M. Wilson, and R. L. Wolman. Current Concepts in the Management of Tendon Disorders. *Rheumatology* (Oxford) 45:508.

5. Naredo, E., P. Aguado, E. De Miguel, et al. Painful Shoulder: Comparison of Physical Examination and Ultrasonographic Findings. *Ann Rheum Dis* 61:132.

6. Kibler, W. B. Rehabilitation of Rotator Cuff Tendinopathy. *Clin Sports Med* 22:837.

Lateral and Medial Epicondylitis

It's Not Tennis Anymore—
It's the Computer!

My transcriptionist Susan, is a young fifty-year-old and has been complaining of weakness and pain in her right elbow and forearm. She has had trouble lifting things with that hand, and her elbow aches at night. NSAIDs, ice, and a wrap have not helped. I finally told her to come see me and found that she had lateral epicondylitis. I showed her some stretches, advised her to make sure her workstation was ergonomically sound, and sent her home with a topical NSAID. She has not complained in weeks, but then again I haven't asked.

Lateral and medial epicondylitis are common causes of elbow pain. Formerly known as *tennis elbow* because it was common in tennis players, lateral epicondylitis involves the tendons on the radial, or outside, part of the elbow originating at the elbow and attaching at the wrist. These tendons perform the function of extending the wrist. Any repetitive extension or pressure against an extended wrist may cause inflammation or tearing of the tendons and pain radiating from the elbow down the forearm. Occasionally, patients will complain solely of forearm pain. These days, overuse of a computer mouse causes this problem, as does carrying heavy shopping bags or briefcases for any length of time.

Medial epicondylitis is the mirror image, involving the tendons originating at the ulnar, or inside, part of the elbow and inserting on the wrist. These tendons perform the function of flexing the wrist. Any forced or repetitive flexion of the wrist will cause inflammation or possibly tears with pain radiating down the forearm. Patients working in the garden with shears or with other instruments can develop these problems. Diagnosis of both forms of epicondylitis is based on the history and pain with pressure on either the medial or lateral epicondyle. I often apply pressure to a wrist locked in flexion or extension to elicit pain at the elbow and confirm the diagnosis.

Treatment starts with correcting the offending activities by either discontinuing or modifying it. At its onset, I suggest ice for twenty minutes three times a day to the area, topical or oral NSAIDs, and either a resting wrist splint or a band around the elbow. Placing the palms of both hands against a wall with elbows straight or completely extended and applying pressure against the wall will stretch those extensor tendons in lateral epicondylitis. Reversing the hands so that their extensor surfaces are against the wall will stretch the flexor tendons in medial epicondylitis. Stretches should be performed two to three times daily and held for one minute. Very occasionally I will inject the tendon sheath with steroids but rarely will repeat the injection, and if I do, I wait at least three months between injections or risk rupture. I will send difficult cases to PT, and after a few months without improvement, I will obtain an MRI looking for tears. I recently treated a very fit fifty-plus-year-old woman who owned a vineyard, picked thousands of grapes, and carried bucketfuls. She had a very resistant medial epicondylitis and after months of treatment was no better. An MRI revealed a partial tear of one of her tendons. She consulted an orthopedic surgeon and decided against surgery. She continued therapy and made adjustments to her picking style, with almost complete resolution of the problem. It's rare that these patients need surgery, but in difficult cases I will seek a surgical opinion.

Pearls

- Pain radiating down the forearm from the elbow may indicate medial or lateral epicondylitis.
- The problem involves the flexor or extensor tendons of the wrist and not the elbow.

- It is usually due to a repetitive motion of the wrist, such as computer use, poor tennis mechanics, or piano playing.
- Ice and stretching help.
- A change in mechanics also is helpful.
- A wrist splint or tennis elbow brace can be helpful.
- Physical therapy for stretches, strengthening, and modalities may be necessary.
- Steroid injections are occasionally curative.
- If all else fails, obtain an MRI and look for tears.

References

1. www.niams.nih.gov>Health_info (Handbook on www.rheumatol-ogy.org/Practice
(Handout on Health: Tendinitis and Bursitis)
2. Anderson, Bob. *Stretching.*
3. Smidt, N., M. Lewis, D. A. van der Windt, et al. Lateral Epicondylitis in General Practice: Course and Prognostic Indicators of Outcome. *J Rheumatol* 33:2053.
4. Haahr, J. P., and J. H. Andersen. Prognostic Factors in Lateral Epicondylitis: A Randomized Trial with One-Year Follow-up in 266 New Cases Treated with Minimal Occupational Intervention or the Usual Approach in General Practice. *Rheumatology* (Oxford) 42:1216.
5. Struijs, P. A., G. M. Kerkhoffs, W. J. Assendelft, and C. N. Van Dijk. Conservative Treatment of Lateral Epicondylitis: Brace versus Physical Therapy or a Combination of Both: A Randomized Clinical Trial. *Am J Sports Med* 32:462.

Trigger Finger

The Finger Lock

Leon is another of my favorite older patients. He is an ex-carpenter who has become a semiprofessional piano player and is taking lessons from a locally famous concert pianist. He complains of cramping or locking of two of his fingers, especially in the morning. At times, he has to literally tear his fingers from his palm. His hands are calloused and leathery, and there is a large nodule on the third flexor tendon. I feel the nodule slide past as he flexes and extends his finger. He's had a similar problem in his other hand and is requesting an injection. I inject his tendon sheath with triamcinolone, a long-acting steroid, and in two weeks, all his symptoms have disappeared.

Trigger fingers are fun and easy. Most patients will complain of their finger locking and needing to forcibly unlock it. Sometimes patients will complain of several contiguous fingers locking, and a good exam and history will find that there is one main offender. The most confusing patients complain of just aching and stiffness of their fingers, and only some skilled questioning and a good exam will discover that they actually have trigger fingers. Diabetes, excessive typing, piano playing, or any repetitive flexion of the fingers may be the cause. Patients have tender nodules attached to one or more of their flexor tendons in the palm of their hand. I have the patients open and close their hand or flex and extend the offending digit, and I can palpate the nodule as it moves up and down. Often the finger will lock during the exam. I find movement is necessary to make the diagnosis. Patients will swear that the problem is farther up their finger at their knuckle, but unless they have significant arthritis, it's unlikely. Treatment is simple and effective. Injection of steroid into the tendon sheath resolves the problem the majority of the time.

Tendons slide through these sheaths, and if there is a bump or nodule in the tendon, it can get hung up or stuck in the sheath while sliding. A steroid shot shrinks the nodule, so it no longer sticks in the sheath. I do have some patients who have recurrences once or twice a year and some who develop other trigger fingers. Again I try not to inject very often, to avoid rupture, and if the patient is recurring more often than once every six months, I send him or her to a surgeon. An ophthalmologist friend of mine who performs thousands of cataract surgeries a year visits me every twelve to eighteen months for an injection of the same tendon sheath, with great results. He knows that if the problem becomes more frequent, I will refer him to my favorite hand surgeon. The need for these referrals is extremely rare.

Pearls

- Look for a nodule on the flexor tendon.
- Inject the steroid proximal to the nodule.
- Surgery is rarely necessary but a consideration if the patient needs more than two injections a year.

References

1. Anderson, B. C. *Office Orthopedics for Primary Care: Diagnosis and Treatment*, 3rd edition. Philadelphia: Elsevier Saunders Company.

Carpal Tunnel Syndrome

When Playing Guitar Can be Hazardous

I love rock and roll, and Brad has been the lead guitarist in several local bands. It has been great hearing his stories and sharing new music. However, when he first saw me, he was depressed and angry and in no mood to talk. He had seen several doctors because of his swollen, painful hands and was becoming despondent because he thought it was the end of his career. There was no life without rock and roll! He was fifty, overweight, and an insulin-dependent diabetic, but as he reminded me, so was Jerry Garcia. I reminded him that Jerry was dead. Strangely, that fact did not lift his spirits. He actually cried as he told me he was losing strength in his fingers and could not perform any more. Although his hands were slightly swollen, the joints were not, often the case in diabetics. I noted that he had lost sensation in the first three fingers of his hand and could not maintain the O sign with his thumb and forefinger when I tried to pull them apart. He complained of tingling when I tapped at the underside of his wrist. I concluded that he had severe carpal tunnel syndrome in both hands, confirmed later by nerve conduction studies. Normally, I would tell most patients to wear wrist splints at night and take NSAIDs, but his case was so severe that I feared permanent nerve damage if he did not have immediate surgery. Three months later, he was in a new band and rocking out. Unfortunately, I am now treating him ten years later for PMR, but that is another story.

Carpal tunnel syndrome is a very common diagnosis in my practice. Most patients will complain of numbness or tingling of their hands at night or when they wake in the morning. Occasionally they will complain of pain or numbness radiating up to their shoulders or just plain aching of their hands. In severe cases they will complain of a weak grip that causes them to drop things. Often there is a history of excessive computer use, bike riding, metabolic problems (such as diabetes, hypothyroidism, or excessive estrogen) or inflammatory diseases (such as rheumatoid arthritis). A good physical exam, including sensory and motor testing and two maneuvers called Tinel's and Phalen's signs that elicit symptoms usually can make the diagnosis. I tell patients to make an O with their thumb and forefinger, and if I can pull the fingers apart, they will need surgery because it indicates weakness of their abductor pollicis longus muscle and major damage to their median nerve, which could be permanent if not treated soon. The carpal tunnel houses the median nerve and several tendons in a sheath between several wrist bones. The median nerve enervates the first three and a half digits of the hand, and when it is swollen or damaged, those fingers become increasingly numb, painful, and weak. If untreated, those fingers can become useless and develop flexion contractures. Most cases are mild and will respond to anti-inflammatories, wrist splints at night, and ergonomic adjustments to activities. If the O can be pulled apart or if the diagnosis is in doubt or if they do not respond to conventional therapy, I send patients to neurology for nerve conduction testing. Be warned however that these tests can be painful. My mother was angry with me for suggesting these tests when she developed carpal tunnel symptoms. I was the guinea pig in medical school for this test and found it very unpleasant. Not only will it confirm the diagnosis and find alternative diagnoses, such as peripheral neuropathy (loss of insulation of the nerves) or cervical radiculopathy (pinched nerve), but it will also measure the severity. Generally, when the test indicates a severe case, I send the patient for surgery, which is almost always successful. In acute cases where the patients cannot tolerate the pain and wait for the surgery, I rarely inject the carpal tunnel with steroids. However, most patients adjust their activities and live with carpal tunnel indefinitely. Personally, I develop carpal tunnel during the cycling season and have to adjust my grip on the handlebars and change my arm and hand position in bed.

Pearls

- Patients may just complain of painful, swollen hands.
- Numbness or tingling in the morning is the most common complaint.
- Wrist splints at night for a mild case are usually sufficient.
- Confirm with nerve conduction study.
- Change ergonomics and rule out underlying causes.
- Once patient is weak and can no longer maintain an O sign against resistance (abductor pollicis longus muscle), surgery is probably necessary.

References

1. Jarvik, J. G., Comstock, M. Kliot, et al. Surgery versus Non-Surgical Therapy for Carpal Tunnel Syndrome: A Randomised Parallel-Group Trial. *Lancet* 374:1074.

2. Bland, J. D. Treatment of Carpal Tunnel Syndrome. *Muscle Nerve* 36:167.

De Quervain's Tenosynovitis

De Quervain's tenosynovitis is a common cause of wrist pain on the radial, or thumb, side of the wrist. It is caused by the inflammation of two tendons (abductor pollicis longus and extensor pollicis brevis) and will cause pain with gripping or grasping. Wrists are usually tender and sometimes swollen along that side of the wrist and at the end of the forearm. It may be mistaken for DJD of the first CMC but is closer to the forearm than the thumb. The Finkelstein test, where patients fold their fingers over their thumb and flick their wrist toward their baby finger, or ulnar side, of their wrist, will often elicit pain. Overuse or repetitive use is usually the cause. Wrist splints, ice, NSAIDs (oral or topical), and modification of activity can be effective, but I find that inevitably I have to inject the tendon sheath with steroids, and it almost always resolves the problem.

Pearls

- Differentiate from DJD of the first CMC.
- Wrist splints, NSAIDs, and icing may be adequate treatment.
- An injection in the tendon sheath with steroids is usually curative, but the repetitive motion (ergonomics) that caused it must be addressed.

References

1. www.rheumatology.org/Practice
(Patient Education—Diseases and Conditions)
2. www.uptodate.com
3. Anderson, B. C. *Office Orthopedics for Primary Care: Diagnosis and Treatment*, 2nd edition. Philadelphia: WB Saunders.
4. Sheon, R. P., R. W. Moskowitz, and V. M. Goldberg. *Soft Tissue Rheumatic Pain: Recognition, Management, Prevention*, 3rd edition. Baltimore: Williams & Wilkins.

Complex Regional Pain Syndrome (CRPS)

This Is Not a Gang in LA

My buddy Larry developed a back problem and had several surgeries, several blood clots in his leg, and now has continuous pain and tenderness, swelling, color changes, coldness, and atrophy of his right leg. He can barely stand to put a sheet on top of his leg; it is so painful. A touch sends him through the roof. Almost certainly he has CRPS. He is a retired rheumatologist and suggested the diagnosis himself. Most physicians cringe at the prospect of treating this syndrome, formerly known as *reflex sympathetic dystrophy*, because it is difficult and can be debilitating. The pain is severe, and the arm, hand, foot, or leg is exquisitely tender to the touch and will develop contractures and become useless if untreated. In the first stages, the limb is cool, dusky, and swollen. Later the skin becomes thickened and brawny, and there is muscle wasting. Finally, the joint or limb becomes stiff, and movement is limited. It is usually precipitated by some sort of trauma, including a heart attack, stroke, orthopedic procedure, fracture, or emotional upset. Early mobilization and aggressive physical or occupational therapy may be preventative or therapeutic. Since chemicals or proteins released by the peripheral nerves are a possible cause, sympathetic nerve blocks or resection of some of the sympathetic nerves are treatments for those patients who do not respond to physical, occupational, or pharmacological therapy or psychological counseling. Early in the disease, I try NSAIDs and tricyclic antidepressants, such as amitriptyline, and then later gabapentin or Lyrica but will quickly move to a moderate or high dose of prednisone for a few weeks. There have been reports of the effectiveness of bisphosphonates, such as alendronate, but I have not used them in this situation as yet. It is important to emphasize the need for movement of the affected limb even if it hurts. Recently, spinal stimulators have had some success. Larry had pushed himself physically more lately, was receiving psychological counseling, and has had some success with a spinal stimulator. After two to three years of extreme disability, he seemed to be rising from the ashes but sadly died of questionable causes just as I was finishing this book. One of my longtime patients with CRPS has done moderately well with physical therapy and medications but cannot make a fist with either hand due to stiffness and pain.

Pearls

- Often occurs after trauma and immobilization.
- The limb(s) is exquisitely tender, cool, and discolored.
- Movement and aggressive physical and occupational therapy, despite the pain, are important.
- Be aggressive early!

Reference

1. www.uptodate.com
2. Sheon, R. P., R. W. Moskowitz, and V. M. Goldberg. *Soft Tissue Rheumatic Pain: Recognition, Management, Prevention*, third edition. Baltimore: Williams & Wilkins, 116.
3. Stanton-Hicks, M., W. Jänig, S. Hassenbusch, et al. Reflex Sympathetic Dystrophy: Changing Concepts and Taxonomy." *Pain* 63:127
4. Quisel, A., J. M. Gill, and P. Witherell. Complex Regional Pain Syndrome: Which Treatments Show Promise?" *J Fam Pract* 54:599.
5. Mellick, L. B., and G. A. Mellick. Successful Treatment of Reflex Sympathetic Dystrophy with Gabapentin. *Am J Emerg Med* 13:96.
6. Price, D. D., S. Long, B. Wilsey, and A. Rafii. Analysis of Peak Magnitude and Duration of Analgesia Produced by Local Anesthetics

Injected into Sympathetic Ganglia of Complex Regional Pain Syndrome Patients. *Clin J Pain* 14:216.

7. Kemler, M. A., G. A. Barendse, M. van Kleef, et al. Spinal Cord Stimulation in Patients with Chronic Reflex Sympathetic Dystrophy. *N Engl J Med* 343:618.

8. Kemler, M. A., H. C. de Vet, G. A. Barendse, et al. Spinal Cord Stimulation for Chronic Reflex Sympathetic Dystrophy—Five-Year Follow-Up. *N Engl J Med* 354:2394.

9. Akkus, S., H. Yorgancigil, and M. Yener. A Case of Recurrent and Migratory Complex Regional Pain Syndrome Type I: Prevention by Gabapentin. *Rheumatol Int* 26:852.

10. Oerlemans, H. M., R. A. Oostendorp, T. de Boo, and R. J. Goris. Pain and Reduced Mobility in Complex Regional Pain Syndrome I: Outcome of a Prospective Randomised Controlled Clinical Trial of Adjuvant Physical Therapy versus Occupational Therapy. *Pain* 83:77.

Bursa

Don't Make It Angry

Bob is a jovial, rotund alcoholic who just can't quite kick his beer habit and still has occasional gout attacks and large white nodules on his elbows and forearms. I am often frustrated with him, but he has an infectious laugh and one of those big personalities. It's hard to stay angry at him. I can almost predict his response to my little lecture about beer and gout: "I am weak, Doc. what can I say?" He failed AA and lost his wife, and I just can't bring myself to fire him as a patient. He has a red-hot, angry-looking fluctuant swelling on his elbow. It almost feels like a baggy filled with a hot liquid. He has olecranon bursitis. I aspirate the bursa and obtain 15 cc of thick, creamy liquid, which is full of white blood cells and urate crystals that are psychedelic under my polarizing microscope. I inject the bursa with steroids, place him on an NSAID, and send him on his way until next time.

Everyone has several bursas, but not everyone has bursitis. There are more than one hundred fifty bursas in the human body. As I mentioned previously, they are fluid-filled sacs distributed through-out the body to protect soft tissue from bony prominences. There are several around the shoulder and upper arm, at the pointy part of the elbow, a large one at the hip, one at the buttocks, and several around the knee. I am just mentioning the ones that seem to become inflamed most often. However, I emphasize that not every new hip or shoulder pain is bursitis. It seems to be a throwaway diagnosis. Inflamed bursas are usually tender and swollen and can be hot and red depending on the cause. Some are inside a joint, such as the subacromial joint (under the tip of the shoulder), and cannot be felt unless very swollen. Others, such as the one at the elbow, are easily visualized and palpated and can be infected or inflamed by gout and other inflammatory diseases. More often they are swollen and slightly inflamed because of trauma. With the use of office ultrasound, almost all these bursas can be easily visualized. Being a dinosaur, I don't have an ultrasound machine, so I can only tell if the easily visualized ones, such as the one at the elbow or knee, are swollen but not many of the others. However, if a bursa is extremely swollen or inflamed, it is obvious by inspection and palpation. These bursas should be aspirated and checked for crystals or infection. If I am not sure I am inserting the needle into the bursa, I will send them for CT-guided aspiration. I may have done so twice in twenty-five years. The gout patient with olecranon or elbow bursitis is one of the most satisfying kinds of patients I see regularly. The elbows will be very red-hot and swollen, with the swelling extending up the arm. It is not hard to determine that the bursa that is subcutaneous is inflamed and not the elbow. It is also easy to stick a needle in the bursa, aspirate the fluid, which is often chalky or milky, and examine it under my polarizing microscope and make a diagnosis of acute gout. Since infection and gout can coexist, I also send the fluid for cultures. If I have a low index of suspicion of infection, I inject the bursa with steroid, and the patient is usually better by the next day, and I am a hero! However, it is important to add one of the ironclad adages of rheumatology—a red-hot bursa or joint is infection until proven otherwise.

Subacromial bursitis is hard to distinguish from rotator cuff tendonitis or subacromial arthritis without ultrasound or MRI. The subdeltoid bursa is right below the deltoid muscle and may cause achiness in the area and is tender to the touch. It can be inflamed or infected, but I am not sure I have ever seen an infection. Local treatments with ice, heat, NSAIDs, and ultrasound are usually enough, but rarely injection with steroids is necessary. Of course if the deltoid is swollen, hot, and red, aspiration is a must.

The majority of patients with bursitis will complain of constant pain exacerbated by pressure on the affected bursa. Hip or trochanteric bursitis is the classic. Patients will complain of pain when lying on that side and with walking or standing. They are exquisitely tender to the touch in the hip area. Unfortunately, fibromyalgia patients are almost always tender there, but hip arthritis and lumbar spondylosis patients are not unless they have coexistent bursitis or nerve problems. Ice, rest, and NSAIDs can be effective, but many of these patients require steroid injections. Again if the area is hot and red and swollen, aspiration is a must under ultrasound or CT guidance. Finally, there are several bursas around the knee. The one just in front of the patella, or knee bone, is particularly susceptible to trauma or the repetitive kneeling necessary in certain professions. Ice, NSAIDs and modification of activities are usually adequate, but again if it is hot and swollen...There is a bursa just below the knee on the big toe side of the leg called the *anserine bursa*. It can become inflamed, especially in endurance athletes with poor mechanics. (That would be me!) The diagnosis can be made by inspection and palpation. A change of shoes, rest, ice, and NSAIDs usually works. By the way, anserine bursitis was first described by two of my teachers and friends. Shout out to Mort and Ed!

Pearls

- Commonly inflamed bursas are olecranon and trochanteric.
- If in doubt, visualize with ultrasound.
- Aspirate and look for crystals or infection.
- If not infected, steroid injection is effective.

References

1. Sheon, R. P., R. W. Moskowitz, and V. M. Goldberg. *Soft Tissue Rheumatic Pain: Recognition, Management, Prevention*, 3rd edition, Baltimore: Williams & Wilkins.

2. Canoso, J. J., and R. A. Yood. Reaction of Superficial Bursae in Response to Specific Disease Stimuli. *Arthritis Rheum* 22:1361.

3. Zimmermann, B., D. J. Mikolich, G. Ho, Jr. Septic Bursitis. *Semin Arthritis Rheum* 24:391.

4. Valeriano-Marcet, J., J. D. Carter, and F. B. Vasey. Soft Tissue Disease. *Rheum Dis Clin North Am* 29:77.

Septic Bursitis

Before leaving the world of bursas, I probably should spend more time on septic bursitis. It is more commonly seen in diabetics, alcoholics, and immunosuppressed patients and usually is the result of direct inoculation of the organism but may be carried through the bloodstream from an infected heart valve. Chronic occupational trauma to a bursa, seen in athletes, miners, plumbers, and so forth, is another predisposing factor. Septic bursas are usually more swollen, redder, and more painful than bursitis from other causes, but gout can be pretty similar. The only way to make a definitive diagnosis is by aspiration. Interestingly, the bursa white blood cell count may be as low as two thousand, as opposed to the much higher counts in septic arthritis, and deceive many an unsuspecting physician. Therefore, the gram stain and culture are keys to the diagnosis. If the inflammation spreads up the extremity and is associated with fever, the prognosis worsens, and that patient probably needs to be hospitalized and started on IV antibiotics and possibly have the bursa incised and drained. Otherwise I treat the patient with oral antibiotics and drain the bursa daily in the office until it is sterile and the volume of fluid is at a minimum or completely gone. Once again, staph aureus is probably the most common bacteria and can be deadly if untreated, and it seeds to the bloodstream. If the infection is mild, I aspirate the bursa daily and treat with dicloxacillin. Clindamycin, trimethoprim-sulfamethoxazole, or doxycycline can be used for MRSA- or penicillin-allergic patients, but by that time, I'm calling my infectious disease specialist, Ruth, or my favorite hospitalist. Once the infection is severe, systemic, or not responding to treatment, it's time for hospitalization and IV antibiotics.

Infections with fungi and TB tend to be a little more indolent and less inflamed but still very problematic. I look for a systemic source by doing a chest x-ray and blood and skin tests, and I refer them to Ruth.

Pearls

- Septic bursas have surprisingly low white blood cell counts.
- Gram stain and cultures are key to diagnosis.
- Aspirate bursa daily until white cells disappear.
- IV antibiotics are necessary once patient has developed cellulitis or fever.
- Consider incision and drainage if not responding after a few days.

References

1. www.rheumatology.org/Practice
(Patient Education—Diseases and Conditions)
2. www.niams.nih.gov>Health_info
(Handout on Health: Tendinitis and Bursitis)
3. Zimmermann, B., D. J. Mikolich, G. Ho, Jr. "Septic Bursitis. *Semin Arthritis Rheum* 24:391.
4. Ho, Jr., G., and E. Y. Su. Antibiotic Therapy of Septic Bursitis: Its Implication in the Treatment of Septic Arthritis. *Arthritis Rheum* 24:905.
5. Valeriano-Marcet, J., J. D. Carter, and F. B. Vasey. Soft Tissue Disease. *Rheum Dis Clin North Am* 29:77.

Plantar Fasciitis

Barefoot-Dancing Days Are Over

I have treated John for years for a variety of overuse injuries. We share a bond or camaraderie of the road; he is a forty-year-old endurance runner. Today, he shares with me his story of woe. He had to drop out of his last marathon at the fourteen-mile mark because each step with his right foot felt like he was stepping on broken glass. Not only can he not run now, but he has trouble walking, and his training is confined to the pool. His right foot is exquisitely tender from the heel to midsole. He has plantar fasciitis and Achilles tendonitis, an injury I have suffered several times. It's the kind of injury that tends to linger and recur, especially in runners. John, as a seasoned runner, has already started the proper therapy with icing, stretching, and abstinence from running. I just need to fine-tune. I remind him never to be barefoot, even around the house, and to wear cushioned shoes at all times. I show him a set of new stretches, with his foot bouncing up and down off the edge of a step, and eventually, I have to send him to physical therapy and recommend a night splint. I suspect he is not completely compliant with the abstinence part. Runners are like that. It may take months, but he will be fine.

As a runner, I've not only experienced the pain of plantar fasciitis but have seen many of my running buddies suffer through long months of inactivity because of it. In my office, I not only see young athletes but many overweight patients with both high arches and flat feet who wear poor shoes. They all describe knife-like pain with each step. Anyone who has suffered from this condition will tell you that the first step out of bed in the morning is excruciating. Walking becomes intolerable.

The plantar fascia is the fibrous band under the skin that extends from the heel of the foot and attaches to the tendon sheaths

305

of the toes on the sole. With each step as the toes extend, the fascia stretches, so it's easy to imagine what it would feel like when it is inflamed. Imagine stepping on an open sore that extends all the way up the bottom of your foot. It stops even a compulsive runner like me dead in his tracks and makes any kind of weight-bearing activity intolerable. Poor shoe wear, sudden increase in miles (especially on hard surfaces), chronic Achilles tendonitis leading to a tight tendon, obesity, flat feet, and high arches are all predisposing conditions. When I first met my wife, we were both running, and I convinced her to run distances to which she was unaccustomed. During a race, she developed sudden, severe foot pain and could not finish. She could barely walk for the next six months and has not run with me since!

Treatment is almost always successful but requires strict discipline. Patients must stop the offending activity until it resolves (or at least is tolerable for those of us running maniacs). Good cushioned shoes must be worn at all times, even around the house, from the first step to the last. The plantar fascia needs to be stretched several times a day. Ice should be applied to the area for about twenty minutes several times a day. NSAIDs, preferably topical, are helpful. If the pain lingers, I advise patients to obtain a special plantar fasciitis foot splint to wear at night, which keeps the foot in extension while you sleep. There are several types, but I find the sock with Velcro seems more comfortable than a hard splint. They can be purchased at some running shoe, drug, or orthopedic supply stores. Physical therapy with ultrasound, phonophoresis with steroids, and stretching are often helpful. Weight loss in obese patients is helpful. I find obese patients with plantar fasciitis are the most likely to become chronic. Education, good shoes, orthotics, proper training, stretching, and weight management are important to prevent recurrences. However, once you've had it, it's easy to get it again, so beware!

Ankylosing spondylitis and psoriatic arthritis can cause inflammation of both the Achilles tendon and plantar fascia. The inflammation needs to be treated aggressively.

Pearls

- Wear good padded shoes at all times, even around the house.
- Stretching, ice, and NSAIDs are helpful.
- Weight loss can be a key.
- PT for stretches and modalities can help.
- Night splints are useful.
- Avoid injections and surgery.

Reference

1. Johnson, Jim. *The Five Minute Plantar Fasciitis Solution.*
2. www.uptodate.com
3. Greene, W. B. (ed.). *Essentials of Musculoskeletal Care*, 2nd edition. Rosemont, IL: American Academy of Orthopaedic Surgeons, 487.
4. Warren, B. L., and C. J. Jones. Predicting Plantar Fasciitis in Runners. *Med Sci Sports Exerc* 19:71.
5. Buchbinder, R. Clinical Practice: Plantar Fasciitis. *N Engl J Med* 350:2159.
6. Powell, M., W. R. Post, J. Keener, and S. Wearden. Effective Treatment of Chronic Plantar Fasciitis with Dorsiflexion Night Splints: A Crossover Prospective Randomized Outcome Study." *Foot Ankle Int* 19:10.

Chapter Twenty-three

Depression

The Dark Vortex

I hadn't seen Sherry in five years. She hasn't changed. Her pretty gray eyes are lifeless, her face is expressionless, and she exerts an energy vacuum on the entire room. She has been on antidepressants and occasional antipsychotics for years and now is taking two types of morphine derivatives. During the exam she almost seems to be dozing off and is irritated by my suggestion she may be overmedicated. She has a generally positive review of systems, which means she has every possible symptom in every organ system. She is off every medication for her lupus and claims she can't possibly exercise for her fibromyalgia.

I can't tell you how many times I walk into a room and the air almost seems heavy. I can almost feel depression instantly. The patient's eyes are clouded—lights are out. Pain can have the same effect, and it may be hard to distinguish which is the cart and which is the horse. It's important to determine whether the patient is depressed and whether the source is their disease, pain, or some external circumstance. Depression in itself can cause somatic pain. Joint and muscle pain may just be a manifestation of their depression. The patient's outside starts to reflect the inside. It changes brain chemistry and may actually exacerbate inflammation and symptoms in any disease. When a stable patient suddenly has an exacerbation, there are a limited number of causes—depression, stress, noncompliance with medications, change in the nature of their disease, or a new complicating problem. The majority of times, stress or depression is the answer. One of the more graphic examples was when one of my favorite rheumatoid arthritis patients who had been stable for years arrived to my office in a wheelchair for the first time. It seemed that every one of her joints had suddenly become inflamed over a two- to three-day period. When I questioned her as to the events that preceded her decline, she admitted to seeing the movie *Schindler's List* on a Saturday and attending her best friend's funeral on a Sunday. By Monday she was in a wheelchair! Not every patient is so forthcoming or obvious. Many patients deny depression while crying uncontrollably or until their spouse contradicts them. It's important to ask pointedly about stress or depression even if they fail to check the box on a questionnaire. If it is not addressed, progress and improvement are unlikely, and the health-care provider is likely to become depressed as well. Chronically depressed patients are among the hardest to treat since they never seem to improve. Fibromyalgia patients are particularly hard because both depression and fibromyalgia amplify pain, so their pain levels seem to go up exponentially. Also, they share many of the same characteristics, and it may be hard to recognize that they coexist. In any case, both depression and the coexisting disease must be treated. I occasionally prescribe antidepressants but prefer psychological counseling for any long-term issues. Many patients are already on a polypharmacy, and adding one more medication just maximizes the chances of adverse reactions. There are patients who are resistant to accepting treatment for financial, cultural, or psychological reasons. I then do my best counseling them and try to remember I am the messenger. Involving a family member is often helpful, and I try to find skilled counselors in each community so that I can refer to the provider who best suits the patient's needs and is close to his or her home.

Pearls

- Be a good observer and listener.
- Depression makes everything worse.
- Medication is not always the answer.
- Discontinue medications that may be making depression worse.
- Involve loved ones if necessary. They may provide objective information and another set of ears.
- Treat any underlying medical problem simultaneously with depression.
- Good counselors may make all the difference.
- Denial is not just a river in Egypt.

References

1. Cepoiu, M., J. McCusker, M. G. Cole, et al. Recognition of Depression by Non-psychiatric Physicians—A Systematic Literature Review and Meta-analysis. *J Gen Intern Med* 23:25.
2. American Psychiatric Association. *Diagnostic and Statistical Manual of Mental Disorders*, fifth edition (DSM-5). Arlington, VA: American Psychiatric Association.

Chapter Twenty-four

Rheumatology Emergencies: Telephone Calls and Hospital Consults

He's Funny, but His Headache Isn't

Steve is seventy-five and a large man with a self-effacing sense of humor. I diagnosed him with giant cell arteritis ten months ago based on the headache from hell and a very high ESR despite the fact he had a negative temporal artery biopsy. He responded immediately to high doses of prednisone but unfortunately had all kinds of problems with the medication. He developed weakness in his hip muscles, irritability, insomnia, and high blood sugars. I finally have tapered his prednisone down to 7 mg, and now he calls and complains of searing left eye pain with hazy vision. I don't bat an eye and tell him to increase his prednisone immediately to 60 mg and see his ophthalmologist and me in the next twenty-four hours.

There are few rheumatology emergencies, but they need to be addressed immediately, or there can be grave consequences. The classic emergency is the polymyalgia rheumatica or giant cell arteritis patient who complains of severe headache or sudden visual loss. These symptoms may signify active inflammation of their arteries and impending stroke or blindness. These patients need to take 60–80 mg of prednisone immediately or risk permanent blindness or stroke. I would apply the same logic to an undiagnosed elderly patient with a severe headache or visual change and a high sedimentation rate or C-reactive protein. I remind you of the story of my sweet elderly polymyalgia patient who developed visual haziness on a Friday and didn't want to bother anyone until Monday, so she remained on 10 mg of prednisone. By Monday she was permanently blind in her right eye, and there was nothing I could do. The first twenty-four to seventy-two hours are critical. So I tell patients to raise their prednisone to 60 mg and then call me. Don't wait until they talk to me. It is better to err on the side of taking an excess of prednisone for a few days than too little. Vision is precious!

References

1. Hunder, G. G. Giant Cell Arteritis and Polymyalgia Rheumatica. In *Textbook of Rheumatology*, 5th edition, edited by W. N. Kelly, E. D. Harris, S. Ruddy, and C. B. Sledge, xx–xx. Philadelphia: WB Saunders.

Beware the Red Eye!

Jimmy, my eight-year-old probable JIA patient, has not seen the pediatric rheumatologist yet, but his mom is calling because he has an intensely painful red eye. I refer him to an ophthalmologist immediately and call the doctor personally to see that he will see Jimmy within twenty-four hours.

A painful red eye is an ophthalmology emergency, especially when associated with diseases such as rheumatoid arthritis, ankylosing spondylitis, juvenile idiopathic arthritis, psoriasis, granulomatosis with polyangiitis, sarcoidosis, lupus, or any other systemic inflammatory process. It may be a symptom of iritis or scleritis and, if untreated, can lead to visual loss. I always have a friendly, skilled ophthalmologist's phone number at my fingertips. A red eye is not a pink eye or a bloodshot eye and is usually associated with photophobia and intense pain.

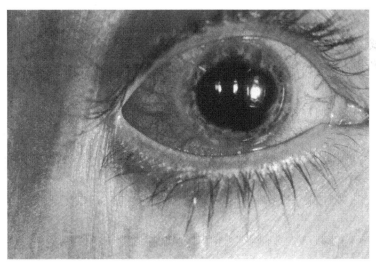

Iritis with synechiae (adhesions)—courtesy of ACR image bank

References

1. Rosenbaum, J. T. Acute Anterior Uveitis and Spondyloarthropathies. *Rheum Dis Clin North Am* 18:143.

2. Rosenbaum, J. T. Uveitis: An Internist's View. *Arch Intern Med* 149:1173.

3. Cassidy, J., J. Kivlin, C. Lindsley, et al. Ophthalmologic Examinations in Children with Juvenile Rheumatoid Arthritis. *Pediatrics* 117:1843.

4. Rothova, A., H. J. Buitenhuis, C. Meenken, et al. Uveitis and Systemic Disease. *Br J Ophthalmol* 76:137.

Hot, Red, and Dangerous

Aaron, the scary anesthesiologist with staph aureus growing out of his finger joint as described in an earlier section, was definitely an emergency. Rather than repeating his story, I refer you back to the section on septic arthritis and repeat that one acutely inflamed joint (monoarticular arthritis) is infection until proven otherwise. Also, infection needs to be diagnosed and treated quickly, or the joint could be totally destroyed, and even worse, the patient could die.

References

1. Goldenberg, D. L. Septic Arthritis and Other Infections of Rheumatologic Significance. *Rheum Dis Clin North Am* 17:149.
2. Goldenberg, D. L., and J. I. Reed. Bacterial Arthritis. *N Engl J Med* 312:764.

Big Heart, Big Pain, and There's the Rub

Anna was a minister's wife and a tough patient. She was young, prim, and proper and wore several layers of clothing. Refusing to get into a gown or shorts, she never allowed me to examine her knees properly. I could never place my stethoscope on her bare skin, and she either refused medications, adjusted the doses as she saw fit, or would disappear for many months. I was on the verge of discharging her for noncompliance, but she had such severe disease I couldn't do it. On this particular day, she visited the office and complained of severe shortness of breath and knife-like chest pain with breathing. She had a creaky sound called a *rub* when I listened to her heart, and the veins in her neck were prominent or bulging. I referred her immediately to the hospital, and as I suspected she had a pericardial effusion, or fluid surrounding her heart, causing tamponade, or the inability for the heart to expand. Ultimately she was hospitalized, and she had to have the fluid drained from around her heart. She then refused any further procedures and left the hospital against medical advice. I discharged her as a patient the following week and have not heard from her since.

Acute shortness of breath or chest pain lasting more than a few minutes is an emergency in any setting—particularly in patients whose immune systems are suppressed or who have systemic inflammatory diseases. Twenty-year-old lupus patients can have heart attacks. Granulomatosis with polyangiitis and Churg-Strauss patients may go into respiratory failure and quickly arrest if not treated aggressively and immediately. Patients on biologics or any immunosuppressive medication may have atypical, serious infections that need immediate attention or can be fatal. Methotrexate can cause inflammation of the lungs, severe shortness of breath, and respiratory failure. Lupus and RA patients may accumulate fluid around their hearts or lungs, causing shortness of breath and sharp pain and leading to cardiac or respiratory arrest if untreated.

References

1. Spodick, D. H. Acute Cardiac Tamponade. *N Engl J Med* 349:684.

2.Searles, G., and R. J. McKendry. Methotrexate Pneumonitis in Rheumatoid Arthritis: Potential Risk Factors: Four Case Reports and a Review of the Literature. *J Rheumatol* 14:1164.

3. Polychronopoulos, V. S., U. B. Prakash, J. M. Golbin, et al. Airway Involvement in Wegener's Granulomatosis. *Rheum Dis Clin North Am* 33:755.

4. Orens, J. B., F. J. Martinez, and J. P. Lynch. Pleuropulmonary Manifestations of Systemic Lupus Erythematosus. *Rheum Dis Clin North Am* 20:159.

Lupus and the Electric Wheelchair

Thelma is in her late sixties and has had lupus for many years. She is short, stocky, and very pleasant. Usually, she has mild symptoms easily treated adequately with Plaquenil and NSAIDs. However, she awoke the morning of her visit with a tingling sensation from her neck down and weakness in all four extremities. When I examined her, she was clearly weak and had lost sensation from her upper neck down. I sent her for an emergency MRI of the cervical and thoracic spinal cord, and she was found to have something called *transverse myelitis* (basically a stroke) of her midcervical cord. She was admitted to the hospital, and despite high-dose prednisone and Cytoxan, she became a quadriplegic. I still see her every few months in her electric wheelchair. Her lupus is stable, but she remains a quadriplegic. Nevertheless, she maintains a great attitude and feels she is getting a little more movement in her hands.

Acute severe neurological symptoms, such as paralysis or severe weakness, the inability to talk, or a change in the level of consciousness, are all emergencies and should be referred to the emergency room. Besides the two young lupus patients who had strokes, I have had two lupus patients who were paralyzed from their midthoracic area downward because of transverse myelitis of their spinal cord. In other words lupus caused inflammation and ultimately a stroke of their spinal cord. Early intensive therapy with high-dose steroids and another immunosuppressive drug may have averted this disaster.

As I mentioned in the RA chapter, weakness of the arms and legs, numbness or tingling, or spasticity in an RA patient should be a red flag for possible cervical disease. If a cervical spine x-ray with flexion and extension views shows significant C-1-C-2 subluxation, an immediate surgical consult is necessary!

References

1. Mok, C. C., C. S. Lau, E. Y. Chan, and R. W. Wong. Acute Transverse Myelopathy in Systemic Lupus Erythematosus: Clinical Presentation, Treatment, and Outcome." *J Rheumatol* 25:467.

2. D'Cruz, D. P., S. Mellor-Pita, B. Joven, et al. Transverse Myelitis as the First Manifestation of Systemic Lupus Erythematosus or Lupus-Like Disease: Good Functional Outcome and Relevance of Antiphospholipid Antibodies. *J Rheumatol* 31:280.

3. Kovacs, B., T. L. Lafferty, L. H. Brent, and R. J. DeHoratius. Transverse Myelopathy in Systemic Lupus Erythematosus: An Analysis of 14 Cases and Review of the Literature. *Ann Rheum Dis* 59:120.

4. Neva, M. H., P. Isomäki, P. Hannonen, et al. Early and Extensive Erosiveness in Peripheral Joints Predicts Atlantoaxial Subluxations in Patients with Rheumatoid Arthritis. *Arthritis Rheum* 48:1808.

5. Chang, D. J., and S. A. Paget. Neurologic Complications of Rheumatoid Arthritis. *Rheum Dis Clin North Am* 19:955.

Pregnant, Lupus, and Bleeding

The telephone call I received from Sally, the doctor who was pregnant and had low platelets, was difficult and definitely an emergency. She was bleeding from her nose, rectum, and vagina and was already on high-dose prednisone. We hospitalized her, found her platelets to be nine thousand, and ordered an emergency splenectomy. The baby and mother survived, and as far as I know, they are both thriving, but she is no longer in my practice.

A sudden drop in red or white blood cell or platelet counts is an emergency in any setting but may be more common in certain rheumatology diseases, such as lupus. These patients may have chronically low numbers, and the urgency to treat will depend on the setting and the exact number. For instance, lupus patients may have platelet counts as low as twenty thousand and be asymptomatic, whereas nonlupus patients would be having nose or GI bleeds. Below twenty thousand and certainly below ten thousand, I start having chest pain.

References

1. Bhatt, A. S., and N. Berliner. Hematologic Manifestations of SLE. In *Lupus Erythematosus: Clinical Evaluation and Treatment*, edited by P. Schur and E. Massarotti, 127–40. New York: Springer.

High Pressures, Bad Kidneys, and Bad Outcomes

Alex has limited scleroderma. He is a thirty-five-year-old fisherman and man-child who was always wrestling with his nicotine addiction. His phone call took me by surprise. He had developed the headache from hell and an unreadable blood pressure. Was he going into a renal crisis? I thought only diffuse scleroderma patients did that? It's one of the most dreaded events in rheumatology and is often quickly fatal. Unfortunately, he was one of the 5 percent of the limited scleroderma patients who did. I sent him immediately to the emergency room, where his blood pressure was critically high, and he was found to be in kidney failure. He briefly lost consciousness, but after his blood pressure was controlled, he recovered but was on dialysis for the next six years. Two years ago, he received a kidney transplant and no longer looks like a concentration camp victim.

Increasing hypertension in a scleroderma patient, especially with some mental status changes, is a dire emergency and needs immediate attention, as I mentioned in the scleroderma chapter.

Most of the rheumatology diseases can have some dire consequences, so when a lupus, vasculitis, scleroderma, polymyositis, or sarcoidosis patient complains of something that seems serious or unusual, I treat it as an emergency until proven otherwise.

Reference

1. www.uptodate.com
2. Traub, Y. M., A. P. Shapiro, G. P. Rodnan, et al. Hypertension and Renal Failure (Scleroderma Renal Crisis) in Progressive Systemic Sclerosis: Review of a 25-Year Experience with 68 Cases. *Medicine* (Baltimore) 62:335.

4.. Guillevin, L., A. Bérezné, R. Seror, et al. Scleroderma Renal Crisis: A Retrospective Multicentre Study on 91 Patients and 427 Controls. *Rheumatology* (Oxford) 51:460.

5. Steen, V. D., and T. A. Medsger, Jr. Case-Control Study of Corticosteroids and Other Drugs That Either Precipitate or Protect from the Development of Scleroderma Renal Crisis. *Arthritis Rheum* 41:1613.

6. Steen, V. D., J. P. Costantino, A. P. Shapiro, and T. A. Medsger, Jr. Outcome of Renal Crisis in Systemic Sclerosis: Relation to Availability of Angiotensin Converting Enzyme (ACE) Inhibitors. *Ann Intern Med* 113:352.

Chapter Twenty-five

Complementary and Alternative Therapies

Rachel was a six-foot fiftyish psychologist with owlish glasses and a pained smile. She had severe rheumatoid arthritis, which had been only moderately stabilized on methotrexate and a TNF inhibitor after one year of trial and error with many combinations of drugs. She was frustrated. After some extensive reading, she decided that she wanted to go off all her medications, go on a retreat, and try six months of Ayurveda (a holistic healing system based on a balance between mind, body, and spirit) with my support and permission. I told her that there were at least two small, blinded, placebo-controlled studies that suggested that an Ayurvedic diet (based on body type) may be as effective as Plaquenil or even methotrexate. The studies were small, and I was a bit skeptical. I also pointed out that methotrexate alone or in combination with several biologics had not controlled her disease at all until we tried the present combination, so I thought that diet alone would be ineffective. Rachel then asked me to describe the worst-case scenario if she adhered to her plan for six months. I told her that one or many of her joints could be destroyed, and she could develop one of the many systemic problems associated with rheumatoid arthritis. She felt her disease was not adequately controlled anyway, so she decided to proceed with her plan.

Six months passed, and Rachel returned from her retreat with a big smile on her face. She shared with me that she hadn't felt better emotionally or physically in years. Her only complaint was that her right wrist had become stiff and painful but not swollen. Her exam just revealed a wrist with little movement; otherwise, she was remarkably swelling free. I decided to order an x- ray of her wrist and compare it to previous ones. Much to our dismay, most of the cartilage or space between her wrist (carpal) bones had disappeared, and there were little erosions in the bones. When I shared this with Rachel, she became angry and accused me of not warning her of the consequences of her "sabbatical." I then gently reminded her that I had. After a brief pause, she burst into tears and asked that I reinstitute her medications or try a new combination. I restarted methotrexate and tried a "new" biologic called *Rituxan*. The combination was very successful. It's been five years; she is happy and doing well but has a stiff wrist.

Not every story involving alternative or complementary medicine ends this way. I prescribe physical and occupational therapy regularly with great success. Diet modification has been shown to be important to maintain health and as a complementary treatment in many disease processes. Small studies have shown the effectiveness of acupuncture in certain chronic pain syndromes, such as fibromyalgia. Chiropractic medicine has been successful in managing neck and back problems, such as SI joint dysfunction. Massage is excellent for relaxation and a variety of musculoskeletal conditions. I often prescribe yoga and Pilates for patients with back, neck, and flexibility issues. Yoga has been found to be effective in improving pain and functional ability in DJD and RA in several small to medium quality studies. There is some evidence that tai chi may be an effective primary therapy for DJD and fibromyalgia and an adjunctive therapy for RA. It improves cardiovascular fitness, muscular strength, balance, coordination, and physical function. Finally, counseling in multiple forms can be critical for the treatment of depression, anxiety, drug dependence, and chronic pain. Medicine is a big tent as long as you choose the right one. Systemic problems usually cannot be treated with any of the above mentioned complementary measures alone, with a few exceptions. When the problem is in the blood or immune system, local measures may help the symptoms but not the disease. Strict diet in gout may bring the uric acid down 0.5–1 mg/dl, but if the uric acid is 10, it's futile. Prayer may help your symptoms, but unless you truly believe in miracles, it is not going to restore your joint space in your knee. Many years ago, a patient with virtually no joint space in either knee (end-stage DJD) asked me to repeat her x-rays after she underwent a prayer healing. She claimed she was cured and felt much better. She even walked better. I told her if she felt better, there was no need to repeat her x-rays, but she insisted. When I eventually showed her that her x-rays were unchanged, she refused to believe that the x-rays were genuine. I did not argue, but she never returned.

The power of placebo, marketing and faith is amazing. It is effective in 30 percent of patients! If a patient believes a therapy is working and there is no potential long-term harm physically or financially, I do not discourage it, especially if it entails a healthy lifestyle change. Aerobic exercise definitely works in fibromyalgia. Mediterranean and Ayurvedic diets seem to be healthy choices for systemic inflammatory diseases, such as lupus and rheumatoid arthritis. I even have a patient who drinks a greenish concoction of vegetables and fruit every morning and claims that it has cured the severe osteoarthritis of his hip. He has thrown away his cane and no longer walks with a limp. Who am I to question success? He has not asked for a new x-ray.

I don't want to be too much of a skeptic, but I have watched patients with a variety of systemic problems exchange their medications for "magic" juices, fruit, herbs, vitamins, and diets only to return months later in a sorry state. I am always impressed by their initial optimism and enthusiasm. Occasionally patients with a mild disease will have spectacular success, and I have to reassess the value of the product. I always find it amusing when the patient starts a new supplement at the same time I prescribe a new medication and inevitably credits the supplement with the success. Marketers and purveyors of pseudoscience seem to empower patients and give them more confidence than their doctors. Unfortunately, there are many people who prey on the weak and desperate. They even involve patients in pyramid schemes selling their products or therapies, thereby indoctrinating them into a belief system that is self-serving. I often tell patients, if a doctor or practitioner is selling you something they are prescribing, don't buy it! Testimonials, especially by paid celebrities, are not good science; neither are studies that are not random, double-blinded, long-term and performed on humans.

In the nineties, alternative and complementary medicine was very big because patients demanded alternatives, and it was big business. The American College of Rheumatology, keeping in step with the times, sponsored many lectures and seminars. New journals and articles on the topic seemed to be flooding the literature almost daily. Since we were not very good at treating many of the diseases at the time, there was a huge need or hole that was being filled. Glucosamine and chondroitin were popular medications, with many studies, especially from Europe, supporting their effectiveness in osteoarthritis. They also were felt to be particularly effective in veterinary medicine. Everyone seemed to have a story about their old limping dog or grandfather suddenly running like a puppy. Then the National Institute of Health published a long-term, randomized, double-blinded, controlled study that failed to show the effectiveness of glucosamine in osteoarthritis of the knee. To this day the debate continues as to the effectiveness of these drugs in DJD. My advice is to buy the cheapest but most reputable formulation of the two and take it for six months, and if it is not effective, stop it. Caution should be used in patients taking warfarin, or Coumadin (a blood thinner).

Other supplements, such as MSM and SAM-e, have virtually no good evidence-based studies supporting their use in rheumatology. In fact, I find it important to educate patients about their disease process and warn them that some supplements may actually exacerbate their disease or have a negative interaction with their medications. For instance, many patients believe that having an autoimmune disease means that their immune system is downregulated. Therefore, they take immune system boosters, like echinacea, which may reduce the effect of their medications. Worse still, they stop their medications all together and replace them with immune boosting supplements.

My knowledge of herbal medicines is limited to reviews of the literature and observation of individual patients. I must emphasize that just because herbs are considered "natural" does not mean they can't have serious adverse effects. For instance, the first Chinese herbal medicine that I read might be effective for RA was thunder god vine (*Tripterygium wilfordii*). Random controlled studies suggested it may reduce inflammation but, because of serious adverse effects, could not be recommended for use. Unfortunately, when a patient asks me to analyze his or her herbal medicine, I am clueless, so I generally leave it to a patient to choose between traditional and

Chinese or herbal medications, fearing that mixing the two may create a dangerous "witch's brew." Of course some patients choose the nontraditional course, as I've mentioned above; some go back and forth, and some hedge their bets and try both surreptitiously. Years ago, I treated a pretty young Asian woman with bad lupus, a scarring skin rash, and bad kidneys and lungs who would have long periods of remission on her medications. However, every few months she needed admission to the ICU for a serious disease flare. It became clear to me that she would stop taking her medications during those periods despite my warnings. Eventually, I discovered that she had a Chinese herbalist in Los Angeles who would intermittently have her take a drug holiday and try Chinese herbs. I finally had to give her a choice, and the next time she stopped her medications, I dismissed her from my practice. There are a few other herbal medications besides thunder god vine whose use has been supported by quality studies. Devil's claw, for DJD and back pain; phytodolor, for arthritis pain; and possibly rose hip (*Rosa canina*), for DJD, are among the few. It's possible there are others, but the evidence supporting their use is sparse or based on testimonials.

Fish oils or omega-3 fatty acids have been studied in a variety of diseases and are popular among patients. They inhibit some of the proinflammatory proteins or cytokines active in RA, lupus, and a variety of other diseases. They are effective in doses between 2.6 and 7.1 g/day and have much the same role as NSAIDs as adjunctive drugs that reduce inflammation but do not actually treat the disease. I find them to be weak, but they have the advantage of cardiovascular benefits and few side effects, except for a fishy aftertaste and gastrointestinal disturbances.

I have already addressed diet in gout and mentioned the Mediterranean and Ayurvedic diets, but I'd like to devote more time to this important but somewhat controversial topic. It's important to understand that adipose tissue secretes a number of inflammatory markers that may cause inflammation, so weight loss in general may reduce inflammation. Therefore, any diet can be anti-inflammatory if you lose enough adipose cells. There have been a few good studies of diet in a variety of rheumatic diseases and a lot of myths. As far as I know, no good study has shown that nightshades are proinflammatory. In osteoarthritis, avocado and soybean unsaponifiables and antioxidant nutrients have been shown to reduce pain in some but not all studies, but no specific diet or dietary measure stands out other than weight loss supplemented by exercise. In RA, a Mediterranean diet has the most support, but vegetarian Aryurvedic diets have been successful in some patients. Elimination diets that remove foods thought to trigger symptoms can be successful but may be hard to design. No diets have been particularly effective in fibromyalgia. I usually recommend the Mediterranean diet for lupus patients.

I don't want to spend much time on medical marijuana because there are not enough good studies to verify its usefulness in rheumatology, although there are several studies suggesting that it does help arthritis pain and some evidence that it does have some anti-inflammatory qualities. In one large but inadequately controlled study in fibromyalgia, it seemed to be helpful in reducing pain but increased the incidence of psychosocial problems.

I admit that I don't practice or prescribe mindful meditation, although my wife insists I need it. Nevertheless, there are some studies that suggest that mindfulness training can have both psychological and possibly physiological effects. It may reduce inflammation and improve coping and growth. My friend Con, the "head-banging" marathoner and gastroenterologist extraordinaire, says "mediation" (as he calls it facetiously) helps reduce or eradicate his depression and the stress of daily life.

References

1. Kolascinski, Sharon L. Complementary and Alternative Medicine in Rheumatology *Rheumatic Disease Clinics of North America* 37, no. 1 (Feb.): xx–xx.

2. Ste.-Marie PA.. et al. Herbal Cannabis Use in Patients Labeled as Fibromyalgia is Associated with Negative Psychosocial Parameters. *Arthritis and Research*, published online 27 July, 2012. DOI.1002/acr.21732

3. Panush, R. S. Diets, Other 'Complementary' and 'Alternative' Therapies, and the Rheumatic Diseases." In *Arthritis and Allied Conditions: A Textbook of Rheumatology*, 14, edited by W. J. Koopman. Baltimore Lippencott, Williams & Wilkins.

4. Panush, R. S. Shift Happens: Complementary and Alternative Medicine for Rheumatologists. *J Rheumatol* 29:656.

5. Sherman, K. J., D. C. Cherkin, R. D. Wellman, et al. A Randomized Trial Comparing Yoga, Stretching, and a Self-Care Book for Chronic Low Back Pain. *Arch Intern Med* 171:2019.

6. Hall, A. M., Maher, P. Lam, et al. Tai Chi Exercise for Treatment of Pain and Disability in People with Persistent Low Back Pain: A Randomized Controlled Trial. *Arthritis Care Res* (Hoboken) 63:**1576**.

7. Chopra, A., P. Lavin, B. Patwardhan, and D. Chitre. Randomized Double Blind Trial of an Ayurvedic Plant Derived Formulation for Treatment of Rheumatoid Arthritis. *J Rheumatol* 27:1365.

8. Furst, D. E., M. M. Venkatraman, M. McGann, et al. Double-Blind, Randomized, Controlled, Pilot Study Comparing Classic Ayurvedic Medicine, Methotrexate, and their Combination in Rheumatoid Arthritis. *J Clin Rheumatol* 17:185.

9. Weinblatt, M. E., A. L. Maier, and P. Emery. Substantial Placebo Response in Active Rheumatoid Arthritis (RA). *Arthritis Rheum* 33:S152.

10. Matthews, D. A. Prayer and Spirituality. *Rheum Dis Clin North Am* 26:177.

Chapter Twenty-six

Medications in Rheumatology

Before I start this section, I have to confess that some of this material is a repetition from previous chapters. I even include a few of the same vignettes or stories. However, I feel that it's important to describe the medications in the context of the diseases and people they treat. I also feel that this chapter more than any other may be read as a separate piece, so to some readers the stories will be fresh. To all the others, I hope that I have included enough new material and stories to keep their interest.

Every specialty has a group of medications that are specific to its patients, and rheumatology is no different. It's important to remember that the common denominator in many of our diseases is inflammation. Often the inflammation is systemic, meaning that the immune system is overproducing certain factors that stimulate inflammatory cells and make them multiply and attack joints, muscles, skin, and other organs. Therefore, many of the medications reduce inflammation or in some way suppress the immune system. No drug is without potential side effects, some more common than others. A good adage to remember is that any drug can do anything as far as adverse effects; it's just that some are well known and more common. Before we choose a medication, we weigh the risks and benefits specific to that patient, and if the risks outweigh the benefits, we don't prescribe them. If there is any question whether an adverse effect is secondary to a medication, stop the medication, and have the patient see the doctor to be examined. Some awful and dangerous mistakes can be made over the phone, even if it involves something as simple as a rash. For instance, you could receive a call from Chloe, the lupus patient who is on a variety of medications, including prednisone. She is crying because she has a painful rash on her back and wants to know if she can increase her prednisone dose. The increase has helped her rashes in the past, so you might be tempted to tell her to do it. However, you would be making a mistake because she has herpes zoster or shingles, and the increase in prednisone would make it worse. That's why it's always better to err on the side of caution and see the patient if in doubt. One look at that rash and you'll breathe a sigh of relief knowing you didn't make it worse by increasing the steroid dose, and you will appropriately prescribe an antiviral med.

Steroids

So let's start our discussion of rheumatology meds with steroids, which the patients will often refer to as "cortisone," which is like referring to fruit as "apple," rather than apple as a "fruit." The most common steroids being used these days include prednisone, triamcinolone (Kenalog), betamethasone, Solu-Medrol, Medrol, and Decadron. Cortisone is one of the earliest corticosteroids and is rarely used any more since it is short acting and not very potent. The proper name for the steroids we use is *corticosteroids*, which are potent anti-inflammatory drugs, as opposed to other steroids, like estrogens and testosterone, which are female and male hormones, or mineralocorticoids, which regulate electrolyte metabolism and fluid regulation. These are not drugs that will make you hit more homeruns or run or cycle faster, although if you have a bad inflammatory disease, you may feel better and perform better.

I often tell patients that the long-term use of steroids is like dancing with the devil—sometimes you just gotta do it, but it is not without consequences. Like every medication, steroids have quite a few potential side effects. Fortunately, most of them occur at higher doses used for periods longer than a few weeks. They include diabetes, hypertension, and glaucoma. Still, easy bruising, poor wound healing, and some weight gain are inevitable after a few months, and when used longer, cataracts and osteoporosis are probable. Fortunately, the latter two are treatable or preventable. Years ago, when I first started practice, many patients would fracture vertebrae or hips because of osteoporosis caused by steroids. It would be painful to watch these older patients become immobile and miserable and then develop complications, such as blood clots, because of their immobility. With new medications for osteoporosis, if used early for prophylaxis, these complications rarely occur. So, if I have a patient older than fifty who I know will be on moderate doses of prednisone for more than three months, I immediately address the potential osteoporosis by ordering a bone density test and placing the patient on vitamin D, calcium, and an antiosteoporosis drug. It makes for happier patients and doctors! Again, these steroids are potent antiinflammatory without any analgesic effects except for those caused by reducing inflammation, swelling, or treating the disease.

There are some instances where a short course of high-dose steroids is preferred, indicated, and even lifesaving. I will give a patient a medium to high dose of triamcinolone or methylprednisolone intramuscularly or intravenously one time only in the office to treat a flare of inflammation in lupus or rheumatoid arthritis for instant relief or to buy time while I adjust the daily medications. The effect often lasts about two weeks but can be more prolonged. Sometimes that's all that's needed. It serves several purposes: patients feel better and can conduct their lives normally immediately; it bridges the time it takes for their disease-modifying drugs to take effect; and sometimes it is a good diagnostic test. If the patient truly doesn't have an inflammatory process, he or she will not respond, although like anything in life or medicine, nothing is absolute, and there are exceptions. What are the potential side effects from these one-time shots? They are rare, but rage, insomnia, transient swelling, and very rarely a paradoxical flare of arthritis or pain can occur. I have had spouses call me in anger and tell me never to prescribe these medications again. God knows what happened at home the night after the shot. Could it be that Dr. Jekyll became Mr. Hyde? I have also had one longtime patient leave my practice because she developed a little dent or crater in her deltoid muscle when she received a shot of triamcinolone. Rarely intramuscular shots of steroids can cause painless fat atrophy at the injection sites. I also have had several black patients develop white spots around joints that I have injected. Steroids can cause depigmentation.

In some severe or serious situations, mostly during hospitalizations but more and more in outpatient settings, three-day pulses of high-dose steroids intravenously will help gain control of a serious situation for a short, intermediate, or long period of time. High-dose steroids (usually prednisone 40–80 mg) may be necessary for two to three months or even longer in very few situations, ones that are life threatening or at high risk for serious consequences. It's not something I like or prefer to do because, as I keep repeating, the drug itself has potential terrible side effects, and the longer the duration and higher the dose, the more likely and the worse the side effect.

One of the most dreaded side effects is called *aseptic* or *avascular necrosis*, which describes bone death secondary to poor circulation. It can occur in any bone but is most common in hips or knees. The bone loses its blood supply and essentially dies and then collapses. There are many causes, but high doses of steroids of any kind, especially for long periods of time, is one of them. The tricky part is that symptoms may begin months after the drug has been stopped. Pain is usually the first symptom, and unfortunately, most cases are only treatable with joint replacement. One such case was the young twenty-year-old Vietnamese woman with lupus whom I described previously. She was deteriorating rapidly after a stroke despite many months of high-dose steroids and multiple chemotherapy agents. We finally tried a new biologic agent called *Rituxan*, which was being used for lymphoma and was eventually approved for rheumatoid arthritis. Over weeks all her findings reversed, and she was tapered off all other drugs, including steroids. It was a real "kick" to see this pretty young woman regain her ability to speak, walk, and lose all the weight she had gained because of months of steroids. Several months later, she had regained her normal lifestyle and was doing well but began experiencing hip pain and was visibly limping. An x-ray was suspicious, but an MRI revealed that both her hips had avascular necrosis and were at risk for collapse. Her pain was from lack of circulation to her femur, or hip bone—in essence her hip was having a heart attack. She now has two artificial hips and continues to do well eight years later. She had danced with the devil and survived but did not do so without paying his toll. Also, the weight gain she experienced during her six months on high-dose steroids was minor compared to some of the patients I have seen. Fifty- to a hundred-pound weight gain is not uncommon. I have watched some really attractive women become disfigured and consequently depressed because of these drugs. Because of this known side effect that usually only occurs at higher doses, it is often hard to convince women, who are the majority of the rheumatology patients, to take steroids.

Steroid-induced diabetes and high blood pressure are other grave side effects, but perhaps the most dramatic one that occurs at higher doses is psychosis. One of my former mentors tells the story of the sweet little lupus patient who was gravely ill in the hospital and placed on high-dose steroids. When he entered her room followed by a group of students, she stood on her bed and stared at him menacingly and told him that he had caused her lupus and she was going to kill him. It may have been funny in some situations, but a rheumatologist had been killed that year by a psychotic lupus patient. I'm not sure, but I think he made a quick exit. Unfortunately, that particular situation was a bit ambiguous because lupus itself can cause psychosis, so the only way you can differentiate is by tapering the steroids. Psychosis is rare even with high-dose steroids, but agitation and insomnia are not and should be addressed and considered when these doses of steroids are prescribed.

High-dose steroids (often prednisone 40–80 mg) are prescribed for more than a few weeks in some of the following instances: grave organ involvement or life-threatening situations in almost any inflammatory or collagen vascular disease, such as severe kidney, brain, skin, lung, or hematological disease in lupus; severe lung, eye, or skin disease in rheumatoid arthritis; severe vasculitis, especially with visual loss; severe headache and jaw pain in temporal or giant cell arteritis; severe polymyositis, especially with lung or other organ involvement; sarcoidosis with severe organ involvement; and a variety of rare situations that may require hospitalizations. I try to avoid prolonged high doses if at all possible, looking for alternatives, but sometimes there are no effective alternatives, such as in giant cell arteritis. Other times, it is the fastest and most effective way of avoiding disaster. The classic example is the patient initially diagnosed with polymyalgia rheumatica who complains of severe headache on the side of the head. Among these patients, 15–20 percent will develop inflammation of the large arteries branching off the aorta, the mother of all vessels pumping blood from your heart. Headache rarely may be the warning sign that their ophthalmic artery is inflamed and blindness is twenty-four hours away. Some patients just become suddenly blind in one eye without warning, and if not treated in twenty-four hours, the blindness will become permanent. Steroid treatment is not always successful, but at least it may prevent blindness in the other eye. Usually, these patients have very high sedimentation rates or C-reactive proteins, which are measures of systemic inflammation. Unfortunately, even those measures are not foolproof since in 10–20 percent of patients they will be normal. These are high-adrenaline situations since time is of the essence and the consequences are so grave, including stroke, heart attack, and other organ damage, as well as blindness. Medicine has a great sense of humor, and sometimes it's a morbid one. Lately, the most common side effect I am seeing from high-dose prednisone is weakness. Ironically, steroids can cause proximal muscle weakness, especially in high doses. Since it's a treatment for polymyositis, weakness from the medication must be distinguished from that caused by the disease. Fortunately, the muscle weakness from steroids does not cause an elevated CPK, whereas that caused by the disease does.

Most of my patients are not on steroids. Rheumatoid arthritis and lupus patients are rarely on prednisone for long if at all. Twenty years ago, we were a lot more liberal with these drugs, but now we have more choices and realize the dangers of long-term steroids even if they are given in low doses. Prednisone is not a long-term solution for either of these diseases, and usually any more than 10 mg of prednisone, especially for arthritis, is overkill unless for just a few days. Sometimes steroids are the lazy doctor's way of dealing with a pesky, difficult disease without really treating the underlying problem. Of course, there are exceptions, such as polymyalgia rheumatica (PMR), the disease mentioned above that causes pain and stiffness in elderly people and is miraculously "cured" within seventy-two hours by 10–20 mg of prednisone. I tell patients that if they are not 80–100 percent better in seventy-two hours, we have the wrong diagnosis, and they should stop the prednisone. The patients should take the initial dose for three months and be tapered slowly over the next year and a half to two years. Luckily, 50–80 percent will never have a recurrence after stopping the steroids.

There are many conditions where prednisone at 15–20 mg for two or three weeks usually does the trick, such as pleurisy (sharp chest pain with breathing) in lupus. Again, I try to avoid long courses of even low doses because of the awful and even fatal side effects. The rate of infections rises dramatically, especially when paired with other immunosuppressive drugs, and skin friability and thinning of the viscera, such as the colon, are inevitable. Occasionally, I encounter patients who are psychologically addicted to steroids and refuse to taper or discontinue their steroids. I understand that it's because of either flares or withdrawal symptoms they've experienced when tapering, but there is almost always another drug to treat their disease, and if they taper slowly and wisely, they can comfortably stop the steroids. Sometimes, as in diseases such as PMR, the taper is over one to two years, and the reduction of prednisone can be in doses as low as 0.5 mg every month. The choice of regimen is part of the art of medicine and has to be tailored to individual needs and responses. Sometimes it's a tango—two steps forward, one step back. There are rare patients who have been on steroids so long that their adrenal glands get lazy and stop secreting the body's own natural steroids. Consequently, they always need to be on steroid supplements, although even these patients can sometimes reactivate their adrenal gland with a slow taper. Most patients can just stop the steroids no matter what the dose after two to three weeks of use, but any longer will require some sort of taper; the speed and duration will depend on the dose and the disease. Prednisone is available in 1, 5, and 20 mg tablets and is probably the easiest of the steroids to taper. If patients are on some other form of steroid, such as Medrol, I usually switch them to an equivalent dose of prednisone and then start the taper. For some older or mentally challenged patients, it may be best to write or print out a day-by-day outline of your proposed regimen; otherwise, the patient will be totally confused. Do not assume patients know simple arithmetic—I often have to show them the taper by counting with my fingers. Many patients have trouble grasping that one 5 mg tablet is different than one 1 mg tablet. For instance, to reduce from 10 to 9 mg, you take four 1 mg tablets and one 5 mg tablet or nine 1 mg tablets. Their inclination is to eliminate one 5 mg tablet since they have been taking two of them. Very concrete thinking, I know, but I think once they grasp the concept that there are 1 mg tablets and 5 mg tablets and that they don't have to find a precise pill cutter to make 1 mg pieces out of the 5 mg tablets, most people are relieved and get it.

Unfortunately, there always will be the patient who refuses steroids or the one who refuses to taper. One of the more tragic cases I encountered a few years ago was a sixty-five-year-old gentleman with psoriasis, arthritis, and hepatitis C. He came to me on 15–20 mg of prednisone, which I considered both unnecessary and excessive, and would double the dose twelve weeks a year when he would vacation in Mexico and wear a bathing suit. He was the nicest and sweetest man you could hope to meet but would just smile and agree when I admonished him about his failure to taper his steroids.

Rudy's Ruminations On **Rheumatology**

During his last visit to Mexico, his colon ruptured, and he died. The autopsy revealed a tissue-thin colon caused by years of steroids. I decided that from then on I would discharge any patient who didn't attempt to taper steroids when it was reasonable to do so. I can't live with the tragedy that often ensues.

Occasionally, I encounter the reverse problem. There are a few patients who insist that they are allergic to even small doses of Prednisone making treatment of diseases like Polymyalgia Rheumatica very frustrating. Initially, I thought these claims were bogus—how could anyone be allergic to Prednisone? There are no 'nevers' in medicine and trial and error proved me wrong in these cases so I have had to become creative. Based on a pearl given to me by Frank Quismiorio, one of my mentors, I treat these patients with Medrol or Methylprednisolone, a more potent steroid similar to Prednisone and have had surprising success. I'm not sure I can quote any studies to support this approach but it has worked for me in a handful of difficult cases. Again, rheumatologists often have to think out of the box.

I think that's enough about steroids. In summary, they are useful tools to be respected and used judiciously, and remember, you are dancing with the devil!

Intra-articular injections of steroids are often very swift and effective treatments for one or two inflamed or irritated joints or tendons, especially in crystal-induced arthritis, such as gout or pseudogout, and also occasionally in RA, DJD, and seronegative spondyloarthritis. Generally, I aspirate and inject the joint with the same needle, screwing off the syringe after the aspiration and replacing it with the steroid-filled syringe. I do not inject joints when I suspect infection, and I wait at least three months between injections of the same joint for fear of damaging it. Triamcinolone and betamethasone are my steroids of choice at doses determined by the size of the joint. After personally experiencing a knee aspiration without anesthesia, I always use topical ethyl chloride and intra-articular lidocaine for the patient's comfort. I also advise patients to minimize use of the joint for at least two days after the injection. Remember that an intra-articular injection, especially into an inflamed joint, will be absorbed systemically, so the patient may have the added benefit of systemic relief.

Pearls

- Corticosteroids, or "steroids," are anti-inflammatory.
- Most rheumatology patients do not need steroids.
- In most cases, low or medium doses (prednisone 5–20 mg) are adequate.
- Most patients do not require long-term steroids.
- There are a few exceptions, such as polymyalgia rheumatic, some vasculitides, and severe organ involvement in lupus.
- When steroids are being prescribed for more than three months, consider prophylaxis for osteoporosis.
- Long-term moderate- to high-dose steroid use (more than 10 mg prednisone) is fraught with danger and rarely justified.
- Any dose of long-term steroids increases the incidence of infection.
- A large pulse dose (IV or IM) may induce remission or buy time in most inflammatory diseases.
- Beware of avascular necrosis, myopathy, psychosis, diabetes, and hypertension.
- Intra-articular and tendon sheath injections of steroids may provide swift and complete relief.
- Beware of the infected joint!
- Do not inject the same joint in less than a three-month interval.
- Repeated injections may destroy the joint or rupture a tendon.
- If patient is Prednisone 'allergic'—try Medrol

References

1. Grossman, J. M., R. Gordon, V. K. Ranganath, et al. American College of Rheumatology 2010 Recommendations for the Prevention and Treatment of Glucocorticoid-Induced Osteoporosis. *Arthritis Care Res* (Hoboken) 62:1515.

2. Buttgereit, F., M. Wehling, and G. R. Burmester. A New Hypothesis of Modular Glucocorticoid Actions: Steroid Treatment of Rheumatic Diseases Revisited. *Arthritis Rheum* 41:761.

3. Schimmer, B. P., and K. L. Parker. Adrenocorticotropic Hormone: Adrenocortical Steroids and Their Synthetic Analogs: Inhibitors of the Synthesis and Actions of Adrenocortical Hormones." In *The Pharmacological Basis of Therapeutics*, 11th edition, edited by L. L. Brunton, J. S. Lazo, and K. L. Parker, 1587. New York: McGraw Hill.

4. Corkill, M. M., B. W. Kirkham, I. C. Chikanza, et al. Intramuscular Depot Methylprednisolone Induction of Chrysotherapy in Rheumatoid Arthritis: A 24-Week Randomized Controlled Trial. *Br J Rheumatol* 29:274.

5. Iglehart, I. W., J. D. Sutton, J. C. Bender, et al. Intravenous Pulsed Steroids in Rheumatoid Arthritis: A Comparative Dose Study. *J Rheumatol* 17:159.

6. Buttgereit, F., D. Mehta, J. Kirwan, et al. Low-Dose Prednisone Chronotherapy for Rheumatoid Arthritis: A Randomised Clinical Trial (CAPRA-2). *Ann Rheum Dis* 72:204.

7. Svensson, B., A. Boonen, K. Albertsson, et al. Low-Dose Prednisolone in Addition to the Initial Disease-Modifying Antirheumatic Drug in Patients with Early Active Rheumatoid Arthritis Reduces Joint Destruction and Increases the Remission Rate: A Two-Year Randomized Trial. *Arthritis Rheum* 52:3360.

8. Paulus, H. E., D. Di Primeo, M. Sanda, et al. Progression of Radiographic Joint Erosion during Low Dose Corticosteroid Treatment of Rheumatoid Arthritis. *J Rheumatol* 27:1632.

9. Blyth, T., JA Hunter, and A. Stirling. Pain Relief in the Rheumatoid Knee after Steroid Injection. A Single-Blind Comparison of Hydrocortisone Succinate, and Triamcinolone Acetonide or Hexacetonide. *Br J Rheumatol* 33:461.

10. Chakravarty, K., P. D. Pharoah, and D. G. Scott. A Randomized Controlled Study of Post-injection Rest following Intra-articular Steroid Therapy for Knee Synovitis. *Br J Rheumatol* 33:464.

11. Owen, D. S. Aspiration and Injection of Joints in Soft Tissue. In *Textbook of Rheumatology*, 4th edition, edited by W. N. Kelley, E. D. Harris, Jr., S. Ruddy, and C. B. Sledge, 545. Philadelphia: WB Saunders.

12. Salvarani, C., F. Cantini, L. Boiardi, and G. G. Hunder. Polymyalgia Rheumatica and Giant-Cell Arteritis. *N Engl J Med* 347:261.

13. Buttgereit, F., G. R. Burmester, R. H. Straub, et al. Exogenous and Endogenous Glucocorticoids in Rheumatic Diseases. *Arthritis Rheum* 63:1.

14. Da Silva, J. A., J. W. Jacobs, J. R. Kirwan, et al. Safety of Low Dose Glucocorticoid Treatment in Rheumatoid Arthritis: Published Evidence and Prospective Trial Data. *Ann Rheum Dis* 65:285.

15. Hoes, J. N., J. W. Jacobs, S. M. Verstappen, et al. Adverse Events of Low- to Medium-Dose Oral Glucocorticoids in Inflammatory Diseases: A Meta-analysis. *Ann Rheum Dis* 68:1833.

The Nonsteroid—Nonsteroidal Anti-inflammatory Drugs (NSAIDS)

NSAIDS are probably the most commonly used medication by our patients, whether it is by prescription or over the counter. They are anti-inflammatory analgesic drugs that are not steroids—thus, they are nonsteroidals. Aspirin is the granddaddy of them all but has little anti-inflammatory effect unless taken in doses that usually exceed more than twelve tablets a day. This dose is both inconvenient and potentially very toxic. The other over-the-counter NSAIDS have similar limitations. Motrin (ibuprofen) is analgesic and not anti-inflammatory in doses less than 1,600 mg daily. Aleve (naproxen) is analgesic and not anti-inflammatory in doses less than 500 mg daily. Newer NSAIDs were designed for less toxicity, more convenient dosing, and better potency. As the science behind their mechanisms of action became better understood, researchers thought they could maximize efficacy and minimize toxicity. Like everything in life, unfortunately perfection was elusive, and some of the modifications created unforeseen new problems and lots of lawsuits. I find that I use much fewer NSAIDs these days because of their known toxicities, especially in the elderly, and because of the controversy caused by Vioxx (rofecoxib) in the early 2000s. Also, now that we have much more effective treatments for diseases such as rheumatoid arthritis, they are often not necessary. Still, used wisely, they are useful drugs. Two of the earliest NSAIDs after aspirin, Indocin (indomethacin) and Butazolodin (phenylbutazone), were two of the more potent anti-inflammatory NSAIDs, but unfortunately they were also two of the more toxic. In fact, phenylbutazone is currently reserved mainly for animals, especially horses. It is rarely used in humans because it can wipe out your supply of white blood cells and cause

Medications in Rheumatology

Stevens-Johnson syndrome, an often fatal skin and mucous membrane reaction. I have only prescribed it once or twice, but it sure is potent and was particularly good for spondyloarthritis, such as ankylosing spondylitis or psoriatic arthritis. Although NSAIDs treat inflammation, there is little evidence that they treat or prevent the progression of any underlying disease. However, there has been some suggestion that they prevent abnormal bone formation in ankylosing spondylitis.

As these drugs were used more and more in the sixties and seventies, it became clear that they had unforeseen toxicities, and new safer NSAIDs were needed. Scientists discovered and studied the prostaglandin and cyclooxygenase (COX-1 and COX-2) inflammatory pathways, and each new NSAID's relative effect on each pathway. They tried to design the perfect NSAID with substantially more potency and efficacy than toxicity. The pharmaceutical companies had a marketing bonanza and introduced one new NSAID after another. Each new drug was marketed as more potent, safer, or as having more convenient dosing. Some were shooting stars—a quick success and an even quicker withdrawal off the market, sometimes accompanied by scandal. Motrin (ibuprofen), Aleve (naproxen), Clinoril (sulindac), Tolectin (tolmetin), Disalcid (salsalate), Feldene (piroxicam), and Meclomen (meclofenamate) were some of the next generation of NSAIDs. The competition for the market was fierce. These medications were being used for everything from menstrual cramps, headaches, fevers, degenerative arthritis to gout, rheumatoid arthritis, and a variety of orthopedic and dental problems. They were extremely effective and seemed much safer than steroids or narcotics. In fact, eventually the FDA approved low-dose nonprescription Aleve (naproxen) and nonprescription low-dose Motrin (ibuprofen). However, like all medications, they had a dark side. They turned out to be toxic to the stomach, kidneys, and liver and inhibited platelets thereby inhibiting coagulation or thinning the blood. All these side effects were manageable, and liver and kidney toxicity were rare and usually occurred with high doses or in patients with already compromised kidney or liver function. Ironically, often patients who were trying to avoid the dangers of narcotics or steroids were the ones who overdosed accidentally on these medications or were not adequately monitored and suffered the worst consequences. There was a famous football player who took handfuls of Motrin instead of narcotics or steroids to help him play through injuries. He eventually was on dialysis. Because of this misconception that NSAIDs are totally benign, I have always been very skeptical of the decision to make them nonprescription. Patients need to be informed and monitored with blood count and liver- and kidney-function blood tests every three or four months.

During the eighties, several studies exposed NSAIDs as a major cause of GI bleeds. They also showed that many patients were asymptomatic before their bleed. In other words, they had no abdominal pain or GI complaints as a warning sign. The findings inspired a large cooperative study that studied the use of Cytotec, or misoprostol, as an adjunctive drug to be paired with NSAIDs to prevent ulcers or GI bleeds. The studies confirmed that misoprostol was effective in preventing ulcers and GI bleeds. However, the drug caused diarrhea and abdominal pain in many patients and had to be taken two to four times a day along with the NSAID. It also was fairly expensive. Imagine paying extra for a drug that did nothing for your symptoms but gave you the trots and cramps. It was not a hit, and the drug companies went back to the drawing board. Interestingly, recently, studies show that proton-pump inhibitors, such as Prilosec (omeprazole), Nexium (esomeprazole), or Prevacid (lansoprazole) are almost as effective at preventing GI bleeds as misoprostol and better tolerated. They add to the expense but less so, and they are usually taken once a day. Unfortunately, long-term use can lead to osteoporosis.

I am getting ahead of myself because by the nineties there was an explosion of research on NSAIDs and especially on the cyclooxygenase (COX) pathways, which regulate inflammation and some important physiologic functions involving the heart, blood pressure, and kidneys. The drug companies first flooded the market with NSAIDs that were relatively COX-2 selective. These drugs selectively inhibited the inflammatory pathways (COX-2) relatively more than the pathways that protected the GI tract, heart, kidneys, and platelet-clotting factors (COX-1). So, depending on the degree they inhibited COX-2 more than COX-1, they were theoretically safer than the older NSAIDs, which were less selective. It was great in theory, but they still had the same problems, and you could not use these drugs with blood thinners because they still had some effects on platelets. The list of these medications included Voltaren (diclofenac), Lodine (etodolac), Daypro (oxaprozin), Relafen (nabumetone), and Ansaid (flurbiprofen).

In the late nineties and early 2000s, we thought we had found the holy grail of NSAIDs—the specifically selective COX-2 inhibitors: Vioxx (rofecoxib), Celebrex (celecoxib), and later Bextra (valdecoxib) and Mobic (meloxicam). The studies showed these drugs had a low incidence of GI bleeds and did not inhibit platelets. They still had the potential kidney and liver problems, but we could live with that. Our patients on Coumadin or other blood thinners could take these drugs, and they seemed better tolerated. Besides, Vioxx seemed to be as potent or effective as Indocin without its toxicity. We were thrilled, and patients just loved these medications. However, in higher doses of Vioxx, we found that certain patients developed hypertension and edema, both known adverse effects of all NSAIDs. It just seemed a little more common with Vioxx, and so we had to be selective in choosing who was a candidate for this drug. Unfortunately, the drug company suppressed some studies that had shown an increased incidence of cardiovascular events with Vioxx—not really surprising and not really on a large scale but enough to attract opportunistic lawyers and create enough lawsuits to make the drug company take a useful drug off the market. My bias is that used judiciously with the right patient, it was a good drug. Bextra was soon withdrawn too, but Celebrex remains on the market because studies failed to draw similar conclusions about its effects on the cardiovascular system. The effect of this scandal and the growing evidence of potential risks of all NSAIDs had its impact on me, as I mentioned above. It also made me wary of drug company spin, even though I confess I still lecture for some of the companies and even lectured about Vioxx just before the scandal broke.

Finally, recently I have been prescribing topical NSAIDs such as Voltaren or Piroxicam (available by compound only) gel, for knee and hand osteoarthritis with fair to good success. Short-term studies have had mixed results and suggest that they may be less toxic than oral NSAIDs, but that remains to be seen. Nevertheless, I tend to use them when one or few joints are involved, especially in elderly patients. In sum, I use NSAIDs much less often, but they remain useful and safe if monitored correctly.

Pearls

- Use them with discretion. They are not necessary in most cases if the underlying disease is treated.
- Beware of the potential for GI bleed—monitor CBC and consider prophylaxis.
- GI bleeds may occur without symptoms.
- Monitor liver and kidney function at least every three to four months.
- Selective COX-2 inhibitors (Celebrex) spare platelets and may be used with warfarin (Coumadin); others can't.

- NSAIDs may inhibit bone formation in ankylosing spondylitis.
- Topical NSAIDs may be effective and less toxic for knee and hand DJD.

References

1. Baum, C., D. L. Kennedy, and M. B. Forbes. Utilization of Nonsteroidal Antiinflammatory Drugs. *Arthritis Rheum* 28:686.

2. Brooks, P. M., and R. O. Day Nonsteroidal Antiinflammatory Drugs—Differences and Similarities. *N Engl J Med* 324:1716.

3. Cryer, B., and M. Feldman. Cyclooxygenase-1 and Cyclooxygenase-2 Selectivity of Widely Used Nonsteroidal Antiinflammatory Drugs. *Am J Med* 104:413.

4. Perazella, M. A., and K. Tray. Selective Cyclooxygenase-2 Inhibitors: A Pattern of Nephrotoxicity Similar to Traditional Nonsteroidal Antiinflammatory Drugs. *Am J Med* 111:64.

5. Pavelka, K., D. P. Recker, and K. M. Verburg. Valdecoxib Is as Effective as Diclofenac in the Management of Rheumatoid Arthritis with a Lower Incidence of Gastroduodenal Ulcers: Results of a 26-Week Trial. *Rheumatology* (Oxford) 42:1207.

6. Simon, L. S., A. L. Weaver, D. Y. Graham, et al. Anti-inflammatory and Upper Gastrointestinal Effects of Celecoxib in Rheumatoid Arthritis: A Randomized Controlled Trial. *JAMA* 282:1921.

7. Leese, P. T., R. C. Hubbard, A. Karim, et al. Effects of Celecoxib, a Novel Cyclooxygenase-2 Inhibitor, on Platelet Function in Healthy Adults: A Randomized, Controlled Trial. *J Clin Pharmacol* 40:124.

8. Solomon, D. H. Selective Cyclooxygenase 2 Inhibitors and Cardiovascular Events. *Arthritis Rheum* 52:1968.

9. Solomon, S. D., J. Wittes, P. V. Finn, et al. Cardiovascular Risk of Celecoxib in 6 Randomized Placebo-Controlled Trials: The Cross Trial Safety Analysis. *Circulation* 117:2104.

10. Tugwell, P. S., G. A. Wells, and J. Z. Shainhouse. Equivalence Study of a Topical Diclofenac Solution (Pennsaid) Compared with Oral Diclofenac in Symptomatic Treatment of Osteoarthritis of the Knee: A Randomized Controlled Trial. *J Rheumatol* 31:2002.

11. "Diclofenac Gel for Osteoarthritis." *Med Lett Drugs Ther* 50:31.

12. Lin, J., W. Zhang, A. Jones, and M. Doherty. Efficacy of Topical Non-steroidal Anti-inflammatory Drugs in the Treatment of Osteoarthritis: Meta-analysis of Randomised Controlled Trials. *BMJ* 329:324.

Antimalarial Drugs

(Plaquenil, Aralen and Quinacrine)

Three old antimalarial drugs, no longer used in malaria, are very effective in lupus and other related diseases and are very inexpensive. They also have relatively favorable adverse-effect profiles. By far, the one most commonly used is Plaquenil (hydroxychloroquine). It inhibits some of the inflammatory factors that are active in lupus. It is a slow-acting drug and takes about six weeks to take effect. I think it's important to advise patients about its slow onset to avoid confusion and premature discontinuation of the drug. It is most effective for the rashes, fatigue, oral ulcers, and joint pain in lupus and has limited or no effect on organ involvement, such as in kidney disease. It is still used in mild forms of arthritis in related diseases, such as rheumatoid arthritis or Sjögren's syndrome, but is not considered a particularly powerful remittive agent. The most common side effect is rash, which can start as just plain itchiness and blossom into the rash from hell involving the whole body if the medication is not stopped promptly. Diarrhea and abdominal pain are rare but again can be quite severe if the medication is not stopped. I have had patients admitted to the hospital for workup of a potentially catastrophic abdominal event until someone stopped the Plaquenil, and the symptoms resolved. The most famous potential side effect is deposits in patients' retinas or corneas leading to visual disturbances. I reassure patients that if they see an eye doctor when starting the medication and then have annual eye examinations, it is extremely safe. Abnormal pigment deposits in the macula can be seen during dilated eye exam years before visual loss might occur. The risk of visual loss is also tied to dose per patient's body weight (not to exceed 6.5 mg/kg) and long-term exposure, and physicians have become good at staying within these limitations. Nevertheless, some patients are so alarmed they refuse the medication. Other adverse effects are also extremely rare, but in my thirty years of rheumatology, I have seen many of them at least once. They include a grayish skin tint, muscle disease, low white count, hypoglycemia, liver abnormalities, and tinnitus and even hearing loss. I have had three or four patients develop ringing in their ears, and at first I did not make the connection. Plaquenil has taught me that any medication can do anything, and before dismissing the possibility that a medication is causing a particular symptom, reread its side-effect profile and consider a drug holiday if in doubt. Overall, Plaquenil is an effective, well-tolerated, safe, and inexpensive drug for the treatment of lupus and occasionally in RA, Sjögren's, and a few other autoimmune diseases. As a bonus, it is safe in pregnancy and during breast-feeding. Several studies over the last three decades have shown that lupus patients who remain on Plaquenil have less frequent and less severe flares.

Quinacrine (Atabrine) is an even older antimalarial that is not even manufactured anymore but may be obtained from compounding pharmacies that can make their own drugs. I use it in lupus patients who can't tolerate Plaquenil or along with Plaquenil in patients who have resistant skin rashes. It is particularly good for patients who have fatigue and cognitive dysfunction. Those who have an allergy or an adverse reaction to Plaquenil usually tolerate quinacrine well. Baseline and annual eye exams are not required with this drug because it does not have the same retinal toxicity. I had never seen a rash caused by quinacrine until recently, but it can cause the skin to turn a reversible color of orange or yellow. Most of my young, female lupus patients who undergo this color change love it because it looks like a good suntan, but not always. I have had one doctor call and inform me that my patient was jaundiced, despite the fact her eyeballs were white. I had one patient stop the medication because she worked in a fast-food restaurant, and the customers started to complain that she might have hepatitis. These patients were the exceptions. Quinacrine is another relatively safe and effective drug, which like Plaquenil does not have to be stopped during an infection or prior to surgery.

Aralen (chloroquine) is similar to Plaquenil but has a higher incidence of eye toxicity. It is probably as effective as Plaquenil and is still used by some rheumatologists. Unlike Quinacrine, it will cross-react with Plaquenil and cause the same allergic reaction. I have only used it once and prefer quinacrine as an alternative to Plaquenil, although some rheumatologists would disagree. Doses higher than 250 mg run a high risk of eye toxicity.

Pearls

- Antimalarials are first-line drugs for lupus.
- They are particularly effective for rashes, oral ulcers, hair loss, fatigue, and joint pain.
- Both hydroxychloroquine and chloroquine can cause pigment to be deposited in the retina and cornea, and patients need annual eye exams.
- Chloroquine is more toxic so hydroxychloroquine is more commonly used.
- Quinacrine does not cause eye toxicity but may cause patients to turn a reversible color of orange.
- Hydroxychloroquine is safe during pregnancy and breast-feeding.
- Hydroxychloroquine rash can be extremely severe and prolonged.

References

1. Gladman, D. D., M. B. Urowitz, J. L. Senécal, et al. Aspects of Use of Antimalarials in Systemic Lupus Erythematosus. *J Rheumatol* 25:983.
2. Wallace, D. J. The Use of Quinacrine (Atabrine) in Rheumatic Diseases: A Reexamination. *Semin Arthritis Rheum* 18:282.
3. Wallace, D. J. Is There a Role for Quinacrine (Atabrine) in the New Millennium? *Lupus* 9:81.

Nonbiologic Remittive Agents

What the hell does that mean? These medications put the disease into remission or treat the underlying problem and not just the symptoms. *Nonbiologic* means they do not target specific molecules or cells of the immune system or their products that are secreted in the joints. In plain language the biologic agents tend to be lasers targeted at specific parts of the immune system that are defective in a particular disease. They use genetic technology and living cells as the "factories" for making the medications. Nonbiologics tend to be shotguns that suppress a whole part of the immune system or a whole cell line (white and red blood cell and platelets) and may affect some innocent bystanders along the way. They tend to be older drugs and are often but not always immunosuppressive. If they are immunosuppressive, they predispose patients to certain infections, although to a surprisingly small degree. Therefore, they should be held during serious infections and prior to major surgeries. Most of them affect the bone marrow and can affect certain blood cell lines.

CellCept (mycophenolate mofetil)

CellCept (mycophenolate mofetil) was first used in organ transplants and has gained wide acceptance for its use in lupus, especially in kidney disease. Recently, it is used occasionally in other diseases, such as granulomatosis with polyangiitis (Wegener's granulomatosis). It is another drug that prevents inflammatory cells from multiplying and has replaced some of the more toxic older chemotherapy drugs we used to use in these situations, such as Cytoxan or Imuran. Most patients tolerate it well, and it is extremely effective in conditions such as kidney disease in lupus, which has a high risk of dialysis or death. I used to cringe when I treated this disease because the treatment of choice was intravenous Cytoxan (cyclophosphamide) monthly for six months and then every three months. Some patients would vomit, lose hair, lose bone marrow function, get infected, become infertile, develop low sodium, bleed into their bladder, and years down the line develop bladder cancer or lymphoma. It seemed worth it at the time, but I always wondered. Patients were miserable, and many of them were also on high-dose steroids and gaining large amounts of weight. You had destroyed these young women's body image with weight gain and hair loss and made them nauseated, vomit, and extremely fatigued. Oh yeah, you also saved their kidneys! Then along came some studies proving that CellCept was at least as effective and much less toxic and could be taken orally. For me, it was a no-brainer. CellCept's most common dose is 2 g, or four pills, a day. I go up to 6 g a day and occasionally taper below 2. Its potential side effects include bone marrow toxicity, liver toxicity, some nausea, and rarely fluid retention and hypertension. If monitored with a complete blood cell count and chemistry panel every four to twelve weeks, it's fairly safe. It is also a steroid-sparing drug and available in generic form. To be fair to Cytoxan, current regimens may be better tolerated, and it can be a life-saving drug, but I still prefer CellCept.

Pearls

- It is the drug of choice for most patients with lupus nephritis.
- Most patients require at least 2 g daily.
- It may cause edema, hypertension, kidney dysfunction, or bone marrow suppression.
- It is better tolerated than Imuran or Cytoxan.

- It may be useful in polymyositis, vasculitis, scleroderma, and interstitial lung disease.
- It should be monitored with complete blood cell count and chemistry panels every four to twelve weeks.

References

1. Lipsky, J. J. "Mycophenolate Mofetil." *Lancet* 348:1357.

2. Riskalla, M. M., E. C. Somers, R. A. Fatica, and W. J. McCune. Tolerability of Mycophenolate Mofetil in Patients with Systemic Lupus Erythematosus. *J Rheumatol* 30:1508.

3. Kingdon, E. J., A. G. McLean, E. Psimenou, et al. The Safety and Efficacy of MMF in Lupus Nephritis: A Pilot Study. *Lupus* 10:606.

4. Haubitz, M., and K. de Groot. Tolerance of Mycophenolate Mofetil in End-Stage Renal Disease Patients with ANCA-Associated Vasculitis. *Clin Nephrol* 57:421.

5. Liossis S. N., A. Bounas, and A. P. Andonopoulos. Mycophenolate Mofetil as First-Line Treatment Improves Clinically Evident Early Scleroderma Lung Disease. *Rheumatology* (Oxford) 45:1005.

6. Pisoni, C. N., M. J. Cuadrado, M. A. Khamashta, et al. Mycophenolate Mofetil Treatment in Resistant Myositis. *Rheumatology* (Oxford) 46:516.

Methotrexate

Methotrexate is the most universally used and reliable of the nonbiologic drugs. It essentially inhibits inflammatory cells and rapidly reproducing cells, such as cancer cells. It has been around for more than a half century and has been used in much higher doses in certain cancers, for example, breast cancer. Importantly, lower doses have much milder and rarer side effects. Methotrexate's use and value in rheumatology have evolved with our knowledge. In the fifties and sixties, it was used for psoriasis (a bad skin disease) and for its sometimes (10–20 percent of patients) associated arthritis. It was very successful, but in a large study, it was found that too many of these patients developed severe liver disease, even cirrhosis. The medical community, especially dermatologists, was spooked, and they stopped using methotrexate, except for certain cancers. During the eighties, new studies rekindled interest in this drug as a treatment for rheumatoid arthritis. Reviews of the old studies in psoriasis revealed that the investigators did not screen out patients who drank excessive amounts of alcohol or had preexisting liver disease. Also, it was felt that monthly or bimonthly monitoring of liver-function tests and consequent dose adjustment or discontinuation of the drug was safe. There was some controversy as to whether blood tests correlated with what was actually going on in the liver. Several large studies of RA patients, which included yearly liver biopsies, indicated that they did. Researchers also found that once-weekly rather than daily doses would decrease toxicity and was extremely effective. They also found that daily folic acid prevented some of the side effects, such as oral ulcers. Still, there was a lot of controversy surrounding this drug. The dermatology community felt that psoriasis patients were different than rheumatoid patients and studies on one did not necessarily correlate with the other. Yet they did not undertake any new, large, long-term study. To this day, dermatologists are reluctant to use methotrexate and feel that patients on this drug should undergo yearly liver biopsies. Most rheumatologists would disagree, but fear of lawsuits and reference to old, flawed studies make some consider liver biopsies in these patients. Also, psoriasis patients are probably more predisposed to liver disease than RA patients, so they may have a point. Still, by 2000, Methotrexate was the gold-standard remittive agent for rheumatoid arthritis and psoriatic arthritis and often used in a variety of other disease, such as lupus, polymyositis, and granulomatosis with polyangiitis (GPA). Lately however, some studies have created doubts about its true effectiveness in psoriatic arthritis. Still, it is a great anti-inflammatory drug that often treats the underlying disease and is considered steroid sparing, allowing patients to lower their doses of steroids or even stop them. If monitored properly, it can be taken for many years without problems. The most common side effects besides liver toxicity and bone marrow toxicity are oral ulcers, nausea, hair loss, and headaches. Uniquely, this drug has an antidote to some of its toxicities—namely, oral ulcers and marrow toxicities—leucovorin, which is actually folinic acid, or the activated form of folic acid.

Early in my rheumatology practice, I had a blind patient with RA who was on twelve aspirin a day and eight methotrexate tablets a week. She mistook her methotrexate for her aspirin and was taking twelve Methotrexate tablets a day for at least a week. She soon developed severe weakness and painful sores in her mouth and vagina. By the time she was seen in our clinic, her lips and mouth were full of open sores, she could barely stand, and we found that she was seriously anemic—her white blood cell and platelet count were dangerously low. Because of her findings, I deduced her mistake, admitted her to the hospital, and thought that her prognosis was grave. However, after two days of intravenous leucovorin, most of her sores had resolved, and all her blood tests had improved dramatically. It was impressive! I don't know of many medications that have such an effective antidote.

A rare but frightening side effect can be severe shortness of breath and possibly respiratory failure caused by inflammation of the lung interstitium (the tissue and space around the air sacs). It probably is caused by an allergic reaction and may require hospitalization, oxygen, and discontinuation of the drug. I have had at least two cases, and both eventually did well, but it was touch and go. It is important to rule out infection and the underlying disease as the cause in these patients. A mistake could be fatal.

Methotrexate is a great long-term drug for many diseases. It is relatively safe as long as it is used in the right patients. Patients who drink excessively, have preexisting liver disease, have severe infections, or are pregnant or trying to become pregnant are not good candidates. Methotrexate can cause miscarriages and fetal abnormalities and should probably be held for six months before pregnancy. We usually request pregnancy tests in child-bearing-age females before starting methotrexate. We also obtain hepatitis B and C tests and instruct patients that they can have a few drinks a week and on special occasions while on the drug. I find that you have to remind people intermittently of this rule because they will either forget or not take you seriously. I am always shocked at how many patients who I see for the first time and are already on methotrexate claim they have never been told of the association of methotrexate, alcohol, and liver toxicity. If patients do not undergo blood tests for liver function and blood count at least every three to four months, I discharge them! Labs should be done every two to four weeks at its initiation until the patient has been stable for several months. Again, methotrexate is a great long-term drug, which is very effective and safe as long as it is used in the right patient and monitored regularly. There are

American College of Rheumatology guidelines for monitoring available. Interestingly, subcutaneous methotrexate may be better tolerated and more effective than the oral form and is less expensive.

Pearls

- It is the drug of first choice for RA and is effective in remitting the disease (preventing progression) in many patients.
- It is effective in polymyositis, many kinds of vasculitis, sclero-derma, lupus, and a variety of other diseases.
- It is effective for psoriasis and questionably effective in psoriatic arthritis.
- It probably has a higher risk for liver-function abnormalities in psoriasis.
- It is usually well tolerated and safe for long-term use if properly monitored.
- CBC and liver function should be drawn every one to three months.
- Folic acid prophylaxis is effective in preventing oral ulcers and hematological side effects.
- Leucovorin is an effective antidote for methotrexate toxicity.
- Patients should minimize alcohol intake to two to three drinks a week or be at high risk for liver problems.
- It can cause a severe subacute pneumonitis and then should be discontinued immediately.
- It may cause severe headache at higher doses.
- It must be stopped at least six months before any pregnancy.
- Subcutaneous methotrexate may be better tolerated and more effective and is less expensive.

References

1. Kremer, J. M., and J. K. Lee. The Safety and Efficacy of the Use of Methotrexate in Long-Term Therapy for Rheumatoid Arthritis. *Arthritis Rheum* 29:822.

2. Cronstein, B. N. Molecular Therapeutics: Methotrexate and Its Mechanism of Action. *Arthritis Rheum* 39:1951.

3. Rich, E., L. W. Moreland, and G. S. Alarcón. Paucity of Radiographic Progression in Rheumatoid Arthritis Treated with Methotrexate as the First Disease Modifying Antirheumatic Drug. *J Rheumatol* 26:259.

4. Saag, K. G., G. G. Teng, N. M. Patkar, et al. American College of Rheumatology 2008 Recommendations for the Use of Nonbiologic and Biologic Disease-Modifying Antirheumatic Drugs in Rheumatoid Arthritis. *Arthritis Rheum* 59:762.

5. Visser, K., Katchamart, E. Loza, et al. Multinational Evidence-Based Recommendations for the Use of Methotrexate in Rheumatic Disorders with a Focus on Rheumatoid Arthritis: Integrating Systematic Literature Research and Expert Opinion of a Broad International Panel of Rheumatologists in the 3E Initiative. *Ann Rheum Dis* 68:1086

6. Bakker, M. F., J. W. Jacobs, P. M. Welsing, et al. Are Switches from Oral to Subcutaneous Methotrexate or Addition of Ciclosporin to Methotrexate Useful Steps in a Tight Control Treatment Strategy for Rheumatoid Arthritis? A Post Hoc Analysis of the CAMERA Study. *Ann Rheum Dis* 69:1849.

7. Saravanan, V., and C. A. Kelly. Reducing the Risk of Methotrexate Pneumonitis in Rheumatoid Arthritis. *Rheumatology* (Oxford) 43:143.

8. Goodman, T. A., and R. P. Polisson. Methotrexate: Adverse Reactions and Major Toxicities. *Rheum Dis Clin North Am* 20:513.

9. Kingsley, G. H., A. Kowalczyk, H. Taylor, et al. A Randomized Placebo-Controlled Trial of Methotrexate in Psoriatic Arthritis. *Rheumatology* (Oxford) 51:1368.

10. Abu-Shakra, M., D. D. Gladman, J. C. Thorne, et al. Longterm Methotrexate Therapy in Psoriatic Arthritis: Clinical and Radiological Outcome. *J Rheumatol* 22:241.

11. Hassan, W. Methotrexate and Liver Toxicity: Role of Surveillance Liver Biopsy. Conflict between Guidelines for Rheumatologists and Dermatologists. *Ann Rheum Dis* 55:273.

12. Newman, E. D., and D. W. Scott. The Use of Low-dose Oral Methotrexate in the Treatment of Polymyositis and Dermatomyositis. *J Clin Rheumatol* 1:99.

13. Metzger, A. L., A. Bohan, L. S. Goldberg, et al. Polymyositis and Dermatomyositis: Combined Methotrexate and Corticosteroid Therapy. *Ann Intern Med* 81:182.

14. Fortin, P. R., M. Abrahamowicz, D. Ferland, et al. Steroid-Sparing Effects of Methotrexate in Systemic Lupus Erythematosus: A Double-Blind, Randomized, Placebo-Controlled Trial. *Arthritis Rheum* 59:1796.

15. Sneller, M. C., G. S. Hoffman, C. Talar-Williams, et al. An Analysis of Forty-Two Wegener's Granulomatosis Patients Treated with Methotrexate and Prednisone. *Arthritis Rheum* 38:608.

16. Specks, U. Methotrexate for Wegener's Granulomatosis: What Is the Evidence? *Arthritis Rheum* 52:2237.

Arava (leflunomide)

Arava (leflunomide) is almost a junior methotrexate. It also inhibits the inflammatory cascade and is used in rheumatoid arthritis, psoriatic arthritis, and sometimes in lupus. It is used solely for arthritis, whereas methotrexate has other uses and is generally more effective. The lone exception may be psoriatic arthritis. It is a daily drug and stays in the system for months after discontinued. When it is absolutely necessary to remove it from a patient's system immediately, there is a medication that will bind to it in the intestinal tract and inactivate it. Liver toxicity is again the main worry, and its interaction with alcohol is even more dangerous. Unlike methotrexate, it can cause hypertension. Diarrhea and abdominal pain can occur. It is toxic to the fetus and again should be discontinued for at least six months before attempting conception. We basically use the same screening procedures and monitoring as with methotrexate. There are some patients who can't tolerate methotrexate who tolerate Arava. Some of its lesser known side effects include severe rash, anorexia, and weight loss. I have a few elderly patients who were wasting away to nothing and have had extensive workups for cancer who immediately regained their appetite and weight when they discontinued Arava. Again it is a good drug when used in the right setting and monitored properly, especially with regular blood pressure readings. I think my most common reason for discontinuing this drug is uncontrolled hypertension.

Pearls

- It is a less effective alternative to methotrexate in many diseases, including RA, lupus, and a variety of other diseases.
- The lone exception may be psoriatic arthritis, where it may be more effective.

- It is more toxic to the liver than methotrexate, and alcohol should be avoided.
- CBC and liver-function tests should be ordered at least every three months.
- Hypertension can be a major side effect.
- Abdominal pain and diarrhea can occur.
- Extreme weight loss occasionally occurs.
- It stays in the system for several months and is extremely toxic to pregnancy.
- There is a medication that binds to it in the intestine and helps wash it out of the system.
- Avoid pregnancy unless discontinued for at least six months.

References

1. Cuchacovich, M., and L. Soto. Leflunomide Decreases Joint Erosions and Induces Reparative Changes in a Patient with Psoriatic Arthritis. *Ann Rheum Dis* 61:942.

2. Tam, L. S., E. K. Li, C. K. Wong, et al. Double-Blind, Randomized, Placebo-Controlled Pilot Study of Leflunomide in Systemic Lupus Erythematosus. *Lupus* 13:601.

3. Sharp, J. T., V. Strand, H. Leung, et al. Treatment with Leflunomide Slows Radiographic Progression of Rheumatoid Arthritis: Results from Three Randomized Controlled Trials of Leflunomide in Patients with Active Rheumatoid Arthritis. Leflunomide Rheumatoid Arthritis Investigators Group. *Arthritis Rheum* 43:495.

4. Scott, D. L., J. S. Smolen, J. R. Kalden, et al. Treatment of Active Rheumatoid Arthritis with Leflunomide: Two Year Follow up of a Double Blind, Placebo Controlled Trial versus Sulfasalazine. *Ann Rheum Dis* 60:913.

1. Narváez, J., C. Díaz-Torné, J. M. Ruiz, et al. Comparative Effectiveness of Rituximab in Combination with Either Methotrexate

or Leflunomide in the Treatment of Rheumatoid Arthritis. *Semin Arthritis Rheum* 41:401.

Azulfidine (sulfasalazine)

Azulfidine is an old medication that combines aspirin with sulfa and magically works as a weak remittive agent in RA, seronegative spondyloarthritis, and inflammatory bowel disease. Although British studies suggest otherwise, I find it to be a weak agent in RA unless combined with Plaquenil and methotrexate. Triple-drug therapy is an effective remittive therapy almost equivalent to biologics and methotrexate. The most common side effects are rash (which can be serious), low white blood cell count (including rarely agranulocytosis, the complete loss of all white cells), low sperm count (reversible), and GI upset. I rarely use it alone, but it is always worth a try in certain circumstances. I have one patient with moderate RA and chronic lung infections who seems to be doing well on this drug alone. It has the advantage of being safe in infected patients.

Pearls
- Best used as part of triple-drug therapy with Plaquenil and methotrexate in RA.
- It is occasionally effective in seronegative spondyloarthritis.

References
1. Amos, R. S. The History of the Use of Sulphasalazine in Rheumatology, supplement. *Br J Rheumatol* 34 (2): S2.
2. Weinblatt, M. E., D. Reda, W. Henderson, et al. Sulfasalazine Treatment for Rheumatoid Arthritis: A Metaanalysis of 15 Randomized Trials. *J Rheumatol* 26:2123.

3. Dougados, M., B. Combe, A. Cantagrel, et al. Combination Therapy in Early Rheumatoid Arthritis: A Randomised, Controlled, Double Blind 52 Week Clinical Trial of Sulphasalazine and Methotrexate Compared with the Single Components. *Ann Rheum Dis* 58:220.

4. Saunders, S. A., H. A. Capell, A. Stirling, et al. Triple Therapy in Early Active Rheumatoid Arthritis: A Randomized, Single-Blind, Controlled Trial Comparing Step-Up and Parallel Treatment Strategies. *Arthritis Rheum* 58:1310.

5. Fuchs, H. A. Use of Sulfasalazine in Rheumatic Diseases. *Bull Rheum Dis* 46:3.

Cytoxan (cyclophosphamide)

Since we mentioned them, let's talk about some of the older che-motherapy drugs that we still use in rheumatology. I guess the gold standard is Cytoxan—maximally effective and toxic, as described above. I remember a well-meaning but misguided supervisor of mine telling a lupus patient who was reluctant to try the drug for her kid-ney disease that she had to think of her kidney disease as Hiroshima and Cytoxan as a nuclear bomb. It would end the war! Needless to say, the patient left the hospital against medical advice never to be seen again, even though in a sense, my old professor was right. Cytoxan destroys many of the renegade inflammatory or cancer cells in your body but takes out a lot of innocent bystanders as well. It basically affects rapidly reproducing cells. We still reserve it for many of our most catastrophic or emergent events, such as hemor-rhaging into a lung in lupus or respiratory or kidney failure in a few of our more serious disease, like GPA (Wegener's) or other vasculitides. It is also used in some cases of scleroderma lung and some seri-ous eye and skin conditions. Many rheumatologists still feel it is the drug of choice for most kidney and brain disease in lupus. It can be prescribed orally or intravenously, daily or monthly or even every six months, according to certain protocols. Amazingly, some patients tolerate it well, but most patients suffer from one of the many short- or long-term side effects described above. There are medications that can prevent the nausea, bladder hemorrhage, or even infertility, but still it's a nasty drug. Thankfully, as the years pass, we are devel-oping safer but equally effective medications, but it's comforting to know that the old nuclear bomb is still available when needed. It is still the 'go-to' drug in vasculitis patients with life-threatening organ involvement.

If IV Cytoxan is used, blood count, urinalysis, and full chemistry panel should be drawn initially after seven to ten days and rechecked two days before the next dose. When oral Cytoxan is used, blood work should be drawn every one to two weeks for the first six weeks. Because bladder cancer is a lifelong risk for patients who have been exposed to long-term (six months or longer) oral more than inter-mittent IV Cytoxan, urinalyses looking for red blood cells should be obtained every three to four months for the rest of their lives.

Recently, one of my very bright lupus patients complained of in-creasing memory lapses. Her MRI revealed white matter lesions or loss of blood flow in certain areas of her brain probably because of inflammation. She researched the best treatment for this kind of problem in lupus and independently suggested monthly IV Cytoxan. Surprisingly after four months of this regimen, she is back to normal with minimal side effects. After two more doses, we will reevaluate her and probably discontinue the Cytoxan and restart CellCept. She will need to have urinalyses done every three to four months for the rest of her life checking for bladder cancer, but she is very satisfied. The possibility of increasing dementia terrified her. Again, in rheuma-tology, sometimes you have to dance with the devil.

Pearls

- Cytoxan is less toxic and perhaps more effective intravenously.
- It is still used in many extreme life-threatening situations, such as extreme cases of vasculitis or acute organ damage.
- In many cases, such as vasculitis and lupus nephritis and CNS disease, there are equally effective and less toxic therapies.
- Monitor CBC, UA, and chemistry panel every one to two months.
- Monitor for lymphoma and bladder cancer for lifetime after com-pletion of therapy.
- Consider bladder- and ovary-protecting therapy.

References

1. Regan, M. J., D. B. Hellmann, and J. H. Stone. Treatment of Wegener's Granulomatosis. *Rheum Dis Clin North Am* 27:863.

2. Balow, J. E., H. A. Austin, G. C. Tsokos, et al. NIH Conference: Lupus Nephritis. *Ann Intern Med* 106:79.

3. Gayraud, M., L. Guillevin, P. Cohen, et al. Treatment of Good-Prognosis Polyarteritis Nodosa and Churg-Strauss Syndrome: Comparison of Steroids and Oral or Pulse Cyclophosphamide in 25 Patients. French Cooperative Study Group for Vasculitides. *Br J Rheumatol* 36:1290.

4. Gourley, M. F., H. A. Austin, D. Scott, et al. Methylprednisolone and Cyclophosphamide, Alone or in Combination, in Patients with Lupus Nephritis. A Randomized, Controlled Trial. *Ann Intern Med* 125:549.

6. Yee, C. S., C. Gordon, C. Dostal, et al. EULAR Randomised Controlled Trial of Pulse Cyclophosphamide and Methylprednisolone versus Continuous Cyclophosphamide and Prednisolone Followed by Azathioprine and Prednisolone in Lupus Nephritis. *Ann Rheum Dis* 63:525.

7. Barile, L., and C. Lavalle. Transverse Myelitis in Systemic Lupus Erythematosus—the Effect of IV Pulse Methylprednisolone and Cyclophosphamide. *J Rheumatol* 19:370.

8. Stojanovich, L., R. Stojanovich, V. Kostich, and E. Dzjolich. Neuropsychiatric Lupus Favourable Response to Low Dose I.V. Cyclophosphamide and Prednisolone (Pilot Study). *Lupus* 12:3.

Imuran (azathioprine)

Imuran is a junior Cytoxan. It is not as effective or toxic. Another old medication that inhibits rapidly reproducing cells, such as inflammatory or bone marrow cells, it is used to maintain remission in many serious diseases, such as GPA or even lupus, and is considered steroid sparing. It has the usual set of adverse effects of drugs of its class, such as nausea and bone marrow toxicity, and the added risk of pancreatitis. I use this drug very rarely these days because of its toxicity and only moderate effectiveness. Also, it has many dangerous drug interactions, such as with allopurinol (see below) and Coumadin (warfarin). There are many better therapies available, but because it is cheap, sometimes the insurances and patients leave me no choice. Again, a blood count and a full chemistry panel should be done every four to eight weeks. Screening for an enzyme called *TPMT* before initiating the drug may predict the probability of a patient developing toxicity.

Pearls

- It is a fair to good steroid-sparing maintenance drug but mediocre remission inducer.
- It may cause macrocytic anemia.
- Beware of drug interactions, such as with allopurinol and warfarin.
- Beware of pancreatitis and lymphoma.
- It is probably safe during pregnancy but questionable for breast-feeding.

References

1. Pagnoux, C., A. Mahr, M. A. Hamidou, et al. Azathioprine or Methotrexate Maintenance for ANCA-Associated Vasculitis. *N Engl J Med* 359:2790.

2. Huskisson, E. C. Azathioprine. *Clin Rheum Dis* 10:325.

3. Moskovitz, D. N., C. Bodian, M. L. Chapman, et al. The Effect on the Fetus of Medications Used to Treat Pregnant Inflammatory Bowel-Disease Patients. *Am J Gastroenterol* 99:656.

4. Henderson, L. K., P. Masson, J. C. Craig, et al. Induction and Maintenance Treatment of Proliferative Lupus Nephritis: A Meta-analysis of Randomized Controlled Trials. *Am J Kidney Dis* 61:74.

Cyclosporine and Tacrolimus

Cyclosporine and tacrolimus also inhibit inflammatory factors, especially interleukin-2. They were initially used for liver and kidney transplants and now are utilized for a variety of diseases, including psoriasis, psoriatic arthritis, rheumatoid arthritis, polymyositis, dermatomyositis, Behcet's, iritis, and many more. A topical form of cyclosporine called *Restasis* is effective as eye drops in some Sjögren's patients. I have used cyclosporine in psoriatic arthritis in combination with a biologic or methotrexate with some success, but toxicity, especially hypertension, has been a problem. I have used tacrolimus in two polymyositis patients with one failure and one success. It also can be used in other special situations where a patient has failed all the usual classes of drug or has a contraindication to them. It is also helpful as a topical cream for resistant rashes in lupus and dermatomyositis. Rheumatologists often have to think "outside of the box" when dealing with patients who have failed, can't tolerate, or can't afford conventional treatment. Cyclosporine and tacrolimus tend to be less bone marrow toxic than the other immunosuppressive drugs but are more toxic to the kidney and have a higher incidence of hypertension. Tremor and other neurological problems can occur. Diabetes has been reported with tacrolimus, and cyclosporine has been reported to cause osteoporosis and hyperuricemia. Like most of the nonbiologic immunosuppressive agents, they can induce nausea and vomiting and other GI issues, but so far I have found these problems to be rare. Paradoxically hair loss and excessive hair growth in undesirable places can be problematic. Like all these medications, regular labs are necessary every two to three months. These drugs are rarely first-line drugs, except in special cases like resistant polymyositis. It's just comforting to know I have two potentially effective medications to pull out of "my box" when I am at wit's end.

Pearls

- Tacrolimus and cyclosporine are second- or third-line choices with a few exceptions.
- Monitor kidney function and blood pressure.
- Cyclosporine may increase uric acid.

References

1. Salvarani, C., P. Macchioni, I. Olivieri, et al. A Comparison of Cyclosporine, Sulfasalazine, and Symptomatic Therapy in the Treatment of Psoriatic Arthritis. *J Rheumatol* 28:2274.

2. Greaves, M. W., and G. D. Weinstein. Treatment of Psoriasis. *N Engl J Med* 332:581.

3. Foulks, G. N. Treatment of Dry Eye Disease by the Non-ophthalmologist." *Rheum Dis Clin North Am* 34:987.

4. Barber, L. D., S. C. Pflugfelder, J. Tauber, and G. N. Foulks. Phase III Safety Evaluation of Cyclosporine 0.1% Ophthalmic Emulsion Administered Twice Daily to Dry Eye Disease Patients for up to 3 Years. *Ophthalmology* 112:1790.

5. Oddis, CV., F. C. Sciurba FC, K. A. Elmagd, and T. E. Starzl. Tacrolimus in Refractory Polymyositis with Interstitial Lung Disease. *Lancet* 353:1762.

6. Wilkes, M. R., S. M. Sereika, N. Fertig, et al. Treatment of Antisynthetase-Associated Interstitial Lung Disease with Tacrolimus. *Arthritis Rheum* 52:2439.

7. Grau, J. M., C. Herrero, J. Casademont, et al. Cyclosporine A as First Choice Therapy for Dermatomyositis." *J Rheumatol* 21:381.

Otezla (Apremilast)

Apremilast is an oral phosphodiesterase-4 inhibitor that suppresses multiple proteins or factors (cytokines) that promote inflammation. In numerous large studies, it has been found to be effective in psoriasis and psoriatic arthritis. . Because it is not a biologic, it does not increase the risk of serious infections, such as TB, and unlike methotrexate or Arava, it does not affect the liver. So it may be ideal for orphan patients who can't find a drug to fit them. However, my one patient on Apremilast became psychotically depressed (a known side effect) and the medication had to be discontinued.

References

1. Schett, G., J. Wollenhaupt, K. Papp, et al. Oral Apremilast in the Treatment of Active Psoriatic Arthritis: Results of a Multicenter, Randomized, Double-Blind, Placebo-Controlled Study. *Arthritis Rheum* 64:3156.

2. Edwards, C. J., F. J. Blanco, J. Crowley, et al. Long-Term (52-Week) Results of a Phase 3, Randomized, Controlled Trial of Apremilast, an Oral Phosphodiesterase 4 Inhibitor, in Patients with Psoriatic Arthritis and Current Skin Involvement (PALACE 3). *Arthritis Rheum* 65:S132.

Biologics

These medications are exciting revolutionary or evolutionary additions to our ability to treat disease. They very specifically target circulating proteins called *cytokines* that trigger inflammatory and sometimes cancer cells. Alternatively, they inhibit specific receptors on inflammatory cells or block the gates on the inflammatory cells that lead to their activating pathways. More and more of these medications are being developed in all the specialties of medicine. Years ago, I would give lectures on what I called "the science fiction of rheumatology." It was the evolving science behind the diseases and potential targets. The science is no longer fiction, and the targets are being hit! In 1998, the first two biologic medications for treatment of rheumatoid arthritis were released—etanercept (Enbrel) and infliximab (Remicade). They ignited the revolution or evolution. Both inhibit tumor necrosis factor alpha (TNF), which is one of the major stimulators of inflammatory cells and plays a major role in rheumatoid arthritis. Studies showed that for the first time we had medications that prevented radiological and clinical progression of the disease. As an offshoot of these long-term studies funded by the drug companies, methotrexate was shown to be pretty effective as well but not quite as good. It is still considered the gold standard against which each new medication in RA is measured. Used in conjunction with TNF antagonists, it adds to the effectiveness while reducing some of their potential side effects. Fifteen years of experience with TNF antagonists have confirmed their long-term effectiveness and their reduction of long-term patient disability. Certainly, they do not work for everybody, but when they do, they make a huge difference in symptoms and disease progression.

Tumor Necrosis Inhibitors

Remicade is infused intravenously every one to two months in an infusion center and has the advantage of adjustable dosing. Enbrel is injected by the patient subcutaneously (under the skin) weekly. Generally, patients feel better within weeks but occasionally it takes months. There are now three other approved TNF antagonists— Humira (adalimumab), Cimzia (certolizumab), and Simponi (golimumab). Humira and Cimzia are injected subcutaneously every two weeks. (Cimzia may be injected monthly at a higher dose.) Simponi is injected subcutaneously or infused intravenously monthly. Remicade and Humira are both antibodies directed at the same part or antigen (a distinctive marker or protein on the surface of the cell) of TNF, but Remicade is a mouse antibody, and Humira is a human one. Simponi and Cimzia are antibodies as well but directed at different parts or antigens of TNF. Enbrel is a fusion protein, or a decoy target, for TNF so that TNF will bind to it rather than the inflammatory cells, thereby taking it out of the system. All these medications have been shown to be effective in RA, ankylosing spondylitis, and psoriasis, but Cimzia is only indicated in RA and AS (and Crohn's disease). Humira and Remicade are effective in iritis and sarcoidosis, whereas Enbrel is not. At this time only Enbrel is approved for juvenile idiopathic arthritis. As I described in my RA chapter, these agents work fairly quickly and have a good safety profile. They make patients feel normal without the "hangover" often experienced with methotrexate and return the patient to normalcy. In other words they often go back to how they felt before the onset of their disease. Joints are no longer painful or swollen, fatigue lifts, psoriasis and psoriatic arthritis clears, and painful red eyes resolve.

However, like all good things, TNF antagonists do have potential dark sides. Those injected subcutaneously can cause painful or itchy redness at the injection site. Intravenous Remicade can cause infusion reactions with wheezing, shortness of breath, and a rise in blood pressure or heart rate. They all can cause the white blood cell count to fall. Minor respiratory tract infections, especially sinusitis, are more common. They can reignite serious dormant "opportunistic" infections, such as TB, hepatitis B, or fungus. There is a risk of multiple sclerosis and other similar neurological problems. They can exacerbate serious heart failure. Paradoxically they can cause psoriasis and other serious rashes and a variety of autoimmune diseases, such as lupus. Finally, there is the controversy over malignancy. There is no evidence that these medications cause solid tumors. There may be a slight increase in nonmelanoma skin cancers. Then there is lymphoma. Unfortunately, many of the diseases we treat have a higher incidence of lymphoma than the normal population, so it's hard to determine whether a medication increases the risk. I have seen studies that go either way. This ambiguity sometimes creates a conundrum for me. I have had one thirty-five-year-old man with ankylosing spondylitis suddenly develop pain going down both legs and a change in his back pain. An MRI showed his vertebrae were filled with tumors. He was on Humira and had previously been injecting Enbrel for several years. Biopsies confirmed lymphoma. Ironically, he was treated with Rituxan and chemotherapy successfully, but I would never offer him a TNF antagonist again despite past successes.

I will close my TNF story with the tale of one of my first Remicade patients. She was a very charming, older Hispanic lady who had fast become one of my favorite patients because of her attitude, feistiness, and strength. She had severe rheumatoid arthritis and had been in a wheelchair or disabled for years, although she maintained her independence. She had chronically swollen and deformed joints and had failed all the conventional drugs, including methotrexate. I started Remicade, and two visits later she walked into my office with a cane and no swollen joints. Her family was ecstatic. She continued to do well for several months until she developed a swollen gland in her neck, which the ear, nose, and throat (ENT) specialist insisted was a bacterial infection and treated with antibiotics. I stopped the Remicade, and her arthritis returned with a vengeance. She begged for Remicade, but the gland remained swollen, although it had shrunk. I suspected TB because she was Hispanic, diabetic, and on drugs that suppressed the immune system. Besides, during my years in East LA, I had seen a fair number of similar patients with scrofula or TB that involved the lymph glands. It looked too similar. The ENT specialists insisted that it wasn't, and her TB skin test was negative, although because she was on prednisone, which suppresses the immune response, the result was in question. Her chest x-ray was unremarkable. Her family met with me en mass and begged me to reconsider. I relented and started Remicade. Two weeks later she was in a coma and died of TB meningitis. The FDA subsequently published a warning that these drugs could ignite latent or dormant TB, and all patients had to be screened for TB before starting these agents and every year thereafter. We now require skin and blood tests and a chest x-ray before starting TNF antagonists and then annually. Oh by the way, these drugs cost between one and two thousand dollars a month!

Pearls

- They all share many of the same qualities and potential adverse effects, but they are not all the same.
- At baseline and every year, patients need a chest x-ray and TB skin test (and QuantiFERON gold) to screen for TB.

- At baseline, patients should be screened for tuberculosis, hepatitis B, and a history of systemic fungus because they can be reignited.
- Multiple sclerosis, chronic infections, and severe congestive heart failure are contraindications.
- Hold before any major surgery or during any major infection.
- They can treat and cause psoriasis.
- They can lower white blood cell count, so CBC should be ordered every several months.
- They should not be managed by physicians unfamiliar with these drugs.
- They can cause elevated antibodies, such as ANA and anti-double-stranded DNA, and rarely drug-induced lupus.
- Enbrel is ineffective in iritis and sarcoidosis, but Remicade and Humira are effective.
- They are very effective in a variety of inflammatory diseases, such as RA, psoriatic arthritis, inflammatory bowel disease, and ankylosing spondylitis but are usually more effective when combined with methotrexate or another drug.
- If one fails, there is over a 30 percent chance a second TNF antagonist will be successful.
- Enbrel may be safe during pregnancy based on preliminary data.
- Enbrel is a fusion protein, or a decoy receptor, whereas all the others are antibodies directed against TNF receptors.

References

1. Weisman, M. H. What Are the Risks of Biologic Therapy in Rheumatoid Arthritis? An Update on Safety, supplement. *J Rheumatol* 65:S33.

2. Moreland, L. W., S. W. Baumgartner, M. H. Schiff, et al. Treatment of Rheumatoid Arthritis with a Recombinant Human Tumor Necrosis Factor Receptor (p75)-Fc Fusion Protein. *N Engl J Med* 337:141.

3. Simsek, I., H. Erdem, S. Pay, et al. Optic Neuritis Occurring with Anti-tumour Necrosis Factor Alpha Therapy. *Ann Rheum Dis* 66:1255.

4. Kwon, H. J., T. R. Coté, M. S. Cuffe, et al. Case Reports of Heart Failure after Therapy with a Tumor Necrosis Factor Antagonist. *Ann Intern Med* 138:807.

5. Gabriel, S. E. Tumor Necrosis Factor Inhibition: A Part of the Solution or a Part of the Problem of Heart Failure in Rheumatoid Arthritis? *Arthritis Rheum* 58:637.

6. Peterson, J. R., F. C. Hsu, P. A. Simkin, and M. H. Wener. Effect of Tumour Necrosis Factor Alpha Antagonists on Serum Transaminases and Viraemia in Patients with Rheumatoid Arthritis and Chronic Hepatitis C Infection. *Ann Rheum Dis* 62:1078.

7. Collamer, A. N., K. T. Guerrero, J. S. Henning, and D. F. Battafarano. Psoriatic Skin Lesions Induced by Tumor Necrosis Factor Antagonist Therapy: A Literature Review and Potential Mechanisms of Action. *Arthritis Rheum* 59:996.

8. Georgescu, L., G. C. Quinn, S. Schwartzman, and S. A. Paget. Lymphoma in Patients with Rheumatoid Arthritis: Association with the Disease State or Methotrexate Treatment. *Semin Arthritis Rheum* 26:794.

9. Askling, J., R. F. van Vollenhoven, F. Granath, et al. Cancer Risk in Patients with Rheumatoid Arthritis Treated with Anti-tumor Necrosis Factor Alpha Therapies: Does the Risk Change with the Time since Start of Treatment? *Arthritis Rheum* 60:3180.

10. Winthrop, K. L., R. Baxter, L. Liu, et al. Mycobacterial Diseases and Antitumour Necrosis Factor Therapy in USA. *Ann Rheum Dis* 72:37.

11. Maini, R. N., F. C. Breedveld, J. R. Kalden, et al. Therapeutic Efficacy of Multiple Intravenous Infusions of Anti-tumor Necrosis Factor Alpha Monoclonal Antibody Combined with Low-Dose Weekly Methotrexate in Rheumatoid Arthritis. *Arthritis Rheum* 41:1552.

12. Moreland, L. W., M. H. Schiff, S. W. Baumgartner, et al. Etanercept Therapy in Rheumatoid Arthritis. A Randomized, Controlled Trial. *Ann Intern Med* 130:478.

13. Kay, J., and J. S. Smolen. Biosimilars to Treat Inflammatory Arthritis: The Challenge of Proving Identity. *Ann Rheum Dis* 72:1589.

14. Weinblatt, M. E., E. C. Keystone, D. E. Furst, et al. Adalimumab, a Fully Human Anti-tumor Necrosis Factor Alpha Monoclonal Antibody, for the Treatment of Rheumatoid Arthritis in Patients Taking Concomitant Methotrexate: The ARMADA Trial. *Arthritis Rheum* 48:35.

15. Kay, J., E. L. Matteson, B. Dasgupta, et al. Golimumab in Patients with Active Rheumatoid Arthritis Despite Treatment with Methotrexate: A Randomized, Double-Blind, Placebo-Controlled, Dose-Ranging Study. *Arthritis Rheum* 58:964

16. Smolen, J., R. B. Landewé, P. Mease, et al. Efficacy and Safety of Certolizumab Pegol plus Methotrexate in Active Rheumatoid Arthritis: The RAPID 2 Study. A Randomised Controlled Trial. *Ann Rheum Dis* 68:797.

17. Heiberg, M. S, C. Kaufmann, E. Rødevand, et al. The Comparative Effectiveness of Anti-TNF Therapy and Methotrexate in Patients with Psoriatic Arthritis: 6 Month Results from a Longitudinal, Observational, Multicentre Study. *Ann Rheum Dis* 66:1038.

18. Saad, A. A., D. P. Symmons, P. R. Noyce, and D. M. Ashcroft. Risks and Benefits of Tumor Necrosis Factor-Alpha Inhibitors in the Management of Psoriatic Arthritis: Systematic Review and Metaanalysis of Randomized Controlled Trials. *J Rheumatol* 35:883.

19. Eder, L., A. Thavaneswaran, V. Chandran, and D. D. Gladman. Tumour Necrosis Factor α Blockers are More Effective Than Methotrexate in the Inhibition of Radiographic Joint Damage Progression among Patients with Psoriatic Arthritis. *Ann Rheum Dis*4; 73:1007

20.Goulabchand, R., G. Mouterde, T. Barnetche, et al. Effect of Tumour Necrosis Factor Blockers on Radiographic Progression of Psoriatic Arthritis: A Systematic Review and Meta-analysis of Randomised Controlled Trials. *Ann Rheum Dis* 73:414.

21. Kavanaugh, A., D. van der Heijde, I. B. McInnes, et al. Golimumab in Psoriatic Arthritis: One-Year Clinical Efficacy, Radiographic, and Safety Results from a Phase III, Randomized, Placebo-Controlled Trial. *Arthritis Rheum* 64:2504.

22. Mease, P. J., R. Fleischmann, A. A. Deodhar, et al. Effect of Certolizumab Pegol on Signs and Symptoms in Patients with Psoriatic Arthritis: 24-Week Results of a Phase 3 Double-Blind Randomised Placebo-Controlled Study (RAPID-PsA). *Ann Rheum Dis* 73:48.

23. Baraliakos, X., J. Brandt, J. Listing, et al. Outcome of Patients with Active Ankylosing Spondylitis after Two Years of Therapy with Etanercept: Clinical and Magnetic Resonance Imaging Data. *Arthritis Rheum* 53:856.

24. van der Heijde, D., M. H. Schiff, J. Sieper, et al. Adalimumab Effectiveness for the Treatment of Ankylosing Spondylitis Is Maintained for up to 2 Years: Long-Term Results from the ATLAS Trial. *Ann Rheum Dis* 68:922.

25. Braun, J., X. Baraliakos, J. Listing, et al. Persistent Clinical Efficacy and Safety of Anti-tumour Necrosis Factor Alpha Therapy with Infliximab in Patients with Ankylosing Spondylitis over 5 Years: Evidence for Different Types of Response. *Ann Rheum Dis* 67:340.

26. van der Heijde, D., J. Sieper, W. P. Maksymowych, et al. 2010 Update of the International ASAS Recommendations for the Use of

Anti-TNF Agents in Patients with Axial Spondyloarthritis. *Ann Rheum Dis* 70:905.

27. Braun, J., X. Baraliakos, K. G. Hermann, et al. The Effect of Two Golimumab Doses on Radiographic Progression in Ankylosing Spondylitis: Results through 4 Years of the GO-RAISE Trial. *Ann Rheum Dis*4; 73:1007.

28. Landewé, R., J. Braun, A. Deodhar, et al. Efficacy of Certolizumab Pegol on Signs and Symptoms of Axial Spondyloarthritis Including Ankylosing Spondylitis: 24-Week Results of a Double-Blind Randomised Placebo-Controlled Phase 3 Study. *Ann Rheum Dis* 73:39.

29. Ulbricht, K. U., M. Stoll, J. Bierwirth, et al. Successful Tumor Necrosis Factor Alpha Blockade Treatment in Therapy-Resistant Sarcoidosis. *Arthritis Rheum* 48:3542.

30.Field, S., A. O. Regan, K. Sheahan, and P. Collins. Recalcitrant Cutaneous Sarcoidosis Responding to Adalimumab but Not to Etanercept. *Clin Exp Dermatol* 35:795.

31. Foeldvari, I., S. Nielsen, J. Kümmerle-Deschner, et al. Tumor Necrosis Factor-Alpha Blocker in Treatment of Juvenile Idiopathic Arthritis-Associated Uveitis Refractory to Second-Line Age nts: Results of a Multinational Survey. *J Rheumatol* 34:1146.

32. Galor, A., V. L. Perez, J. P. Hammel, and C. Y. Lowder. Differential Effectiveness of Etanercept and Infliximab in the Treatment of Ocular Inflammation. *Ophthalmology* 113:2317.

33. Simonini, G., A. Taddio, M. Cattalini, et al. Prevention of Flare Recurrences in Childhood-Refractory Chronic Uveitis: An Open-Label Comparative Study of Adalimumab versus Infliximab. *Arthritis Care Res* (Hoboken) 63:612.

B-cell inhibitors

Benlysta (belimumab)

Benlysta (belimumab) is the first new medication specifically designed for lupus in fifty-plus years. It is an antibody directed against B-lymphocytes, which are a type of white cell. Interestingly, some of the cells in this lineage produce antibodies, major players in lupus. Administered intravenously monthly, it is effective for most of the manifestations of lupus, but its effectiveness in kidney and neurological disease has not been confirmed. Anecdotally, three of my patients with cognitive problems have improved. At this point, it is reserved for patients who have failed antimalarial drugs, as well as CellCept, methotrexate, or other nonbiologic medications. So far, I have been impressed by its effectiveness in six to seven patients, and like all biologics, we are talking one to two thousand dollars a month. Adverse effects include minor infections, such as sinusitis and bronchitis, nausea, diarrhea, insomnia, pain in the extremities, headaches, and fever. Rarely serious infections can occur.

Pearls
- It is effective in lupus, but no good studies show its effectiveness in kidney disease or neurological problems.
- It may take at least three months to produce symptomatic relief

References
1. Wallace, D. J., W. Stohl, R. A. Furie, et al. A Phase II, Randomized, Double-Blind, Placebo-Controlled, Dose-Ranging Study of Belimumab in Patients with Active Systemic Lupus Erythematosus. *Arthritis Rheum* 61:1168.

2. van Vollenhoven, R. F., O. Zamani, D. J. Wallace, et al. Belimumab, a BlyS-Specific Inhibitor, Reduces Disease Activity and Severe Flares in Seropositive SLE Patients: BLISS-76 Study, supplement. *Ann Rheum Dis* 69 (3): S74.

Rituxan (rituximab)

Rituxan is another B-cell inhibitor used in rheumatoid arthritis, ANCA-associated vasculitis, and lymphoma and off-label for lupus, polymyositis, and a variety of other diseases. I have found it to be lifesaving in some cases. The Vietnamese patient with lupus who had a stroke and failed all conventional medications recovered miraculously after two Rituxan infusions. She continues to receive Rituxan when she shows any evidence of a flare about every two years. I have had several lupus patients, particularly those with severe inflammatory arthritis, who responded to Rituxan after failing other medications. It has not been proven to be effective in lupus kidney disease, but there is some suggestion it may have some effect. It can be spectacularly effective in rheumatoid arthritis, which is its primary indication, and is usually reserved for patients who have failed TNF inhibitors. However, I use it instead of TNF inhibitors at the outset in certain cases, such as patients who have multiple sclerosis (MS) since TNF inhibitors are contraindicated. In fact, I have a patient who has RA, Sjögren's, and MS who has had improvement in all three conditions with Rituxan. Of course there is my patient with Sjögren's who could not sit or stand because autonomic neuropathy made his blood pressure drop dangerously when he was upright. With biannual infusions of Rituxan, he is riding his motorcycle!

Rituxan was first used to treat lymphoma, a cancer of the lymphatic system. In RA it is given in two six-hour infusions two weeks apart. Patients may respond and remain under control for six to twelve months. The earliest I can reinfuse them is after six months. Patients are often ecstatic with the results, especially after months or years of medication failures and frustration. They will insist there is no need for a repeat infusion until there is. Then it becomes urgent. I have patients who last eight and nine months on one set of infusions and one who lasted a year and a half. Like all the biologics, this medication has some rare but major risks, especially infections and infusion or allergic reactions. It may deplete antibodies or immunoglobulins, and occasionally I will give patients monthly immunoglobulins if they are having recurrent infections. Rituxan has some advantages that make it more attractive than TNF antagonists for some patients. It is used to treat lymphoma, and RA has an increased incidence of lymphoma. It is only given at the most every six months and can last longer. It is effective in some sorts of vasculitis and is approved for ANCA-associated vasculitis. In these cases it is given in smaller doses weekly for four weeks every six months or longer. It has shown some promise in Sjögren's and polymyositis.

Adverse effects include infusion reactions with wheezing, cough, shortness of breath, and tachycardia. These reactions are rare and occur less frequently with each infusion. Infections, especially upper respiratory, are a little more common, although as in all the biologic medications, some serious ones, such as TB, can occur. Patients should be screened for hepatitis B before starting Rituxan because the drug can reactivate the infection. Headache, abdominal pain, fever, sweating, itchiness, and diarrhea may occur for a few weeks after the infusion. Low white counts can occur. Conveniently, Rituxan is an effective treatment for thrombocytopenia, or low platelet count, common in lupus. There is also a very rare risk of progressive multifocal leukoencephalopathy, an extremely dangerous brain infection that has occurred mainly in cancer patients who are also on chemotherapy. All in all it's a great drug but even more expensive than TNF inhibitors.

Pearls

- Rituxan is effective in RA and ANCA-associated vasculitis.
- It is an effective and much less toxic alternative to Cytoxan in granulomatosis with angiitis.
- The interval between each set of infusions in RA is not less than six months but varies with the clinical course. Some patients do well with longer intervals (eight months, one year, etc.).
- It may be effective in polymyositis, lupus, Sjögren's, cryoglobuli-nemia, and a few other diseases but is not FDA approved for any of them.
- If an infusion reaction is going to occur, the likelihood diminishes with each infusion.
- Rituxan may often reduce IGM and rarely IGG antibodies.
- If IGG is reduced significantly and patients experience an in-creasing number of infections, consider IVIG, although there are no large studies to support its use in this situation.
- Don't worry about IGM.
- Screen patients for TB and hepatitis B before initial dose.
- The rare cases of PML associated with Rituxan are mainly can-cer patients on chemotherapy.

References

1. Tieng, A. T., and E. Peeva. B-Cell-Directed Therapies in Systemic Lupus Erythematosus. *Semin Arthritis Rheum* 38:218.

2. Edwards, J. C., and G. Cambridge. Sustained Improvement in Rheumatoid Arthritis Following a Protocol Designed to Deplete B Lymphocytes. *Rheumatology* (Oxford) 40:205.

3. Keogh, K. A., M. E. Wylam, J. H. Stone, and U. Specks. Induction of Remission by B Lymphocyte Depletion in Eleven Patients with Refractory Antineutrophil Cytoplasmic Antibody-Associated Vasculitis. *Arthritis Rheum* 52:262.

4. Edwards, J. C., L. Szczepanski, J. Szechinski, et al. Efficacy of B-Cell-Targeted Therapy with Rituximab in Patients with Rheumatoid Arthritis. *N Engl J Med* 350:2572.

5. Smith, K. G., R. B. Jones, S. M. Burns, and D. R. Jayne. Long-Term Comparison of Rituximab Treatment for Refractory Systemic Lupus Erythematosus and Vasculitis: Remission, Relapse, and Re-treatment. *Arthritis Rheum* 54:2970.

6. Fleischmann, R. M. Progressive Multifocal Leukoencephalopathy Following Rituximab Treatment in a Patient with Rheumatoid Arthritis. *Arthritis Rheum* 60:3225.

7. Pyrpasopoulou, A., S. Douma, T. Vassiliadis, et al. Reactivation of Chronic Hepatitis B Virus Infection Following Rituximab Administration for Rheumatoid Arthritis. *Rheumatol Int* 31:403.

8. Meijer, J. M., P. M. Meiners, A. Vissink, et al. Effectiveness of Rituximab Treatment in Primary Sjögren's Syndrome: A Randomized, Double-Blind, Placebo-Controlled Trial. *Arthritis Rheum* 62:960.

9. Gottenberg, J. E., L. Guillevin, O. Lambotte, et al. Tolerance and Short Term Efficacy of Rituximab in 43 Patients with Systemic Autoimmune Diseases. *Ann Rheum Dis* 64:913.

10. Ramos-Casals, M., F. J. García-Hernández, E. de Ramón, et al. Off-Label Use of Rituximab in 196 Patients with Severe, Refractory Systemic Autoimmune Diseases. *Clin Exp Rheumatol* 28:468.

11. Stone, J. H., P. A. Merkel, R. Spiera, et al. Rituximab versus Cyclophosphamide for ANCA-Associated Vasculitis. *N Engl J Med* 363:221.

12. Jones, R. B., J. W. Tervaert, T. Hauser, et al. Rituximab versus Cyclophosphamide in ANCA-Associated Renal Vasculitis. *N Engl J Med* 363:211.

13. Oddis, C. V., A. M. Reed, R. Aggarwal, et al. Rituximab in the Treatment of Refractory Adult and Juvenile Dermatomyositis and Adult Polymyositis: A Randomized, Placebo-Phase Trial. *Arthritis Rheum* 65:314.

14. Brulhart, L., J. M. Waldburger, and C. Gabay. Rituximab in the Treatment of Antisynthetase Syndrome. *Ann Rheum Dis* 65:974.

15. Noss, E. H., D. L. Hausner-Sypek, and M. E. Weinblatt. Rituximab as Therapy for Refractory Polymyositis and Dermatomyositis. *J Rheumatol* 33:1021.

Actemra (tocilizumab)

Actemra is an antibody that inhibits IL-6, a proinflammatory factor that is reflected in the CRP, one of the principle measures of inflammations. IL-6 is also elevated in obesity and a variety of inflammatory diseases. Actemra is approved for RA and is one of the infusions that have been shown to be effective alone. It is particularly effective in types of juvenile idiopathic arthritis (systemic) and has shown promise in adult-onset Still's disease, PMR, and giant cell arteritis. It has many of the classic adverse reactions of biologics, especially risk of infection, and has the added risks of raising cholesterol levels and causing liver abnormalities and emptying wallets. I have had trouble maintaining one patient's absolute neutrophil (a type of white blood cell) count above two thousand. The infusion should not be given at any levels lower than this number, so the patient is constantly missing doses, although she is doing well.

Pearls

- CRP measures IL-6.
- Obesity elevates IL-6.
- Actemra is effective and FDA approved for RA and systemic JIA and may be effective in crystal-induced arthritis, giant cell arteritis, and PMR.
- It can be effective alone (without methotrexate).
- It may cause lipid or liver abnormalities.

References

1. Emery, P., E. Keystone, H. P. Tony, et al. IL-6 Receptor Inhibition with Tocilizumab Improves Treatment Outcomes in Patients with Rheumatoid Arthritis Refractory to Anti-tumour Necrosis Factor

Biologicals: Results from a 24-Week Multicentre Randomised Placebo-Controlled Trial. *Ann Rheum Dis* 67:1516.

2. Emery, P. Optimizing Outcomes in Patients with Rheumatoid Arthritis and an Inadequate Response to Anti-TNF Treatment, supplement. *Rheumatology* (Oxford) 51 (5): v22.

3. Gabay, C., P. Emery, R. van Vollenhoven, et al. Tocilizumab Monotherapy versus Adalimumab Monotherapy for Treatment of Rheumatoid Arthritis (ADACTA): A Randomised, Double-Blind, Controlled Phase 4 Trial. *Lancet* 381:1541.

4. Inaba, Y., R. Ozawa, T. Imagawa, et al. Radiographic Improvement of Damaged Large Joints in Children with Systemic Juvenile Idiopathic Arthritis following Tocilizumab Treatment. *Ann Rheum Dis* 70:1693.

5. De Benedetti, F., H. I. Brunner, N. Ruperto, et al. Randomized Trial of Tocilizumab in Systemic Juvenile Idiopathic Arthritis. *N Engl J Med* 367:2385.

6. Beyer, C., R. Axmann, E. Sahinbegovic, et al. Anti-interleukin 6 Receptor Therapy as Rescue Treatment for Giant Cell Arteritis. *Ann Rheum Dis* 70:1874.

7. Salvarani, C., L. Magnani, M. Catanoso, et al. Tocilizumab: A Novel Therapy for Patients with Large-Vessel Vasculitis. *Rheumatology* (Oxford) 51:151.

8. Perdan-Pirkmajer, K., S. Praprotnik, and M. Tomšič M. A Case of Refractory Adult-Onset Still's Disease Successfully Controlled with Tocilizumab and a Review of the Literature. *Clin Rheumatol* 29:1465.

Orencia (abatacept)

Orencia is a selective costimulator modulator. What the hell does that mean? It's a drug that blocks two proteins on the membrane of some key immune system cells that are usually activated during the inflammatory process. It can be administered in RA or JIA subcutaneously or intravenously. It has a slow onset but seems to be the safest drug for those prone to infection, including TB, although it has a similar safety profile to the other biologic agents. I have had some spectacular long-term successes with this drug in difficult RA patients, although my subjective bias is that it is not as potent as some of the others. It has been studied in a variety of other diseases, and (except for possibly lupus) RA and JIA seem to be the only diseases it effectively treats.

Pearls
- It has a slow onset (up to three months).
- It is one of the safer biologics, especially in terms of infection.
- It is effective and approved for RA and JIA.

References

1. Genovese, M. C., J. C. Becker, M. Schiff, et al. Abatacept for Rheumatoid Arthritis Refractory to Tumor Necrosis Factor Alpha Inhibition. *N Engl J Med* 353:1114.
2. Schiff, M., C. Pritchard, J. E. Huffstutter, et al. The 6-Month Safety and Efficacy of Abatacept in Patients with Rheumatoid Arthritis Who Underwent a Washout after Anti-tumour Necrosis Factor Therapy or Were Directly Switched to Abatacept: The ARRIVE Trial. *Ann Rheum Dis* 68:1708.
3. Mease, P., M. C. Genovese, G. Gladstein, et al. Abatacept in the Treatment of Patients with Psoriatic Arthritis: Results of a Six-Month,

Multicenter, Randomized, Double-Blind, Placebo-Controlled, Phase II Trial. *Arthritis Rheum* 63:939.

4. Ruperto, N., D. J. Lovell, P. Quartier, et al. Abatacept in Children with Juvenile Idiopathic Arthritis: A Randomised, Double-Blind, Placebo-Controlled Withdrawal Trial. *Lancet* 372:383.

5. Ruperto, N., D. J. Lovell, T. Li, et al. Abatacept Improves Health-Related Quality of Life, Pain, Sleep Quality, and Daily Participation in Subjects with Juvenile Idiopathic Arthritis. *Arthritis Care Res* (Hoboken) 62:1542.

Kineret (anakinra)

Kineret inhibits IL-1, another proinflammatory factor. It is administered subcutaneously daily and is not as potent as the other biologics
in RA but is particularly good for certain kinds of juvenile idiopathic
arthritis, especially Still's disease. I have used it with great success
in adult-onset Still's disease, and it seems to be also effective (but
not FDA approved) for acute gout and pseudogout. Nevertheless, it
is rarely used these days, although it may be the safest of the biologic agents because of its short duration in the bloodstream. TB
does not seem to be a problem as it is with all the other biologics,
especially the TNF antagonists. Its commonest adverse effect in my
practice years ago was an intense injection site reaction—a painful,
red bump. It is also surprisingly expensive. I am prescribing it for two
RA patients with a history of multiple infections in the past, hoping
that it can be cleared from their bloodstream quickly if they have a
recurrence of their infections. It should not be used in conjunction
with another biologic.

Ilaris another IL-1 inhibitor was just approved for Still's disease or
JIA and is infused intravenously every two months. It may be effective for gout and pseudogout but has not been approved for them
by the FDA.

Pearls

- They are effective for Still's disease and a few other periodic fe-
  ver syndromes.
- They are effective for acute crystal-induced arthritis but not FDA
  approved.
- Because Kineret is short acting, it may be the safest biologic.
- Kineret is a fairly weak treatment for RA.

References

1. Vasques Godinho, F. M., M. J. Parreira Santos, and J. Canas da Silva. Refractory Adult Onset Still's Disease Successfully Treated with Anakinra. *Ann Rheum Dis* 64:647.

2. Lequerré, T., P. Quartier, D. Rosellini, et al. Interleukin-1 Receptor Antagonist (Anakinra) Treatment in Patients with Systemic-Onset Juvenile Idiopathic Arthritis or Adult Onset Still Disease: Preliminary Experience in France. *Ann Rheum Dis* 67:302.

3. Kalliolias, G. D., P. E. Georgiou, I. A. Antonopoulos, et al. Anakinra Treatment in Patients with Adult-Onset Still's Disease Is Fast, Effective, Safe and Steroid Sparing: Experience from an Uncontrolled Trial. *Ann Rheum Dis* 66:842.

4. Schlesinger, N., R. E. Alten, T. Bardin, et al. Canakinumab for Acute Gouty Arthritis in Patients with Limited Treatment Options: Results from Two Randomised, Multicentre, Active-Controlled, Double-Blind Trials and Their Initial Extensions. *Ann Rheum Dis* 71:1839.

5. Ruperto, N., H. I. Brunner, P. Quartier, et al. Two Randomized Trials of Canakinumab in Systemic Juvenile Idiopathic Arthritis. *N Engl J Med* 367:2396.

6. Chen, K., T. Fields, C. A. Mancuso, et al. Anakinra's Efficacy is Variable in Refractory Gout: Report of Ten Cases. *Semin Arthritis Rheum* 40:210.

7. So, A., M. De Meulemeester, A. Pikhlak, et al. Canakinumab for the Treatment of Acute Flares in Difficult-to-Treat Gouty Arthritis: Results of a Multicenter, Phase II, Dose-Ranging Study. *Arthritis Rheum* 62:3064.

Stelara (ustekinumab)

Stelara (ustekinumab) inhibits interleukin-17 (IL-17) and IL-23 and is effective in the treatment of psoriasis and psoriatic arthritis. It is injected subcutaneously at week zero, week four, and then every three months. Adverse effects are similar to other biologics—minor infections and occasional inflammation at the injection site. It requires all the usual pretreatment screening (TB and hepatitis B) and vaccinations. So far, I have had moderate success in treating arthritis and skin lesions in two patients. It may be used alone or in combination with methotrexate.

Pearls
- It is effective for both psoriasis and psoriatic arthritis.
- It may be used alone or in combination with methotrexate.

References
1. Ritchlin, C., A. B. Gottlieb, I. B. McInnes, et al. Ustekinumab in Active Psoriatic Arthritis Including Patients Previously Treated with Anti-TNF Agents: Results of a Phase 3, Multicenter, Double-Blind, Placebo-Controlled Study. *Arthritis Rheum* 64:S1080.
2. Gottlieb, A., A. Menter, A. Mendelsohn, et al. Ustekinumab, a Human Interleukin 12/23 Monoclonal Antibody, for Psoriatic Arthritis: Randomised, Double-Blind, Placebo-Controlled, Crossover Trial. *Lancet* 373:633.

Cosentryx (Secukinamab)

It is an IL-17 antagonist and is effective in treating both skin and joint disease in psoriasis. In 2015, it is only approved in the U.S. for skin disease. It is injected 300 mg. subcutaneously week 0, 1, 2, 3, 4 and then every 4 weeks.

References

1. Paul C, Lacour JP, Tedremets L, et al. Efficacy, safety and usability of secukinumab administration by autoinjector/pen in psoriasis: a randomized, controlled trial (JUNCTURE). J Eur Acad Dermatol Venereol 2015; 29:1082.

2. Blauvelt A, Prinz JC, Gottlieb AB, et al. Secukinumab administration by pre-filled syringe: efficacy, safety and usability results from a randomized controlled trial in psoriasis (FEATURE). Br J Dermatol 2015; 172:484.

3. Thaçi D, Blauvelt A, Reich K, et al. Secukinumab is superior to ustekinumab in clearing skin of subjects with moderate to severe plaque psoriasis: CLEAR, a randomized controlled trial. J Am Acad Dermatol 2015; 73:400.

Cosentryx (Secukinamab)

It is an IL-17 antagonist and is effective in treating both skin and joint disease in psoriasis. Recent studies have shown its effectiveness in Ankylosing Spondylitis. However, as of early 2016, it is only approved in the U.S. for skin disease.

References

1. Paul C, Lacour JP, Tedremets L, et al. Efficacy, safety and usability of secukinumab administration by autoinjector/pen in psoriasis: a randomized, controlled trial (JUNCTURE). J Eur Acad Dermatol Venereol 2015; 29:1082.

2. Blauvelt A, Prinz JC, Gottlieb AB, et al. Secukinumab administration by pre-filled syringe: efficacy, safety and usability results from a randomized controlled trial in psoriasis (FEATURE). Br J Dermatol 2015; 172:484.

3. Thaçi D, Blauvelt A, Reich K, et al. Secukinumab is superior to ustekinumab in clearing skin of subjects with moderate to severe plaque psoriasis: CLEAR, a randomized controlled trial. J Am Acad Dermatol 2015; 73:400.

4. Baerte D., Sieper J. et al. Secukinumab, an Interleukin-17A inhibitor, In Ankylosing Spondylitis. NEJM 2015 373:26. P.2534-2547

Xeljanz (tofacitinib)

The new biologic Xeljanz is an oral agent that inhibits JAK kinase, the pathway along which the activating signals of certain inflammatory cells travel. It may be used alone or in combination with other remittive medications but not other biologics. I have had little experience with it yet, but one patient with a particularly difficult case of inflammatory arthritis has responded spectacularly to it after years of suffering. Two others with severe disease are doing well, and another could not tolerate it because of diarrhea. It has many of the same side effects as all biologics, but diarrhea, abnormal liver tests, elevated lipid profiles, and low white counts seem to be more prominent. Atypical infections, such as TB and fungus, are also worries, as is lymphoma. Much to my disappointment and dismay, it is at least as expensive as the injectable biologics.

Pearls

- It may be used alone.
- It is the first oral biologic.
- It has the same risks as most biologics, but it is important to check lipids and liver function tests intermittently.

References

1. Fleischmann, R., J. Kremer, J. Cush, et al. Placebo-Controlled Trial of Tofacitinib Monotherapy in Rheumatoid Arthritis. *N Engl J Med* 367:495.
2. van Vollenhoven, R. F., R. Fleischmann, S. Cohen, et al. Tofacitinib or Adalimumab versus Placebo in Rheumatoid Arthritis. *N Engl J Med* 367:508.

Biologic Screening, Rules, and Cautionary Measures

Before starting a biologic, I always obtain a chest x-ray, a TB skin and blood test, and hepatitis B blood tests including core antibody. The chest x-ray and TB tests are repeated yearly. I carefully question the patients about previous systemic fungal infections, such as valley fever, which can be reactivated by these drugs. I avoid prescribing these drugs to patients with any chronic infection or those undergoing treatment for cancer, although sometimes there is a gray zone with drugs such as Rituxan. Anti-TNF agents are contraindicated in MS and severe congestive heart failure patients. I recommend non-live vaccinations, including flu and pneumococcal, prior to starting the medications and then seasonally. Live vaccines, like herpes zoster or shingles, may be administered fourteen to thirty days prior to initiation of therapy. They are to be avoided once therapy has been initiated, and to make it even more complicated, patients should not be exposed to anybody who had a recent live-virus vaccine, or they may get the virus! Also, there have been some strange reports of patients being infected by weird bacteria contained in brie cheese they have eaten. Despite all this fearmongering, with the right precautions and in the right patients, biologics are very safe.

Pearls

- Always screen for TB, hepatitis B, fungus, and chronic infections before initiating therapies.
- Vaccinate (pneumovax, flu, hepatitis B) regularly, but avoid live-virus vaccines.
- Monitor patients at least every two to three months with blood counts and liver panels.

References

1. Furst, D. E., E. C. Keystone, J. Braun, et al. Updated Consensus Statement on Biological Agents for the Treatment of Rheumatic Diseases, 2010," supplement. *Ann Rheum Dis* 70 (1): i2.

2. Gardam, M. A., E. C. Keystone, R. Menzies, et al. Anti-tumour Necrosis Factor Agents and Tuberculosis Risk: Mechanisms of Action and Clinical Management." *Lancet Infect Dis* 3:148.

3. Saag, K. G., G. G. Teng, N. M. Patkar, et al. American College of Rheumatology 2008 Recommendations for the Use of Nonbiologic and Biologic Disease-Modifying Antirheumatic Drugs in Rheumatoid Arthritis. *Arthritis Rheum* 59:762.

4. Lee, J. H., N. R. Slifman, S. K. Gershon, et al. Life-Threatening Histoplasmosis Complicating Immunotherapy with Tumor Necrosis Factor Alpha Antagonists Infliximab and Etanercept. *Arthritis Rheum* 46:2565.

5. Bergstrom, L., D. E. Yocum, N. M. Ampel, et al. Increased Risk of Coccidioidomycosis in Patients Treated with Tumor Necrosis Factor Alpha Antagonists. *Arthritis Rheum* 50:1959.

Osteoporosis Meds

Bisphosphonates

Alendronate (Fosamax) or risedronate (Actonel) are both bisphos-phonates, a class of drugs that inhibits osteoclasts, the "Pac-Men" or termite-like cells in bones described previously. Both are oral drugs that have been found to increase bone density in both the hip and spine. A third drug, ibandronate, which is available in intravenous and oral forms, has been found to be effective only in increasing bone density in the spine, not the hip, so I don't prescribe it. These medications are very effective and have changed the course of osteo-porosis treatment dramatically over the last two decades. However, these medications are not without their drawbacks or controversy. A few years ago, there was a big furor about these drugs causing aseptic necrosis of the jaw, which, as you remember, means that the jaw bone would die because of poor circulation. This complication occurred mainly in patients with gum disease and poor dentition and mostly in the cancer population who were receiving these medica-tions in much higher doses in an intravenous form. Its incidence was one in ten thousand patients. Nevertheless, patients were being told by their dentists about the risks and often stopped the medication despite the fact they had little gum or dental disease. I had several patients who immediately began to complain of jaw pain and swell-ing and demanded x-rays and MRIs. Fortunately, none were positive. I believe I have seen one case over the last twenty years picked up by a dentist. It was one of those times that I wished I had a handout depicting the risks of osteoporosis. Ted Pincus, one of the giants in rheumatology, has said that he gives patients handouts outlining the risks of the disease before giving them a handout outlining the risks of a medication. Patients seem to be more concerned about potential risks of medication than the terrible risks of a disease. Before starting patients on a bisphosphonate, I screen for gum or dental disease and will try another class of drug if it's a problem. The most common side effect of oral bisphosphonates is acid reflux (GERD), and patients are told to avoid lying down while taking these meds and to take them thirty minutes before breakfast with a full glass of water, so they are absorbed well. If the patient already has a problem with GERD or develops it while on therapy, I switch to zoledreonic acid (Reclast), which is an intravenous bisphosphonate, or try Prolia or Forteo. Other rare side effects include flu-like symptoms with muscle and bone pain, painful red eyes, low calcium, and atrial fibrillation. I do not use these drugs in patients with moderate to severe kidney malfunction.

Reclast may be more effective than the oral alternatives, and because it is a fifteen-minute infusion every twelve months, it leads to better compliance. There is some evidence that patients are not very compliant in taking the oral bisphosphonates. I prescribe Reclast when patients have failed oral bisphosphonates, have GERD, or have compliance problems. The most recent controversy regarding this class of drug is atypical hip fractures, another rare event, but the media was all over it. Understandably, patients wanted to stop their bisphosphonate immediately since they thought that they were taking these drugs to prevent fractures, not create them. The studies indicate that these atypical fractures occur in patients who have been taking these medications for more than five years, and the risks of osteoporotic fractures off these medications much outweigh the risks of these atypical fractures. Because of these findings, most physicians are advocating at least one year of drug holiday after three to five years of therapy. I choose three years.

Finally, bisphosphonates are effective and approved for osteoporosis in men and steroid-induced osteoporosis. They also are effective and recommended as prophylaxis in patients over fifty on long-term steroids.

Pearls

- Bisphosphonates are first-line drugs for osteoporosis and are relatively safe and effective.
- Fosamax and Actonel have been shown to prevent vertebral and nonvertebral fractures.
- They should be taken when upright and thirty minutes before food to prevent GERD and promote good absorption.
- Screen patients for bad teeth or gum disease to avoid jaw necrosis.
- Jaw necrosis is very rare and typically occurs in cancer patients on high-dose IV bisphosphonate therapy.
- To prevent the adverse effect of atypical fractures, patients should be given a drug holiday after three to five years of therapy.
- Avoid bisphosphonates in patients with severe kidney disease (creatinine clearance of less than 30 cc).
- Zoledronic acid is a good choice for noncompliant patients and those with GERD.
- It may be more effective than oral bisphosphonates.
- There have been no good studies in premenopausal women.
- They are effective and approved for osteoporosis in men.
- Bisphosphonates are effective for steroid-induced osteoporosis.
- A drug holiday should be given every three years, and then give drug every other year.

References

1. Liberman, U. A., S. R. Weiss, J. Bröll, et al. Effect of Oral Alendronate on Bone Mineral Density and the Incidence of Fractures in Postmenopausal Osteoporosis. The Alendronate Phase III Osteoporosis Treatment Study Group. *N Engl J Med* 333:1437.
2. Chesnut, C. H., M. R. McClung, K. E. Ensrud, et al. Alendronate Treatment of the Postmenopausal Osteoporotic Woman: Effect of

Multiple Dosages on Bone Mass and Bone Remodeling. *Am J Med* 99:144.

3. Bone, H. G., D. Hosking, J. P. Devogelaer, et al. Ten Years' Experience with Alendronate for Osteoporosis in Postmenopausal Women. *N Engl J Med* 350:1189.

4. Harris, S. T., N. B. Watts, H. K. Genant, et al. Effects of Risedronate Treatment on Vertebral and Nonvertebral Fractures in Women with Postmenopausal Osteoporosis: A Randomized Controlled Trial. Vertebral Efficacy with Risedronate Therapy (VERT) Study Group." *JAMA* 282:1344.

5. Delmas, P. D., M. R. McClung, J. R. Zanchetta, et al. Efficacy and Safety of Risedronate 150 mg Once a Month in the Treatment of Postmenopausal Osteoporosis. *Bone* 42:36.

6. Silverman, S. L., N. B. Watts, P. D. Delmas, et al. Effectiveness of Bisphosphonates on Nonvertebral and Hip Fractures in the First Year of Therapy: The Risedronate and Alendronate (REAL) Cohort Study. *Osteoporos Int* 18:25.

7. Reid, I. R., J. P. Brown, P. Burckhardt, et al. Intravenous Zoledronic Acid in Postmenopausal Women with Low Bone Mineral Density. *N Engl J Med* 346:653.

8. Black, D. M., P. D. Delmas, R. Eastell, et al. Once-Yearly Zoledronic Acid for Treatment of Postmenopausal Osteoporosis. *N Engl J Med* 356:1809.

9. Fedele S., S. R. Porter, F. D'Aiuto, et al. Nonexposed Variant of Bisphosphonate-Associated Osteonecrosis of the Jaw: A Case Series. *Am J Med* 123:1060.

10. Khan, A. A., G. K. Sándor, E. Dore, et al. Bisphosphonate Associated Osteonecrosis of the Jaw. *J Rheumatol* 36:478.

11. Heckbert, S. R., G. Li, S. R. Cummings, et al. Use of Alendronate and Risk of Incident Atrial Fibrillation in Women. *Arch Intern Med* 168:826.

12. Karam, R., J. Camm, M. McClung. Yearly Zoledronic Acid in Postmenopausal Osteoporosis. *N Engl J Med* 357:712.

13. Lenart, B. A., D. G. Lorich, and J. M. Lane. Atypical Fractures of the Femoral Diaphysis in Postmenopausal Women Taking Alendronate. *N Engl J Med* 358:1304.

14. Schilcher, J., K. Michaëlsson, and P. Aspenberg. Bisphosphonate Use and Atypical Fractures of the Femoral Shaft. *N Engl J Med* 364:1728.

15. Watts, N. B., R. A. Adler, J. P. Bilezikian, et al. Osteoporosis in Men: An Endocrine Society Clinical Practice Guideline. *J Clin Endocrinol Metab* 97:1802.

16. Boonen, S., J. Y. Reginster, J. M. Kaufman et al. Fracture Risk and Zoledronic Acid Therapy in Men with Osteoporosis. *N Engl J Med* 367:1714.

17. Saag, K. G., E. Shane, S. Boonen, et al. Teriparatide or Alendronate in Glucocorticoid-Induced Osteoporosis. *N Engl J Med* 357:2028.

18. de Nijs, R. N., J. W. Jacobs, W. F. Lems, et al. Alendronate or Alfacalcidol in Glucocorticoid-Induced Osteoporosis. *N Engl J Med* 355:675.

19. American College of Rheumatology Ad Hoc Committee on Glucocorticoid-Induced Osteoporosis. Recommendations for the Prevention and Treatment of Glucocorticoid-Induced Osteoporosis: 2001 Update. *Arthritis Rheum* 44:1496.

Prolia (denosumab)

Prolia is a biologic and is an antibody against RANKL, a protein that stimulates osteoclast receptors. It can be used as mentioned previously in kidney failure patients, may be effective in patients who fail bisphosphonates, and just recently became FDA approved for men. It is injected subcutaneously (under the skin) every six months and may lead to better compliance. Rash, hypocalcemia, and joint or bone pain are occasional adverse effects. Also, because it does inhibit RANKL function in the immune system, there is some controversy regarding whether there is an increased incidence of serious infections. Finally, as in bisphosphonates, there is a less than 2 percent chance of aseptic necrosis of the jaw, and the same screening precautions should be taken. I have used it with some success in patients who have failed bisphosphonates, and it is my drug of choice in postmenopausal patients with poor kidney function.

Pearls
- It is an antibody directed against RANKL and inhibits osteoclasts.
- It is given subcutaneously every six months so not associated with GERD.
- It is relatively safe in kidney failure patients.
- Use same precautions as in bisphosphonates to avoid jaw necrosis.
- Give a drug holiday every three years for one year.
- It is approved for osteoporosis in men.

References
1. Cummings, S. R., J. San Martin, M. R. McClung, et al. Denosumab for Prevention of Fractures in Postmenopausal Women with Osteoporosis. *N Engl J Med* 361:756.

2. McClung, M. R., E. M. Lewiecki, Cohen, et al. Denosumab in Postmenopausal Women with Low Bone Mineral Density. *N Engl J Med* 354:821.

3. Orwoll, E., C. S. Teglbjærg, B. L. Langdahl, et al. A Randomized, Placebo-Controlled Study of the Effects of Denosumab for the Treatment of Men with Low Bone Mineral Density. *J Clin Endocrinol Metab* 97:3161.

Forteo (teriparatide)

Many patients have needle phobias and won't consider daily subcutaneous injections. However, Forteo is the only available medication that stimulates osteoblasts (the bone "bricklayers") and is especially good for patients with multiple fractures. In fact, I recommend it for osteoporosis patients with a fracture because an increase in bone density occurs much quicker than it does with bisphosphonates. Its major side effects include high calcium, nausea, dizziness, joint pain, weakness, and runny nose.

Pearls

- Forteo stimulates osteoblasts and builds bone the fastest.
- It is ideal in patients with osteoporosis and fractures.
- It often is effective in patients who have failed or can't tolerate bisphosphonates.
- It is only approved for one two-year course.
- There is a study that suggests that Forteo given twelve weeks on and twelve weeks off for two years is just as effective as a daily regimen over the same duration.
- It is effective for steroid-induced osteoporosis.

References

1. Neer, R. M., C. D. Arnaud, J. R. Zanchetta, et al. Effect of Parathyroid Hormone (1-34) on Fractures and Bone Mineral Density in Postmenopausal Women with Osteoporosis. *N Engl J Med* 344:1434.

2. Finkelstein, J. S., A. Hayes, J. L. Hunzelman, et al. The Effects of Parathyroid Hormone, Alendronate, or Both in Men with Osteoporosis. *N Engl J Med* 349:1216.

3. American College of Rheumatology Ad Hoc Committee on Glucocorticoid-Induced Osteoporosis. "Recommendations for the Prevention and Treatment of Glucocorticoid-Induced Osteoporosis: 2001 Update." *Arthritis Rheum* 44:1496.
4. Cosman, F., J. Nieves, M. Zion, et al. Daily and Cyclic Parathyroid Hormone in Women Receiving Alendronate. *N Engl J Med* 353:566.

Medications in Rheumatology

I no longer prescribe the other medications used in osteoporosis such, as SERMs (raloxifene), estrogen, and calcitonin except in certain situations because they are not as effective. Calcitonin has also been associated with cancer.

Gout Medications

Nonsteroidals and steroids can be used for acute attacks or prophylaxis. For details about their uses and mechanisms, see my chapter on gout and an earlier section in this chapter.

Colchicine

Colchicine is an extremely old oral drug that inhibits the activation and migration of neutrophils (an inflammatory white blood cell) and inhibits the activation of IL-1 (interleukin-1 beta) a proinflammatory factor. Given orally at a dose of 1.2 mg and then 0.6 mg one hour later, it often effectively terminates an acute attack. Years ago, physicians used to tell patients to take it hourly until they developed diarrhea or the attack was aborted, but a recent study showed that the above mentioned regimen was equally effective and much less toxic. Many older gout patients have bad memories of colchicine and refuse to take it. Can you blame them? In addition to diarrhea and abdominal cramps, it occasionally wiped out the white blood cells in the bone marrow, which could be life threatening. In fact, colchicine was sometimes administered intravenously to hospitalized patients, but the incidence of dangerously low white blood cell counts (neutropenia and agranulocytosis) was so high that the medical community stopped using it. Finally, recently because of a wily move by a drug company, colchicine is no longer generic and is extremely expensive. The drug company actually performed the above mentioned study and claimed that since it was the first of its kind, it allowed them to patent the drug for use in gout. Wow! Finally, colchicine must be used with caution in patients with kidney or liver problems. Nevertheless, it is still an option and is also used as a prophylactic drug at either 0.6 mg daily or twice a day, protecting against acute attacks as the uric acid is being lowered to the appropriate level for maintenance over the course of three to six months.

Pearls

- Colchicine may be used for acute attacks of gout or for prophylaxis until uric acid is below 6.0 mg/dl. (after three to six months).

- The best colchicine regimen for treatment of acute gout is 1.2 mg and 0.6 mg one mg./dl. hour later.
- It does not lower uric acid and is not a long-term drug.
- Do not use IV colchicine for fear of agranulocytosis.
- Avoid in severe renal or liver insufficiency.

References

1. Zhang, W., M. Doherty, T. Bardin, et al. EULAR Evidence Based Recommendations for Gout. Part II: Management. Report of a Task Force of the EULAR Standing Committee for International Clinical Studies Including Therapeutics (ESCISIT). *Ann Rheum Dis* 65:1312.

2. Terkeltaub, R. A., D. E. Furst, K. Bennett, et al. High versus Low Dosing of Oral Colchicine for Early Acute Gout Flare: Twenty-Four-Hour Outcome of the First Multicenter, Randomized, Double-Blind, Placebo-Controlled, Parallel-Group, Dose-Comparison Colchicine Study. *Arthritis Rheum* 62:1060.

3. Terkeltaub, R. A. Colchicine Update: 2008. *Semin Arthritis Rheum* 38:411.

Uric-Acid-Lowering Medications

Benemid (probenecid)

The majority of patients underexcrete uric acid in the urine, so uricosuric drugs, such as probenecid (the only one approved in the United States), which increase the output of uric acid in the urine, are the drugs of choice in many cases. Often before starting Benemid, I will have the patient collect his total urine output over twenty-four-hours and measure the uric acid produced in the urine over that period of time. I will only choose benemid as therapy if the value is significantly lower than 1,000 mg/day. Otherwise, there is a risk of kidney stones and damage.

Benemid is also not as effective in patients with kidney disease and should not be used in patients with tophi or uric acid kidney stones. Its adverse effects are rare, but recently I had one patient develop fairly severe liver abnormalities while taking it.

Pearls

- Benemid increases urinary excretion of uric acid.
- It is probably effective in many patients.
- Titrate the doses up slowly every one to two weeks until uric acid is below 6 mg./dl..
- Use prophylaxis while titrating over three to six months.
- It is contraindicated in patients with uric acid stones and patients taking aspirin.
- It may not be effective in moderate to severe renal insufficiency.
- It has many drug interactions.
- Flares during titration stage may be because of change in uric acid levels and lack of prophylaxis.

References

1. Reinders, M. K., E. N. van Roon, T. L. Jansen, et al. Efficacy and Tolerability of Urate-Lowering Drugs in Gout: A Randomised Controlled Trial of Benzbromarone versus Probenecid after Failure of Allopurinol. *Ann Rheum Dis* 68:51.
2. Fam, A. G. Difficult Gout and New Approaches for Control of Hyperuricemia in the Allopurinol-Allergic Patient. *Curr Rheumatol Rep* 3:29.
3. Perez-Ruiz, F., H. Inaki, and A. M. Herrero-Beites. Uricosuric Therapy. In *Crystal-Induced Arthropathies: Gout, Pseudogout and Apatite-Associated Syndromes*, edited by R. L. Wortmann, H. R. Schumacher, Jr., M. A. Becker, and L. M. Ryan, 369. New York: Taylor & Francis.
4. Harris, M., L. R. Bryant, P. Danaher, and J. Alloway. Effect of Low Dose Daily Aspirin on Serum Urate Levels and Urinary Excretion in Patients Receiving Probenecid for Gouty Arthritis. *J Rheumatol* 27:2873.

Leisenurad

Leisenurad (Zurampic) is a drug approved by the FDA in 2015. It helps the kidney excrete uric acid by by inhibiting the function of transportation proteins invovolved in the reabsorption of uric acid. Lesinurad is prescribed in combination with Allopurinol or Uloric (xanthine oxidase inhibitors). When prescribed alone, kidney failure is more common.

Pearls

- Decreases uric acid by inhibiting reabsorption in urine
- Used only in combination with Uloric or Allopurinol

Medications in Rheumatology

1. Saag K, Fitz-Patrick, Kopicko, et al; Leisenurad, a selective uric acid reabsorption inhibitor in combination with Allopurinol: Results from a phase 3 study in gout patients having an inadequate response to standard of care (clear 1). Ann. Rheum Dis. 2015, June; 74 (sup. 2): 540. Abstract. Fr 10320. Doi: 10.136/Ann. Rheum Dis.—2015. Eular. 3273.

2. Bardiaa T, Keenan R, Khanna P, et al. Leisenurad, a selective uric acid reabsorption inhibitor in combination with Allopurinol: Results from a phase 3 study in gout patients having an inadequate response to standard of care (clear 2). Ann. Rheum Dis. 2015, June; 74 (sup. 2): 545. Abstract Fr 10333. Doi: 10.1136/ AnnRehumdisease—2015— Eular. 1238

Allopurinol

The most popular and inexpensive drug that lowers production of uric acid is allopurinol. It is effective in most cases. I use it in doses between 100 mg and 800 mg, but most physicians never use doses higher than 300 mg. The medication needs some adjustment in kidney disease, but rheumatologists are a little less timid about increasing doses even in patients with impaired kidney disease. Allopurinol strikes fear in many physicians because of a small but significant incidence of Stevens-Johnson syndrome associated with it. Once you have seen a patient with it, you never want to see one again. It is an allergic reaction that starts with a rash and quickly turns into a blister-like eruption on the body, oral cavity, GI and GU tract, and even the eyes. These lesions weep large amounts of fluid, and patients can go into shock. The blisters and subsequent scars on the eyes can lead to blindness. I have seen two cases, and they both died. It's a horrible hideous death. Fortunately, it is rare, and if a patient on allopurinol tells me they have a rash, I tell them to stop it immediately. I also warn all patients of the risks before starting the drug and tell them to stop it if they develop any oral ulcers. Occasionally, allopurinol can cause abnormal liver functions or an allergic reaction with a rash and fever. The liver abnormality just needs to be monitored, and if it continues to worsen, then I would consider discontinuing the medication, but I would probably not rechallenge the patient who has had the allergic reaction, particularly since we now have good alternatives.

Pearls

- Allopurinol doses needed to lower uric acid blow 6 mg./dl. are between 100 mg and 800 mg.

- Start at 100 mg and increase the dose every one to two weeks by 100 mg until uric acid is below 6.
- Never start or stop it or change dose during an acute attack.
- Always use prophylaxis during titration period until uric acid has been below 6 mg./ dl. for a few months.
- Beware of rash and Stevens-Johnson syndrome, and stop allopurinol immediately if rash occurs.
- Flares during titration stage may be because of change in uric acid levels and lack of prophylaxis.
- Hypersensitivity reaction to drug may include fever, abnormal liver-function tests, and high eosinophil count.
- Slight elevations of liver-function tests may occur and are benign.
- Beware of interactions with Imuran and Coumadin.

References

1. Perez-Ruiz, F., A. Alonso-Ruiz, M. Calabozo, et al. Efficacy of Allopurinol and Benzbromarone for the Control of Hyperuricemia. A Pathogenic Approach to the Treatment of Primary Chronic Gout. *Ann Rheum Dis* 57:545.

2. Webster, E., and R. S. Panush. Allopurinol Hypersensitivity in a Patient with Severe, Chronic, Tophaceous Gout. *Arthritis Rheum* 28:707.

3. Wallace, S. L., and J. Z. Singer. Therapy in Gout. *Rheum Dis Clin North Am* 14:441.

Uloric (febuxostat)

Recently, we have the first two new drugs introduced for the treatment of gout in over forty years—Uloric and Krystexxa. The former is similar to allopurinol in that it inhibits similar pathways (xanthine oxidase) but is structurally a different drug and has a few different actions, so it doesn't cross-react with allopurinol and can be used in patients who have had allergic reactions to allopurinol. It is safer in patients with mild to moderate kidney disease and seems to be more effective. Cost and newness make this the drug of second or third choice. Maybe when it is generic and has a longer track record, it may surpass allopurinol. Liver function abnormalities and dizziness seem to be the most common side effects. It should be avoided with Imuran but is safe with Coumadin.

Pearls

- Uloric may be effective in patients who are allergic to allopurinol.
- It may be effective in patients who have failed allopurinol, but attempts to maximize allopurinol dose should be made first.
- Slight elevations of liver-function tests may occur and are usually benign.
- It may be safer than allopurinol in mild to moderate kidney disease.
- Flares during titration stage may be because of change in uric acid levels and lack of prophylaxis.
- It should be avoided with Imuran.
- It is safe with Coumadin

References

1. M.A. Becke, H. R. Schumacher, Jr., R. L. Wortmann, et al. Febuxostat Compared with Allopurinol in Patients with Hyperuricemia and Gout. *N Engl J Med* 353:2450.

2. M.A. Becker, H. R. Schumacher, Jr., R. L. Wortmann, et al. Febuxostat, a Novel Nonpurine Selective Inhibitor of Xanthine Oxidase: A Twenty-Eight-Day, Multicenter, Phase II, Randomized, Double-Blind, Placebo-Controlled, Dose-Response Clinical Trial Examining Safety and Efficacy in Patients with Gout. *Arthritis Rheum* 52:916.

Krystexxa (pegloticase)

Krystexxa is a biweekly intravenous drug that works on a completely different pathway converting uric acid to allantoin, a benign compound. Birds and other nonmammals have an enzyme similar to this drug (uricase) that does it naturally. The drug lowers the uric acid quickly and dramatically, but there is a significant incidence of scary infusion or allergic reactions, especially if the uric acid is high any time after the first infusion. So it's important to draw a uric acid the day before each infusion and discontinue the infusions if it is high. G6PD deficiency must be ruled out before starting these infusions. Also, the drug is expensive and has to be given every two weeks. For those patients with a large load of uric acid who are resistant to the other agents, regardless of their kidney function, it is a good choice and a breakthrough. I have little experience with Krystexxa thus far but have had excellent results with one out of three patients. There have been studies and reports of spectacular results and complete resolution of tophi in short periods of time.

Pearls

- Krystexxa is effective in patients who have large uric acid loads and have failed or not tolerated Uloric, allopurinol, and Benemid.
- It is safe in renal failure.
- Patients must not have G6PD deficiency.
- It must be administered by IV every two weeks.
- Uric acid should be drawn prior to each infusion, and if it has risen above 6 mg./dl. two consecutive times, discontinue Krystexxa because of the risk of infusion reaction.
- If there has been an interval longer than four weeks between infusions, the risk of infusion reaction increases.

- It can bring uric acid level down to close to zero and melt tophi rapidly over months.
- Use prophylaxis during the first six months of therapy.
- Do not administer during an acute attack.

References

1. Sundy, J. S., H. S. Baraf, R. A. Yood, et al. Efficacy and Tolerability of Pegloticase for the Treatment of Chronic Gout in Patients Refractory to Conventional Treatment: Two Randomized Controlled Trials. *JAMA* 306:711.

Fibromyalgia Medications

There are three FDA-approved medications for fibromyalgia—Lyrica, Cymbalta, and Savella. I find them to be effective in about 60 percent of patients if they can tolerate or afford them. Patients have usually read about them or seen their commercials and request them. They all can reduce pain and fatigue and in some patients work like magic and allow them to start exercising and resume a normal life. Lyrica may be the most effective for insomnia and pain; Savella, for fatigue; and Cymbalta, for depression.

Lyrica

Lyrica blocks calcium channels in the brain and therefore slows down the pain pathways, which are in hyper drive in fibromyalgia. The most common side effects are fluid retention, fatigue, dizziness, loss of balance, tremor, and the most bothersome fluid weight gain. I have had at least two patients who have suffered from amnesia from this drug. I try to avoid using it in patients who are obese or have a tendency to retain fluid.

Pearls

- Lyrica may be used twice a day or just at nighttime.
- It may be sedative and may help insomnia.
- It is also effective for paresthesia or nerve pain.
- It may be effective for restless leg syndrome.
- Fluid retention and weight gain can be major problems.
- Dizziness and lack of balance are associated as well.
- Beware of memory loss and amnesia.
- It should be weaned off slowly when discontinued.

References

1. L.J. Crofford, M. C. Rowbotham, P. J. Mease, et al. Pregabalin for the Treatment of Fibromyalgia Syndrome: Results of a Randomized, Double-Blind, Placebo-Controlled Trial. *Arthritis Rheum* 52:1264.

Neurontin (gabapentin)

Another medication that may be helpful in some patients is gabapentin. It has a somewhat similar mechanism of action as Lyrica but is not identical and is not FDA approved for fibromyalgia. There are some studies supporting its effectiveness at doses of 1,800 mg daily, but the results have been lukewarm. Since it is inexpensive and fairly well tolerated (similar side effects as Lyrica), it's worth a try. Recently, a study showed that it may be effective as a sleep aid in these patients at doses of 600 mg nightly.

Pearls

- It may be effective at doses of 600 mg at nighttime or 600 mg three times a day.
- It may be sedative and may help insomnia.
- It is also effective for paresthesia or nerve pain.
- It may be effective for restless leg syndrome.
- Fluid retention and weight gain can be major problems.
- Dizziness and lack of balance are associated as well.
- Beware of memory loss and amnesia.
- It should be weaned off slowly when discontinued.

References

1. Arnold, L. M., D. L. Goldenberg, S. B. Stanford, et al. Gabapentin in the Treatment of Fibromyalgia: A Randomized, Double-Blind, Placebo-Controlled, Multicenter Trial. *Arthritis Rheum* 56:1336.

Cymbalta (duloxetine) and Savella (milnacipran)

Cymbalta and Savella are serotonin norepinephrine receptor antagonists (SNRIs). Cymbalta increases serotonin more than norepinephrine, and the reverse is true for Savella, and Cymbalta minimally increases dopamine. Since norepinephrine is an adrenaline-like substance, one can imagine that taking these drugs is like an adrenaline rush—Savella more so than Cymbalta. There is a norepinephrine and serotonin imbalance in fibromyalgia in at least some patients (other chemical imbalances have been noted as well). Therefore, theoretically these drugs should help some patients. These imbalances are also found in depressed and chronic pain patients as well. Cymbalta is FDA approved for depression, neuropathy, and chronic pain, and Savella is approved in the United Kingdom for depression. The medications work magically in some patients, especially those who have an element of depression. They are expensive (as is Lyrica) and have some worrisome side effects. Cymbalta can cause headaches, fatigue, sweats, dry mouth, nausea, and constipation. Savella may increase the heart rate or blood pressure and cause palpitations but also can cause tremor, nausea, dizziness, sweats, and difficulty urinating, which can be particularly problematic in older men. I try to avoid Savella in patients with any kind of heart or blood pressure problem. I have also had many older women tell me that they feel they are going through menopause again, with night sweats and hot flashes, with both these drugs.

Another SNRI that has been prescribed with mixed success in fibromyalgia is Effexor (venlafaxine). It also weakly increases dopamine and has even less effect on norepinephrine than Savella or Cymbalta. I find it to be ineffective, and it is approved only for depression. All three of these medications need to be weaned off slowly and not abruptly discontinued. In quite a few cases, patients can use these medications as bridge therapy to a healthy lifestyle with exercise and eventually be medication free.

Pearls

- Cymbalta is effective for fibromyalgia, depression, neuropathy, and chronic pain.
- Both are often effective for the fatigue element of fibromyalgia (Savella a little more).
- Avoid in cardiac patients.
- They may increase blood pressure and heart rate.
- Sweating and hot flashes are common problems.
- They may cause tremors.
- Since they increase serotonin, beware of serotonin syndrome when mixing with other drugs that increase serotonin, such as SSRIs or tramadol.
- They must be weaned off slowly.

References

1. L. M. Arnold, Y. Lu, L. J. Crofford, et al. A Double-Blind, Multicenter Trial Comparing Duloxetine with Placebo in the Treatment of Fibromyalgia Patients with or without Major Depressive Disorder. *Arthritis Rheum* 50:2974.

2. L. M. Arnold, A. Rosen, Y. L. Pritchett, et al. A Randomized, Double-Blind, Placebo-Controlled Trial of Duloxetine in the Treatment of Women with Fibromyalgia with or without Major Depressive Disorder. *Pain* 119:5.

3. Gendreau, R. M., M. D. Thorn, J. F. Gendreau, et al. Efficacy of Milnacipran in Patients with Fibromyalgia. *J Rheumatol* 32:1975.

4. L. M. Arnold, R. M. Gendreau, R. H. Palmer, et al. Efficacy and Safety of Milnacipran 100 mg/day in Patients with Fibromyalgia:

Results of a Randomized, Double-Blind, Placebo-Controlled Trial. *Arthritis Rheum* 62:2745.

5. K. Sayar, G. Aksu, I. Ak, and M. Tosun. Venlafaxine Treatment of Fibromyalgia. *Ann Pharmacother* 37:1561.

Tricyclics

There are a variety of medications that are not FDA approved but have some efficacy in fibromyalgia. They include tricyclic antidepressants (amitriptyline, imipramine, desipramine, and nortriptyline), which are usually used as sleep aids but in some patients at high doses can alleviate many of their symptoms. Unfortunately, most patients can't tolerate the higher doses. They can cause dizziness, fatigue, voracious appetites with weight gain, compulsive gambling, and very dry mouth. Nevertheless, they can be very effective in some patients and are very inexpensive. Early in my career, they were really the only drugs available that had any effect. I did see one woman go on a gambling spree and one gain fifty pounds in a several-month period. I rarely use these medications as anything more than a sleep aid these days. These medications can be toxic in elderly patients and increase dementia, dizziness, and the risk of falling. They increase norepinephrine and serotonin, so use with caution with SNRIs or SSRIs since they can cause serotonin syndrome, which can be quite nasty, even fatal, and also can increase blood pressure and heart rate. Just think of norepinephrine as adrenaline, and you can imagine what it could do in high doses to someone with a shaky cardiovascular system. Tricyclics also have an anticholinergic or atropine-like affect. What does that mean? I was taught that these patients become mad as a hatter, red as a beet, and dry as a bone. I know these drugs sound nasty, but in the right setting and the right patient, they are very helpful for central pain, including fibromyalgia.

Pearls

- Tricyclics increase serotonin, norepinephrine, and dopamine and are anticholinergic.
- They may be helpful as sleep aids and reduce some of the pain.

- Beware of mixing with other antidepressants, especially in the elderly.
- They might cause confusion, weight gain, urinary retention, dizziness, compulsive gambling, dry mouth, and tachycardia.
- In low doses, they may be helpful for peripheral neuropathy.

References

1. Goldenberg, D. L., D. T. Felson, and H. Dinerman. A Randomized, Controlled Trial of Amitriptyline and Naproxen in the Treatment of Patients with Fibromyalgia. *Arthritis Rheum* 29:1371.

2. R. M. Bennett, R. A. Gatter, S. M. Campbell, et al. A Comparison of Cyclobenzaprine and Placebo in the Management of Fibrositis: A Double-Blind Controlled Study. *Arthritis Rheum* 31:1535.

3. N. Uçeyler, W. Häuser, and C. Sommer. A Systematic Review on the Effectiveness of Treatment with Antidepressants in Fibromyalgia Syndrome. *Arthritis Rheum* 59:1279.

Tramadol (Ultram)

Tramadol is another medication that some studies have shown to be effective, and that would make sense since it has some SNRI effects, so it is similar to Cymbalta and Savella but less potent. It is also a partial opiate agonist, so it is a narcotic despite some misconceptions to the contrary. In some respects, it is a very dangerous drug because practitioners unaware that it increases norepinephrine and serotonin will mix it with an SNRI or SSRI and increase the possibility of toxicity. I saw a pregnant young lady who was taking an SSRI, tramadol, and Elavil (all not good in pregnancy) and had a grand mal seizure because of serotonin syndrome on this combination. Patients are often under the false impression that tramadol is not an opiate and not addicting. Its major adverse effects include flushing, dizziness, fatigue, nausea, and constipation. I try to stay away from this drug if I can, but occasionally I will only give it for a short term, but that can be difficult.

Pearls

- Tramadol is a partial opiate agonist (narcotic) and an SNRI (increases norepinephrine and serotonin).
- Beware of serotonin syndrome when combining with SSRIs or SNRIs.
- It can cause seizures.
- It is subject to abuse and dependence.
- It must be withdrawn slowly.

References

1. R. M. Bennett, M. Kamin, R. Karim, and N. Rosenthal. Tramadol and Acetaminophen Combination Tablets in the Treatment of

Fibromyalgia Pain: A Double-Blind, Randomized, Placebo-Controlled Study. *Am J Med* 114:537.

2. Tofferi, J. K., J. L. Jackson, and P. G. O'Malley. Treatment of Fibromyalgia with Cyclobenzaprine: A Meta-analysis. *Arthritis Rheum* 51:9.

Cyclobenzaprine (Flexeril)

Cyclobenzaprine is a muscle relaxant that has been useful in the insomnia associated with fibromyalgia. There have been some small studies supporting it, and it is inexpensive, but I have been receiving more and more "Dear Doctor" letters warning of its toxicity in elderly people.

References

1. Reynolds, WJ., H. Moldofsky, P. Saskin, and F. A. Lue. The Effects of Cyclobenzaprine on Sleep Physiology and Symptoms in Patients with Fibromyalgia. *J Rheumatol* 18:452.
2. Quimby, L. G., G. M. Gratwick, C. D. Whitney, and S. R. Block. A Randomized Trial of Cyclobenzaprine for the Treatment of Fibromyalgia, supplement. *J Rheumatol* 19:S140.
3. Moldofsky, H., H. W. Harris, W. T. Archambault, et al. Effects of Bedtime Very Low Dose Cyclobenzaprine on Symptoms and Sleep Physiology in Patients with Fibromyalgia Syndrome: A Double-Blind Randomized Placebo-Controlled Study. *J Rheumatol* 38:2653.

Sjögren's Syndrome Medications

Plaquenil, methotrexate, Rituxan, and prednisone are all used for the systemic manifestations of Sjögren's, such as fatigue and arthritis. We told you the story of our patient with autonomic neuropathy who responded dramatically to Rituxan. All these medications have been described previously.

Evoxac (Cevimeline) and Salagen (Pilocarpine)

The two drugs I most commonly prescribe for Sjögren's are Evoxac (cevimeline) and Salagen (pilocarpine). Both are effective in treating dry mouth and less so dry eyes. They stimulate certain receptors (muscarinic) on glands that induce them to produce more fluids. I have some patients who can barely talk or swallow because of dryness until they take the medications. They also can help with vaginal dryness. Unfortunately, patients may overproduce saliva and drool, and they may sweat profusely. It can be especially bad in a woman already having hot flashes. I also imagine it would be embarrassing to drool spontaneously. Nevertheless, these drugs can really improve quality of life for some patients. I particularly like Evoxac because it seems to be more effective for the eye dryness, although not great, and seems to be a more potent drug. It is taken three times a day. Nausea, visual blurriness, and upper respiratory problems are some of the other adverse effects. The advantage of Salagen is that it is available in two doses so that you can always titrate up. It is less expensive but less potent and potentially more toxic. Flushing, dizziness, and urinary frequency are some of the other adverse effects. They are contraindicated in asthma, narrow angle glaucoma, and severe liver disease.

Pearls

Evoxac and pilocarpine are helpful for dry mouth.

Evoxac is particularly effective and may even increase moisture in the eyes.

Drooling, sweating, and dizziness are the main side effects.

They are contraindicated in narrow angle glaucoma, asthma, and severe liver disease.

References

1. Petrone, D., J. J. Condemi, R. Fife, et al. A Double-Blind, Randomized, Placebo-Controlled Study of Cevimeline in Sjögren's Syndrome Patients with Xerostomia and Keratoconjunctivitis Sicca. *Arthritis Rheum* 46:748.

2. Papas, A. S., Y. S. Sherrer, M. Charney, et al. Successful Treatment of Dry Mouth and Dry Eye Symptoms in Sjögren's Syndrome Patients with Oral Pilocarpine: A Randomized, Placebo-Controlled, Dose-Adjustment Study. *J Clin Rheumatol* 10:169.

3. Tsifetaki, N., G. Kitsos, C. A. Paschides, et al. Oral Pilocarpine for the Treatment of Ocular Symptoms in Patients with Sjögren's Syndrome: A Randomised 12 Week Controlled Study. *Ann Rheum Dis* 62:1204.

4. Leung, K. C., A. S. McMillan, M. C. Wong, et al. The Efficacy of Cevimeline Hydrochloride in the Treatment of Xerostomia in Sjögren's Syndrome in Southern Chinese Patients: A Randomised Double-Blind, Placebo-Controlled Crossover Study. *Clin Rheumatol* 27:429.

5. Yamada, H., Y. Nakagawa, E. Wakamatsu, et al. Efficacy Prediction of Cevimeline in Patients with Sjögren's Syndrome. *Clin Rheumatol* 26:1320.

6. Nusair, S., and A. Rubinow. The Use of Oral Pilocarpine in Xerostomia and Sjögren's Syndrome. *Semin Arthritis Rheum*; 28:360.

Chapter Twenty-six

Narcotics

THIS IS A NON-NARCOTIC OFFICE is written boldly on my office entrance and exit doors and in my introductory brochure. It is mostly a fact and reflects my philosophy and bias. I do not believe long-term narcotics have a role in most chronic diseases. In fact, as mentioned before, long-term-narcotic therapy may paradoxically cause a hyperalgesia syndrome which lowers the pain threshold and increases pain, especially in fibromyalgia patients. Short-term therapy, especially for acute events, such as fractures or herniated discs, may be effective and necessary, and I will prescribe a few weeks' supply of a short-acting narcotic, such as Vicodin or hydrocodone or tramadol. I also will give some patients thirty tablets of these medications for breakthrough pain to last for several months. Rarely has a patient abused this agreement. Most of the diseases I treat are chronic and can last a lifetime. I believe that by treating the underlying disease usually I can alleviate the pain. Alternatively, I can find nonpharmaceutical methods, which are much more enduring and less potentially toxic, to treat problems such as chronic back pain. Finally, there are more and more alternative medications to narcotics that are sometimes more effective and benign in the long term. Cymbalta, Lyrica, Neurontin, and NSAIDs are just a few. The pendulum keeps swinging back and forth in the medical community's attitudes toward pain and narcotics. When I was in training, we were very cautious about prescribing narcotics. Addiction was just one problem we considered. In the last few decades, studies often funded by drug companies have suggested that long-acting and long-term narcotics were not only benign but effective in most chronic pain syndromes. Most of these studies were, at the most, of one year's duration but usually much shorter. As more and more long-acting narcotics, such as MS Contin and Oxycontin, were developed and approved, the enthusiasm for prescribing them grew, as did the pain management specialty. There seemed to be a "no pain" philosophy. In fact, some families and patients won lawsuits for inadequate pain management.

Pain specialists are usually anesthesiologists trained specially in pain management. They use effective invasive procedures, mainly injections, and often manage chronic narcotic therapy with expertise that many of us lack. It's great passing this role to someone else. Dealing with patients on narcotics can be a tiring, frustrating experience for the whole office, especially if you are the prescriber. However, placing patients on long-term narcotics is fraught with dangers. It sometimes diverts the patient from a healthier and better treatment, such as exercise for fibromyalgia and low back pain or anti-inflammatories in inflammatory diseases. It also can exacerbate depression, cause severe fatigue and brain fog, and paralyze the bowels, causing severe constipation or even obstruction. Fifteen years ago when I first arrived in Ashland, I remember having heated discussions with fellow physicians about chronic narcotic therapy. The few of us who opposed it were greeted with derision. Since that time the pendulum has been swinging again. I have had one elderly lady with lupus and on methadone who passed out twice behind the wheel, once landing in a ditch and the second time hitting another car and causing multiple injuries. After an extensive negative work-up, we concluded that methadone caused these events. Her primary care and prescribing doctor was insulted and wanted to attribute it to the 10 mg of prednisone that I prescribed. The patient, who weighed less than one hundred pounds, could barely stay awake during her visits and slurred her words. I reported her to the DMV, and she lost her license. In anger, she stopped seeing me for a year but returned when she could not remember the reason why she had left the practice.

I have also seen two or three fibromyalgia patients in their twenties and thirties who required pacemakers placed in their GI tracts because their stomachs and colons had become permanently paralyzed by chronic narcotic therapy. I find it sad to see twenty-year-olds who have already been on morphine or morphine-like drugs for years because of back pain. What will these patients do in twenty years? I have heard pain specialists say that they only continue these medications if it keeps these patients functional, but I have seen no studies that look at these patients five to ten years down the line. In fact, I see many patients who tell me they have ten out of ten pain and can't function but insist that their narcotics allow them to get out of bed in the morning and are extremely effective. They are resistant to any suggestion to the contrary. Other patients have actually thanked me for treating their underlying disease and suggesting that they wean off narcotics. I believe many physicians prescribe narcotics with good intentions but often in frustration because they don't know what else to do. It is a short-term fix that satisfies the patients, but as time passes there is often a dose creep until the patients are no longer satisfied. It's then that I often see them.

I am all for treating someone with cancer or for postoperative pain with narcotics. They have their role. In the last few years, as the abuse of these medications has become obvious, I feel confident that the medical community is starting to reassess the use of narcotics long term for chronic pain. In the meantime, I will adhere to my philosophy and bias. The only narcotics I have prescribed in the last fifteen years are tramadol and Vicodin, and these prescriptions have been few and far between.

Pearls

- Narcotics are rarely long-term solutions.

References

1. Painter, J. T., and L. J. Crofford. Chronic Opioid Use in Fibromyalgia Syndrome: A Clinical Review. *Journal of Clinical Rheumatology* 19 (2): 72–77.

2. Crofford, L. J. *Nat. Rev Rheumatology* 6 (4 Apr.): 191–97.

Narcotics

Well, that's it folks! You've just read my take on rheumatology, the patients, the practice, the successes, and the tragedies. Over the years I have read thousands of journal articles and many textbooks and attended hundreds of conferences. I drew on my assimilation of all that information and thirty years of rheumatology to write this book and referred often to the online textbook *Uptodate*. In the end, these words are my subjective ruminations or one man's opinion based on his experiences. I hope it was an enjoyable and informative read. Thanks for your attention.

Chapter Twenty-seven

Heroes and Celebrities with Rheumatic Diseases

I consider many of my patients heroes for their courage and attitudes. The rheumatic diseases can affect people of any age, class, race, or stature. I have had several big celebrities in my practice and found them to be incredibly grateful, humble, and interesting. I can't reveal their identities, but I can list some famous people who have or have had these diseases.

Rheumatoid Arthritis:
1. Artists—Pierre Auguste Renoir, Raul Dufy, Peter Paul Rubens
2. Actors—Kathleen Turner, Rosalind Russell, James Coburn
3. Singer—Edith Piaff

Lupus:
1. Singer—Toni Braxton
2. Journalist—Charles Kuralt
3. Actor—Nick Cannon

4. Major League Baseball Player—Tim Raines
5. Dog—George and Barbara Bush's dog Millie

Discoid Lupus:
Singer—Seal

Polymyositis:
Pro Football Player—Ricky Bell

Sjögren's Syndrome:
Pro Tennis Player—Venus Williams

Psoriatic Arthritis:
Pro Golfer—Phil Mickelson
Founding Father—Benjamin Franklin
Dictator—Josef Stalin

Gout:
1. King—Henry VIII
2. Opera Singer—Luccio Pavarotti
3. Actor—Jim Belushi
4. Artist—Ansel Adams

Scleroderma:
Artist—Paul Klee

Ankylosing Spondylitis:
Variety Show Host—Ed Sullivan

Sarcoidosis:
Comedian—Bernie Mac

Osteoporosis:

1. Actor—Sally Field
2. Comedian—Joan Rivers

Chapter Twenty-eight

Glossary

Aciphex (rabeprazole)—Proton pump inhibitor used for acid reflux and important in scleroderma patients

Actemra (tocilizumab)—Intravenous (IV) IL-6 inhibitor that treats rheumatoid arthritis

Actonel (risedronate)—Oral medication for osteoporosis

Allopurinol—Uric-acid-lowering drug for gout

Amitriptyline (Elavil)—Tricyclic antidepressant used for insomnia, fibromyalgia, and neuropathy

Amyloidosis—A multisystem disease often involving joints, kidneys, and heart, caused by deposition of an abnormal protein in the tissues; it may be associated with a blood cancer or chronic inflammatory diseases; there are several kinds of amyloid proteins with predilections for different organs and therefore associated with different clinical pictures

ANCA (antineutrophil cytoplasmic antibody)—It is an antibody associated with certain kinds of vasculitides and inflammatory bowel disease.

Ankylosing Spondylitis—A systemic inflammatory disease that usually starts in the teens or early twenties; it may affect the whole spine and be associated with inflammatory arthritis of large joints, such as knees and hips; iritis, inflammatory bowel disease, and psoriasis may be associated; there is also a hereditary component with a characteristic histocompatibility gene (HLA-B27) in 90 percent of patients; however, the majority of people with HLA-B27 gene do not get the disease

Antimalarials—Include Plaquenil, quinacrine, and chloroquine; used in the past to treat malaria and now used for lupus

Apremilast (Otezla)—A twice-daily oral phosphodiesterase-4 inhibitor approved for psoriasis and psoriatic arthritis

Aralen (chloroquine)—Old antimalarial drug used in lupus

Aspirin—the granddaddy of all nonsteroidal anti-inflammatory drugs

Atabrine (quinacrine)—Old antimalarial drug used in treatment of lupus

Glossary

Baker's Cyst—cyst or swelling in the back of knee, which can rupture and cause swelling of the whole leg

Behcet's Disease—A vasculitis characterized by oral and genital ulcers and multisystem disease; milder variants seem to be becoming more common; classically seen in Middle Eastern races, but that may be changing

Benemid (probenecid)—Oral drug that increases urinary excretion of uric acid and used in gout prevention

Benlysta (belimumab)—Biologic drug that inhibits B-lymphocytes (a kind of white blood cell) and is approved for treatment of lupus

Biologics—They inhibit particular factors (called *cytokines*) that trigger inflammatory and sometimes cancer cells; they may also block their receptors or activating pathways

Bisphosphonates—Class of drugs used for osteoporosis; they inhibits osteoclasts, the "Pac-Men" or termite-like cells in bones

Buspar (buspirone)—An antianxiety drug

Canakinumab (Ilaris)—An interleukin (IL-1) beta inhibitor approved for JIA and possibly useful in other inflammatory arthritides, such as gout

Carpal Tunnel Syndrome—Numbness, burning, tingling, and eventually weakness of the hand caused by pressure on the median nerve

Celebrex (celecoxib)—A nonsteroidal anti-inflammatory drug (NSAID) that is selective for COX-2 inhibition

Celexa (citalopram)—A serotonin reuptake inhibitor (SSRI) that treats depression

CellCept (mycophenolate mofetil)—Oral immunosuppressive drug used in lupus and a variety of other diseases

Certolizumab—See *Cimzia*

Churg-Strauss Disease—see *Eosinophilic Angiitis with Granulomatosis*

Cimzia (certolizumab)—Tumor necrosis factor inhibitor indicated for treatment of Crohn's disease and rheumatoid arthritis

Circulating Anticoagulants, or Antiphospholipid Antibodies— They cause the blood to clot easily and lead to blood clots, strokes, and miscarriages; their effect can be inconsequential or catastrophic

Clinoril (sulindac)—A nonsteroidal anti-inflammatory drug (NSAID)

Colchicine—An oral agent used for acute gout or as prophylaxis while lowering the uric acid below 6; it is not meant for chronic use except in a few other disease states

Cosentryx (Secukinumab) —It is an IL-17A inhibitor that is effective in Psoriasis, Psoriatic arthritris and Ankylosing Spondylits but as of early 2016 is FDA approved only for Psoriasis

Glossary

Complex Regional Pain Syndrome (CRPS)—A chronic pain syndrome associated with an extremely painful, exquisitely tender, swollen, cold, and discolored appendage

CREST—A form of limited scleroderma

Cryoglobulinemia—A disease in which abnormal proteins or immunoglobulins (antibodies) precipitate out in blood vessels when exposed to the cold; it can cause skin, lung, kidney, or neurological disease and often severe Raynaud's phenomenon; drawing blood specimens for testing must follow a strict protocol to be accurate

Crystal-Induced Arthritis—Usually refers to gout, pseudogout, or hydroxyapatite deposition disease (HADD)

Cyclosporine (Sandimmune, Neoral)—Oral immunosuppressive agent used as a second-line drug in certain diseases, such as psoriatic arthritis, and certain conditions, such as macrophage activation syndrome

Cymbalta (duloxetine)—A serotonin-norepinephrine reuptake inhibitor (SNRI) used in fibromyalgia, neuropathy and depression

Cytoxan (cyclophosphamide)—Potent and toxic immunosuppressive drug used in severe lupus, vasculitis, and a few other severe conditions, such as scleroderma lung

Daypro (oxaprosin)—An NSAID

Depression—Ubiquitous and deflating

Rudy's Ruminations On **Rheumatology**

Dermatomyositis—An inflammatory autoimmune muscle disease associated with weakness and characteristic skin findings

Dexlansoprazole (Dexilant)—A proton inhibitor used for GERD

Diltiazem (Tiazac, Cardiazem)—A calcium channel blocker used mainly in hypertension but also Raynaud's and pulmonary hypertension

DMARDs—Disease modifying agents in the rheumatic diseases

Effexor (venlafaxine)—A serotonin-norepinephrine reuptake inhibitor (SNRI) used in depression

Eosinophilic Fasciitis—Swollen, painful, inflamed extremity or extremities with a tight orange-peel appearance; it is associated with overexertion or extreme activity and high eosinophil count in blood and tissue

Eosinophilic Polyangiitis with Granulomatosis (Churg-Strauss Disease)—A vasculitis associated with asthma, lung infiltrates, upper respiratory symptoms, and potentially other organ involvement; high eosinophil counts in the blood and tissues are characteristic; often have positive ANCAs

Elavil (amitriptyline)—Tricyclic antidepressant used for insomnia, fibromyalgia, and neuropathy

Enbrel (etanercept)—A tumor necrosis factor inhibitor injected subcutaneously to treat rheumatoid arthritis, psoriasis, psoriatic arthritis, reactive arthritis, ankylosing spondylitis, juvenile idiopathic arthritis, and occasionally off-label for other inflammatory diseases

Epicondylitis (medial and lateral)—It is a tendonitis involving the tendons on the pinky or thumb side of the elbow, which either flex or extend the wrist, respectively.

Evoxac (cevimeline)—Drug that stimulates salivary and tear flow and prescribed in Sjögren's

Feldene (piroxicam)—NSAID available orally or topically (if compounded); it has a long half-life, so it lasts a long time in the system and may be potentially more toxic than other NSAIDs, especially in the elderly

Fibromyalgia—A condition characterized by diffuse aches and pains, fatigue, brain fog, and tender points on both sides of the body, above and below the waist; it is caused by an abnormality in the part of the brain that processes all sensory input so that there is a chemical imbalance and the volume on all sensory input is turned up

Flolan (epoprostenol)—An IV prostanoid that dilates blood vessels and treats pulmonary hypertension

Forteo (teriparatide)—Daily subcutaneous drug approved for osteoporosis; it stimulates osteoblasts that make bone; it's a truncated but active form of parathyroid hormone

Fosamax (alendronate)—Oral bisphosphonate used for osteoporosis treatment

Rudy's Ruminations On **Rheumatology**

Giant Cell Arteritis (Temporal Arteritis)—Vasculitis characterized by visual loss, headache from hell in the temporal area, sometimes jaw pain and fever; it can cause extremity pain, stroke, and
organ failure, may be associated with polymyalgia rheumatica, and
is typically seen in seventy- to eighty-year-olds

Gout—A systemic disease caused by the accumulation of uric
acid in tissues, causing severe inflammatory destructive arthritis,
kidney stones, and kidney disease; it may seem intermittent but is
actually chronic, and key to treatment is keeping serum uric acid
levels below 6 mg./dl.

Granulomatosis with Polyangiitis (Wegener's Granulomatosis)—
Vasculitis characterized by sinus, upper respiratory, scleritis, and in-
ner/middle ear inflammation and, in severe cases, life-threatening lung
and kidney disease; 90 percent of patients will have positive ANCAs,
a very distinctive antibody

Humira (adalimumab)—A tumor necrosis factor inhibitor injected
subcutaneously to treat rheumatoid arthritis, psoriasis, psoriatic arthritis, reactive arthritis, ankylosing spondylitis, Crohn's disease, ulcerative
colitis, and occasionally off-label for other inflammatory diseases

Hyluronate—see *Synvisc-One*

Hypersensitivity Vasculitis, or Henoch-Schonlein Purpura—
Vasculitis associated with purpuric skin lesions, arthritis, and kidney
and sometimes gastrointestinal disease; it may be seen in children
and is often self-limited

Glossary

Ibandronate (Boniva)—Oral or intravenous bisphosphonate used for osteoporosis

Ilaris (canakinumab)—An interleukin (IL-1) beta inhibitor approved for JIA and possibly useful in other inflammatory arthritides, such as gout

Indocin (indomethacin)—An old and potent NSAID

IVIG—Intravenous immunoglobulins used for resistant polymyositis for forms of thrombocytopenia (low platelets), for immunoglobulin deficiency and for a variety of diseases such as Susacs that are resistant to other medications

Imuran (Azothiaprine)—A junior Cytoxan or immunosuppressive agent used in a variety of diseases such as lupus, vasculitis, polymyositis (not my favorite)

Kawasaki Disease—Often starts after viral illness and is a vasculitis seen in infants and small children, associated with fever, red eyes, cracked lips, strawberry tongue, rash, and sometimes coronary artery aneurysms due to vasculitis hands and feet swelling are early signs; coronary artery aneurysms often can be prevented with early treatment (the babies are usually very sick!)

Kenalog (triamcinolone)—an intramuscular, intra-articular (injected into joints), or topical anti-inflammatory steroid used in a variety of inflammatory diseases, such as rheumatoid arthritis and lupus

Rudy's Ruminations On **Rheumatology**

Kineret (anakinra)—An IL-1 inhibitor approved for treatment of rheumatoid arthritis and effective for Still's disease and acute gout; it is injected subcutaneously daily

Krystexxa (pegloticase)—An IV drug given every two weeks for severe chronic tophaceous gout

Leisenurad (Zurampic)—An oral drug that lowers uric acid It helps the kidney excrete uric acid by by inhibiting the function of transportation proteins invovolved in the reabsorption of uric acid. Lesinurad is prescribed in combination with Allopurinol or Uloric (xanthine oxidase inhibitors). When prescribed alone, kidney failure is more common.

Letairis (ambrisentan)—An endothelin receptor antagonist that dilates blood vessels and treats pulmonary hypertension

Lexapro (escitalopram)—A serotonin reuptake inhibitor (SSRI) that treats depression

Leukocytoclastic Vasculitis—Involves small vessels of the skin; patients usually have a characteristic rash on their legs, sometimes skin ulcerations, and it is often caused by drug reactions

Lodine (etodolac)--An NSAID

Lupus (Systemic Lupus Erythematosus)—A systemic autoimmune disease where inflammatory cells attack a variety of organs, especially joints, skin, kidneys, lungs, heart, and nervous system; patients may have characteristic butterfly rash, oral ulcers, fatigue, arthritis, and low white blood cell and platelet counts; usually starts at an early age but has onset in teens to midthirties; occasionally first appears at extremes of age spectrum; it affects predominantly females

Lyme Disease—It is a tick-borne infection by an organism called a *spirochete* that can cause arthritis and multisystem disease

Lyrica (pregabalin)—It blocks calcium channels in the brain and noradrenergic and serotonin pathways in the spinal cord; it is approved for fibromyalgia

Magnesium Trisalicylate—A weak NSAID

Meclomen (meclofenamate)—An NSAID

Medrol (methylprednisolone)—It ia an anti-inflammatory steroid used in a variety of diseases and situations; occasionally patients that are resistant to prednisone will respond to this drug

Methotrexate—Potent anti-inflammatory remittive agent, given orally, intramuscularly or subcutaneously, approved primarily for rheumatoid arthritis, juvenile idiopathic arthritis, psoriasis, and granulomatous angiitis but often used in lupus, polymyositis, dermatomyositis, psoriatic arthritis, reactive arthritis, and a variety or other diseases; it is often the first and primary drug

Microscopic Polyangiitis—It is a vasculitis associated with the ANCA antibodies, nasal or oral inflammation, and kidney disease

Mixed Connective Disease—It is a systemic autoimmune disease with features of lupus, scleroderma, polymyositis, and Sjögren's but usually spares the kidneys; it is associated with a specific antibody (anti-RNP); some patients will develop scleroderma after decades

Mobic (meloxicam)—An NSAID

Morphea—Scleroderma skin changes confined to a certain part of the body without systemic or organ involvement

Motrin (ibuprofen)—An NSAID that is anti-inflammatory at doses above 1,600 mg daily

Naprosyn (naproxen, Aleve)—An NSAID that is anti-inflammatory at doses above 500 mg daily

Neurontin (gabapentin)—It blocks calcium channels in the brain and is approved for treatment of neuropathy but is sometimes effective in fibromyalgia

Nexium (esomeprazole)—A proton pump inhibitor used for acid reflux and important in scleroderma patients; it is often used to treat ulcers, gastritis, and esophagitis

Nifedipine (Procardia)—It is a calcium channel blocker used mainly in hypertension but also Raynaud's and pulmonary hypertension

Nonsteroidals (NSAIDs)—class of anti-inflammatory drugs; aspirin is the granddaddy; Motrin, Celebrex, and others

Norpramin (desipramine)—It is a tricyclic antidepressant used for insomnia and fibromyalgia

Glossary

Norrvasc (amilodopine)—It is a calcium channel blocker used mainly in hypertension but also Raynaud's and pulmonary hypertension

Orencia—A selective costimulator modulator, a drug that blocks two proteins on the membrane of some key immune system cells that are usually activated during the inflammatory process; it is approved for RA and JIA; it is administered IV monthly or subcutaneously weekly

Orudis (ketoprofen)—An NSAID available orally or topically (if compounded)

Osteoarthritis—Wear-and-tear arthritis; cartilage wears down; it is not very inflammatory or systemic and is associated with aging and trauma; no one escapes it as they age

Osteoporosis—Low bone mass causing bone fragility and fracture risks

Pamelor (nortriptyline)—Tricyclic antidepressant used for insomnia, fibromyalgia, and neuropathy

Paxil (paroxetine)—A serotonin reuptake inhibitor (SSRI) that treats depression, anxiety, and panic attacks

Polyarteritis Nodosum—It is the prototypical vasculitis with multiorgan involvement, especially skin, kidney, neurological, gastrointestinal, and musculoskeletal

Polymyalgia Rheumatica—It is a systemic disease associated with pain and stiffness around shoulders and/or hips but sometimes other joints; patients generally feel weak and tired, have high ESRs and CRPs, and are fifty-five to sixty years old or older; 20 percent may develop giant cell arteritis; the disease is very responsive to low to medium doses of prednisone

Polymyositis—An inflammatory muscle disease associated with proximal muscle weakness (hips and shoulders); sometimes patients can have severe lung disease and skin changes (see *Dermatomyositis*)

Plaquenil (hydroxychloroquine)—Old antimalarial drug used mostly for lupus but occasionally for rheumatoid arthritis, Sjögren's, and a few other diseases

Prilosec (omeprazole)—A proton pump inhibitor used for acid reflux and important in scleroderma patients

Procardia (nifedipine)—A calcium channel blocker used mainly in hypertension but also Raynaud's and pulmonary hypertension

Prolia (denosumab)—Subcutaneous drug given every six months for osteoporosis

Prozac (floxetine)-- It is a serotonin reuptake inhibitor (SSRI) that treats depression

Pseudogout—It is an inflammatory arthritis that can mimic gout and is caused by deposition of calcium pyrophosphate crystals in the joints; often causes inflammation and swelling of knees or wrists

Psoriatic Arthritis—A systemic inflammatory arthritis associated with psoriasis; it may be very mild or extremely destructive and can involve tendons and ligaments; it is a member of the seronega-tive spondyloarthritis family, along with ankylosing spondylitis

Prednisone—It is an anti-inflammatory steroid used in many diseases and situations. It is a staple of rheumatology, but some-times it's like dancing with the devil

Prevacid (lansoprazole)—A proton pump inhibitor used for acid reflux and important in scleroderma patients

Protonix (pantoprazole)—It is a proton pump inhibitor used for acid reflux and important in scleroderma patients

Raynaud's Phenomenon—Spasm of the small arteries of the hands, feet, nose, or whole extremities causing white, blue, and red color changes and cold and numb fingers and toes; in extreme cas-es, it causes extreme pain, skin ulcers, and even loss of digits or extremities; it is common in diseases such as scleroderma but may stand alone

Reactive Arthritis (formerly Reiter's Syndrome)—A member of the seronegative spondyloarthritis family and causes inflammatory arthritis involving large joints, such as knees or hips; it is an au-toimmune reaction to an infection and may also cause sacroiliitis, conjunctivitis or iritis, urethritis, rash (circinate balanitis, keratoder-mia blenhorragica), and oral ulcers; it is usually triggered by specific infectious agents, such as chlamydia, campylobacter, salmonella, or shigella

Reclast (zoledronic acid)—Intravenous drug given yearly as treatment for osteoporosis

Rudy's Ruminations On **Rheumatology**

Relapsing Polychondritis—It is a systemic inflammatory disease associated with inflammation of ear, eye, nasal, upper respiratory, and joint cartilage; patients often complain of intermittent, painful ear swelling; it may involve multiple organs; involvement of the tracheal cartilage and major bronchi in severe cases can lead to life-threatening airway obstruction

Relafen (nabumetone)—An NSAID

Remicade (infliximab)—A tumor necrosis factor inhibitor infused intravenously to treat rheumatoid arthritis, psoriasis, psoriatic arthritis, reactive arthritis, ankylosing spondylitis, Crohns disease, ulcerative colitis, and occasionally off-label for other inflammatory diseases

Remittive Agent—Medication that induces remission in a disease

Restasis—Immunosuppressive (cyclosporine) eye drops approved for Sjögren's

Revatio (Viagra, sildenafil)—A phosphodiesterase-5 inhibitor that dilates blood vessels and is used to treat pulmonary hypertension

Rheumatoid Arthritis—It is a systemic inflammatory disease that causes severe destructive arthritis of large and small joints on both sides of the body; heart, lungs, eyes, and skin may also be severely affected; it is the classic autoimmune disease with a genetic predisposition and is eminently treatable

Rituxan (rituximab)—A medication that inhibits B-lymphocyte, which is a type of white blood cell; it is approved for treatment of rheumatoid arthritis, granulomatosis with polyangiitis, microscopic angiitis, and allergic granulomatosis but may be helpful in lupus, Sjögren's, and a few other diseases

Salagen (pilocarpine)—Drug that stimulates salivary and tear flow that is prescribed for Sjögren's

Salsalate—A weak NSAID with perhaps less effect on platelets

Sarcoidosis—A multiorgan granulomatous disease that involves lungs, eyes, skin, joints, and muscles; liver, lymph nodes, and the central nervous system, especially the spinal cord, can also be involved; it is a strange disease that can be very mild or deadly

Savella (milnacipran)—A serotonin-norepinephrine uptake inhibitor (SNRI) used in fibromyalgia, neuropathy, and depression

Scleroderma—It means "hardened skin" and comes in two forms, limited and diffuse; the first is a slowly progressive disease, and the second is often explosive and fatal; the hallmark of this disease is progressive swelling of skin, leading to a leathery tightness; it is an autoimmune inflammatory disease causing inflammation of small blood vessels in the skin and other organs leading to poor blood flow and dysfunction; Raynaud's, difficulty swallowing, poor intestinal motility, severe lung disease, pulmonary hypertension, digital ulcers and resorption are common; sudden malignant hypertension and kidney failure may be fatal, mostly in the diffuse form; diffuse disease is very scary, but we now have good treatments for individual manifestations

Secukinumab (Cosentryx)—It is an IL-17A inhibitor that is effective in Psoriasis, Psoriatic arthritris and Ankylosing Spondylits but as of early 2016 is FDA approved only for Psoriasis

Rudy's Ruminations On **Rheumatology**

Septic Arthritis—Infection of a joint; often a medical emergency

Seronegative Spondyloarthritis, or Spondyloarthropathy—*Seronegative* means patients with these diseases test negative for rheumatoid arthritis; *spondyloarthritis* means that they have an inflammatory arthritis that typically involves the axial skeleton or spine (but not always); the four major diseases associated with this category are ankylosing spondylitis, psoriatic arthritis, reactive arthritis, and inflammatory bowel disease

Simponi (golimumab)—It is a tumor necrosis factor inhibitor injected subcutaneously to treat rheumatoid arthritis, psoriatic arthritis, and ankylosing spondylitis

Sinequan (doxepin)—A tricyclic antidepressant used for insomnia and fibromyalgia

Sjögren's Disease—Autoimmune systemic disease causing inflammation of salivary and lacrimal (tear ducts) glands; classic symptoms are dry eyes and dry mouth often associated with fatigue and joint pain; occasionally causes lung, skin, and neurological problems; usually associated with other autoimmune diseases but may stand alone and is then called *primary Sjögren's syndrome*; it carries a significant risk for lymphoma (a blood cancer)

SNRI (Serotonin-Norepinephrine Reuptake Inhibitor)—Class of antidepressants also used in fibromyalgia; Cymbalta and others

SSRI (Serotonin Reuptake Inhibitor)—Class of antidepressants; Prozac and others

Glossary

Stelara (ustekinumab)—Inhibits interleukin-17 (IL-17) and IL-23 and is effective in treatment of psoriasis and psoriatic arthritis.

Still's Disease—A form of rheumatoid arthritis usually seen in children but may occur in adults; it causes daily fevers, high white blood cell counts, high ferritin, arthritis, rash, and swollen glands; it may cause enlarged liver or spleen and inflammation of the lung and heart lining; it is rarely associated with macrophage activating syndrome, which can be life threatening

Synvisc-One (hyaluronate)—A gel injected once into the knee to treat osteoarthritis; it reduces pain but does not reverse disease process; it is my preferred form of hyaluronate because it is a one-time injection that lasts for at least six months; other forms include Synvisc, Euflexxa, Orthovisc (three weekly injections), and Supartz (five weekly injections)

Tacrolimus (Prograf, Advagraf, Protopic)—An immunosuppressive drug given orally or topically; similar to cyclosporine and used for resistant forms of polymyositis and rarely for lupus and a variety of other diseases; it is an effective topical in some resistant rashes; developed to prevent rejection of organ transplants

Takayasu's Arteritis ("Pulseless Disease," Aortic Arch Syndrome)—A vasculitis seen in young women that causes inflammation, occlusion, and dissection of the aorta and the major blood vessels coming off of it; fever and joint pain are common early symptoms; pulmonary, cardiac, gastrointestinal, and neurological involvement may occur; it is a serious disease

Rudy's Ruminations On **Rheumatology**

Tocilizumab (Actemra)—Intravenous IL-6 inhibitor that treats rheumatoid arthritis

Tofranil (imipramine)—A tricyclic anti-inflammatory used for insomnia and fibromyalgia

Tolectin (tolmetin)—An NSAID

Tracleer (bosentan)—It is an endothelin receptor antagonists that dilates blood vessels and treats pulmonary hypertension

Tramadol—see *Ultram*

Trazodone (Oleptro)—It is a serotonin reuptake inhibitor used mainly for insomnia and depression and occasionally for ibromyalgia

Tricyclics—Old class of antidepressants used more for sleep aids, neuropathy, and fibromyalgia; Elavil and others

Uloric (febuxostat)—It is an oral agent that lowers uric acid levels and is approved for preventative treatment of gout only

Ultram (tramadol)—It is a weak narcotic and weak serotonin nor-epinephrine uptake inhibitor used to treat pain

Undifferentiated Connective Disease—It has features of a variety of autoimmune diseases, such as lupus, rheumatoid arthritis, polymyositis, and so forth, but lacks the specific antibodies of mixed connective disease and does not meet the criteria for any specific diagnosis

Glossary

Ustekinumab (Stelara)—Inhibits interleukin-17 (IL-17) and IL-23 and is effective in treatment of psoriasis and psoriatic arthritis

Vasculitis—Inflammation of big, medium and/or small sized blood vessels; it may be confined to skin but can be systemic and very serious

Ventavis (iloprost)—A subcutaneously injected prostanoid, or prostacyclin analogue, that dilates blood vessels and treats pulmonary hypertension

Voltaren (diclofenac)—An NSAID available orally or topically

Wegener's Granulomatosis—See *Granulomatosis with Polyangiitis*

Wellbutrin (bupropion)—Inhibits the reuptake of dopamine and norepinephrine (increases their levels) and treats depression

Xeljanz (tofacitinib)—Inhibits enzyme JAK kinase and treats rheumatoid arthritis

Zoloft (sertraline)—A serotonin reuptake inhibitor (SSRI) that treats depression